AF829577

Atopic Dermatitis

Johannes Ring

Atopic Dermatitis

Eczema

Foreword by Jon M. Hanifin

Springer

Johannes Ring
Department of Dermatology and Allergology Biederstein
Technische Universitaet Muenchen (TUM)
Munich, Bavaria
Germany

Christine Kuehne Center for Allergy Research and Education (CK-CARE)
Hochgebirgsklinik (High Altitude Hospital)
Davos
Switzerland

Translation from the German language edition: Neurodermitis - Atopisches Ekzem by Johannes Ring, © Georg Thieme Verlag 2012. All rights resevered

ISBN 978-3-319-79384-9 ISBN 978-3-319-22243-1 (eBook)
DOI 10.1007/978-3-319-22243-1

Springer Cham Heidelberg New York Dordrecht London

Softcover reprint of the hardcover 1st edition 2016

Printed on acid-free paper

Springer International Publishing AG Switzerland is part of Springer Science+Business Media (www.springer.com)

Preface

Atopic dermatitis (atopic eczema, eczema, endogenous eczema, Besnier's prurigo, neurodermitis constitutionalis, etc.) is one of the most common—in childhood *the* most common—noncontagious inflammatory skin disease. Although easily recognizable by the experienced physician, the disease poses a variety of problems and difficulties in diagnosis due to its diversity and variability, with poorly defined morphology.

Affected individuals suffer considerably, not only from the disfigurement when face and hands are involved, but especially from the excruciating and tormenting itch. This sensation causes sleeplessness, fatigue, reduction of daily achievements, and a considerable impairment in quality of life not only for the patient but also for his familial and social environment.

Many physicians are helpless and talk about an "incurable" disease. There are only few other fields in medicine where so many "alternative," "complementary," or "unconventional" procedures are used as in atopic dermatitis. Many affected individuals can report an odyssey of visits to doctors and healers in search for a "miracle" ointment or pill!

The disease is frequent: 10–20 % of 5–6-year-old children are affected, and this is the case in many countries of the world. This was different 50 years ago, when in high school I first heard about this condition, and later as a medical student from the unforgettable Professor Alfred Marchionini in Munich. Early epidemiological data from the 1950s reported a prevalence of ca. 1–2 %.

The disease is part of the atopic triad, together with bronchial asthma and hay fever; however, it differs in essential aspects especially with regard to the understanding of the mechanisms involved in pathogenesis, which are better established in hay fever and allergic asthma.

For the dermatologist, atopic dermatitis does not belong to the classical diseases with a very characteristic, ideally pathognomonic, typical "beautiful" skin lesion as primary lesion—as for example in psoriasis as red, scaly, and sharply margined patches, or hexagonal slightly elevated red papules as in lichen planus, or grouped vesicles as in herpes simplex. Atopic dermatitis shows a rather diffuse morphology with unprecise lesions, mostly characterized by secondary changes due to bouts of scratching for strong itch.

It is understandable that 40 years ago the interest in dermatological research in this disease was not very pronounced. Other fields of dermatology were more attractive for research, which holds true even today in many countries.

In the World Congress for Dermatology (Congressus Mundi Dermatologiae), which takes place every 5 years—since recently every 4 years—in various places in the world, there was in 1977 in Mexico City, among 1,000 presentations, only *one* "workshop" dealing with "atopic dermatitis," chaired by the masters Jon Hanifin and Georg Rajka together with 12 participants. Most of these became famous personalities in the field of atopic dermatitis later on and are still good friends.

The interest in this disease obviously has increased tremendously in recent decades, in parallel with the increase in prevalence.

What attracted me to become engaged in this disease? In Germany, the majority of allergists are originally dermatologists, followed by pediatricians, ENT specialists, pneumologists, and other physicians. I was already an established immunologist, having written a PhD thesis on anaphylaxis due to dextran infusions for volume substitution or horse-anti-human lymphocyte globuline (ALG) for immunosuppression in the Institute for Surgical Research (Prof. Walter Brendel). Then I continued research with a stipend from the Deutsche Forschungsgemeinschaft in the laboratory of Prof. Eng Tan at Scripps Clinic and Research Foundation in La Jolla, California.

I already had decided to join—after returning to Germany—the Department of Dermatology at Ludwig Maximilians University in Munich (Prof. Otto Braun-Falco). So in La Jolla, Prof. Eng Tan sent me to the library to find a topic on which it was worthwhile to do 2 years of research, aimed at connecting the previous work in immunology and allergy with the future in dermatology. I wrote a short research grant on the role of vasoactive mediators in atopic dermatitis and started—not knowing that I would be caught by this disease for decades over my professional life. In the 1970s, the progress in the field was very slow. It was not like jumping onto a moving train into a glorious future! It required high frustration tolerance to keep going. One motivation was the surprising and obvious increase in the prevalence of this disease all over the world.

As representatives for many others, I would like to thank the above-mentioned teachers, as well as my predecessors as directors of the Allergy Department (Prof. Karlheinz Schulz) and the Department of Dermatology at the University Hospital Eppendorf (Prof. Theodor Nasemann) and the Department of Dermatology and Allergy Biederstein (Prof. Siegfried Borelli) at the Technical University Munich.

When a researcher is asked to write or edit a book on his favorite topic, this means work and fun at the same time. The field is so extensive and rich that it would be easy to edit a new edition of a handbook—as we have done in the past involving over 50 authors!

However, I personally like books that have been written by *one person* as responsible author; there one can see a red thread, unnecessary repetitions are avoided, and contradictory statements will be rare. Of course, this goes along with the disadvantage of less actual objectivity. I believe that it is attractive for the reader not only to find, as in an encyclopedia, a collection of the newest publications but rather a painting of the whole disease with its many facets, and how it became apparent in the experience of a researcher and physician over decades. Thus, I apologize and ask the reader, as though he/she was traveling on holiday, to trust my more or less experienced guidance with all its subjectivity in the selection and accentuation of various facts, hypotheses, and arguments, in the hope that the reader may not be bored!

It is obvious that many other distinguished individuals could have written this book equally well or probably better: therefore it makes sense—here and now—to say thank you to people who have helped me on the long and difficult path of dealing with atopic dermatitis/eczema.

There is in the first place my experimental teacher Walter Brendel who brought me to transplantation research, immunology, and via antilymphocyte serum towards allergic skin reactions. Eng Tan from Scripps Clinic in La Jolla should be thanked for the openmindedness with which he supported my humble starts in eczema research.

I thank my respected clinical teacher Otto Braun-Falco for his masterly education in dermatology and for the absolute freedom he gave me in research, which was quite different from the structured hierarchy in clinical responsibilities of a university department.

I thank my predecessor as founder and director of the Biederstein Department of Dermatology Siegfried Borelli for his early work in atopic dermatitis ("neurodermitis") and his manifold support for the activities in Davos, Switzerland. Without my friend Bernhard Przybilla as co-resident on the children's ward and longtime co-worker in allergy, many things would have been impossible. Thomas Bieber was a case of good luck for dermatology and allergy, and I am proud that I was allowed to superficially guide him for some time and carry out research with him. It is wonderful that this research has been continued by Andreas Wollenberg. Along with Dieter Vieluf and Barbara Kunz from Hamburg, it was Ulf Darsow and Knut Brockow who brought the eczema research to our department in Munich. At this juncture, Heidelore Hofmann, Dietrich Abeck, and Christina Schnopp should also be mentioned for holding up the flag of pediatric dermatology, together with Claudia Kugler in Munich and Martina Premerlani, Daniela Münch, and Matthias Möhrenschlager in Davos for excellent care for children with eczema and for development of the "eczema school."

Without Torsten Schäfer and Ursula Krämer, the epidemiology of atopic dermatitis in various parts of Germany would not have been written. Marcus Ollert as master of in vitro allergy diagnosis and Bernadette Eberlein in skin physiology have contributed considerably.

Real research in a clinical department is only possible with good cooperation with an experimental unit. This was the case and the good luck we had at the Biederstein campus in cooperation with the newly established Zentrum Allergie und Umwelt – ZAUM (Center for Allergy and Environment) founded in 1998 by Heidrun Behrendt and directed by her until 2010, then later by Carsten Schmid-Weber; here, the experimental immunologic–allergologic together with dermatologic research allowed real progress and was connected to the names of Thilo Jakob, Martin Mempel, Claudia Traidl-Hoffmann, Johannes Huss-Marp, Florian Pfab, Jan Gutermuth, Kilian and Stephanie Eyerich, Stefan Weidinger, Wen-Chie Chen, Jeroen Buters, and many others.

I want to thank Andreas Mauermayer for the excellent clinical photographs, and Brigitte Engelmann, Eleonora Enderlein, Daniela Bolocan, and Sybille Walter for excellent secretarial work.

No research group can stand on its own; among the attractive things in research are the national and international contacts and friendships which refresh thinking and which via the exchange of experiences but also materials lead to new paths. In this sense, I want to thank Thomas Platts-Mills in Charlottesville/Virginia, Donald Leung in Denver, Jon Hanifin in Portland, Ikutaro Yoshida in Nagasaki, Hirohisa Takegawa in Matsumotu, Matsutaka Furue in Kumamoto, Hideyoki Ogawa in Tokio, José Caraballo in Bogota, Yoshiky Miyachi in Kyoto, Kenji Kabashima in Kyoto, Jean-Hilaire Saurat in Geneva, Brunello Wüthrich in Zürich, Alain Taieb in Bordeaux, John Harper in London, Agostin Alomar in Barcelona, Alberto Gianetti and Stefania Seidenari in Modena, Carlo Gelmetti in Milano, Kristian Thestrup-Pedersen and Mette Deleuran in Aarhus, Georg Stingl in Vienna, Alexander Kapp and Thomas Werfel in Hannover, Margitta Worm and Torsten Zuberbier in Berlin, Uwe Gieler in Giessen, Yves DeProst in Paris, Anne Broberg in Goeteborg, Carla Bruijnzel in Utrecht, Jan Bos in Amsterdam, Peter Schmid-Grendelmeier in Zürich, and many others.

I would also like to thank Georg Rajka, who created the tradition of international symposia on the disease "atopic dermatitis" which contributed considerably to progress in the field. It is reassuring that these ideas are taken up and still alive in the regular organization of these symposia under the International Society of Atopic Dermatitis (ISAD).

Finally, I want to thank Dr. Engeli from Thieme, Stuttgart, who gave the permission for an English version of this book, and Mr. Klemp from Springer Science who made the contract. Finally, I want to thank Mrs. Kayalvizhi for her excellent lecturing and final work in the book production.

Whenever medical doctors try to write something in an understandable way, this often does not mean that many people—even physicians of other specialities—will really understand. Yet I hope that this book may find readers also among individuals affected by atopic dermatitis and their caregivers, who might find interesting information for dealing practically with this difficult disease.

Munich, Bavaria, Germany Johannes Ring
December 2015

Foreword

Atopic dermatitis is a common and troublesome inflammatory skin disease, especially during childhood. For those affected and their families, this condition presents an extreme burden of personal suffering, impaired quality of life, and high direct and indirect costs.

While clearly described in the nineteenth century, atopic dermatitis continues to present a complicated puzzle for researchers, doctors, and patients. Even moreso than asthma and hay fever, the "sister" diseases in the atopic triad, the pathomechanisms are considerably more complex. In addition to the epidermal barrier dysfunction and the Th2-deviated inflammatory and immune responses, the frequent IgE-mediated allergic reactions, neurogenic inflammation, pruritus, and an imbalance in the autonomic nervous system seem to play a role.

This book covers the wide spectrum of atopic dermatitis from epidemiology, pathophysiology, and clinical aspects to modern diagnostics and therapy. It is written by one person, namely Professor Johannes Ring, a dermatologist who has focused particularly on the puzzling relationship of allergy and irritancy in eczematous skin reactions.

He has been coeditor and editor of two editions of *Handbook of Atopic Eczema* and given lectures on national and international congresses both in dermatology, pediatric dermatology, and allergy. He was a friend and participant in George Rajka's international symposia on atopic dermatitis and has become president of the International Society of Atopic Dermatitis (ISAD) organizing the valuable research conferences which foster participation and knowledge exchange from many nations. He has also been active in several scientific societies, serving as president of the European Academy of Dermatology and Venerology (EADV) and the Collegium Interationale Allergologicum (CIA) and has organized several outstanding events like the European Dermatology Congress in 2001 and the World Allergy Congress in 2005 both in Munich. More recently, he has hosted a series of international symposia "New Trends in Allergy" taking place every 5 years.

A single-author book has both advantages and disadvantages. One disadvantage is that no individual can have full knowledge of a complex condition like atopic dermatitis, resulting in a certain degree of subjectivity in the selection and accentuation of topics. Such weaknesses may well be offset by the advantage to the reader who will get *one* clear opinion of an expert without the distracting contradictions and redundancies often found in multiauthor books.

Although I personally do not share every opinion of Johannes Ring – and we have a long history of debating our often varied concepts – I enjoy reading his views such as those presented in this book. He provides a well-planned and comprehensive description of this complex disease, combining basic scientific knowledge and good clinical pragmatism for practitioners, be they primary care physicians, pediatricians, dermatologists, or allergists.

November 2015

Jon Hanifin
Department of Dermatology
Oregon Health & Science University
Portland, OR, USA

Contents

Abbreviations

ADHD	Attention deficit hyperactivity disorder
APT	Atopy patch test
ASIT	Allergen-specific immunotherapy
BHR	Bronchial hyperreactivity
CFU	Colony-forming units
CLA	Cutaneous lymphocyte antigen
CMV	Cytomegalovirus
DC	Dendritic cells
DLQI	Dermatology Life Quality Index
DMSO	Dimethyl sulfoxide
DTH	Delayed type hypersensitivity
EAACI	European Academy for Allergy and Clinical Immunology
EBV	Epstein-Barr virus
ECP	Eosinophil cationic protein
EDC	Epidermal differentiation complex
ETFAD	European Task Force Atopic Dermatitis
FcγRI	High-affinity receptor for immunoglobulin G
FcεRI	High-affinity receptor for immunoglobulin E
FDA	Food and Drug Administration
GALT	Gut-associated lymphoid tissue
GM-CSF	Granulocyte monocyte colony-stimulating factor
GvHD	Graft-versus-host disease
GWAS	Genome-wide association study
HIV	Human immunodeficiency virus
HPV	Human papillomavirus
HSV	Herpes simplex virus
IBD	Inflammatory bowel disease
IDDM	Insulin-dependent diabetes mellitus
IDEC	Inflammatory dendritic epidermal cell
Ig	Immunoglobulin
IL	Interleukin
IR	Index of Reactivity
LTT	lymphocyte transformation test
MHC	Major histocompatibility complex
MMF	Mycophenolate mofetil
NMF	Natural moisturizing factor
PDE	Phosphodiesterase

PLD	Polymorphous light dermatosis
PUFA	Polyunsaturated fatty acids
RAST	Radio-allergo-sorbent test
SALT	Skin-associated lymphoid tissue
SCF	Stem cell factor
SCID	Severe combined immunodeficiency
SCORAD	Scoring Atopic Dermatitis
SPT	Skin prick test
TCI	Topical calcineurin inhibitor
TDT	Transmission disequilibrium test
TEWL	Transepidermal water loss
TGF	Tumor growth factor
TLR	Toll-like receptor
TNF	Tumor necrosis factor
TRAC	Thymus and activation-regulated chemokine
VOC	Volatile organic compound
WAO	World Allergy Organization

1 General Introduction and Epidemiology

1.1 Introduction

Allergic diseases are among the major health problems of our time. Especially the so-called atopic diseases, namely, asthma, rhinoconjunctivitis (hay fever), and eczema (atopic dermatitis, atopic eczema), have increased in prevalence during the last decades dramatically (Alfvén et al. 2006; Borelli and Schnyder 1962; Rajka 1989; Schultz Larsen and Hanifin 1992; Williams 2000; Wüthrich 2001; UCB European Allergy Whitebook 1997). Atopic eczema as skin manifestation of the atopic trait represents today the most common chronic noncontagious inflammatory skin disease in childhood (Ring et al. 2006; Wüthrich 1975; Leung and Bieber 2003). Atopic dermatitis usually starts in childhood or early adolescence and is characterized by intense pruritus und disfiguring inflammatory skin lesions. The disease is associated with a dramatic impairment in quality of life. In times when economic reasons only consider mortality statistics measurable in dollars, we have to be the advocates of our patients suffering from chronic skin diseases. The skin as the surface and frontier organ of the human organism is characterized by a multitude of physical and chemical biological functions important for the integrity of human beings. Skin diseases lead to an impairment of self-confidence (Gieler 2006). When skin diseases start in childhood, they may influence the whole life history of a person in a long-lasting way.

At the beginning of this book, I want to start with some very personal reflections: since 1977 I have been engaged scientifically and clinically with this disease, when I performed a postdoctoral fellowship to do research with a grant of the Deutsche Forschungsgemeinschaft at the Scripps Clinic and Research Foundation in La Jolla, California, USA, in the Division of Allergy and Immunology under the guidance of Dr. Eng M. Tan. When I had told him that after this postdoctoral fellowship I most likely would join the Dermatology Department in Munich, he sent me to the library to decide in what field I would like to spend the 2 years.

I found that in those days many other and markedly rarer diseases attracted more attention than atopic dermatitis. So I decided to start here. Later my teacher in clinical dermatology, Prof. Otto Braun-Falco, tolerated this decision although he himself focused on psoriasis; he probably did not like atopic dermatitis so much, since the disease was too unprecise and "diffuse." However, he always gave me the freedom to follow my scientific interests, and he accompanied the progress of my work very intensively and critically.

At the World Congress of Dermatology (Congressus Mundi Dermatologiae) 1977 in Mexico City, there was only one workshop to the subject "atopic dermatitis" among a program with over thousand lectures and posters, chaired by Professors Georg Rajka and Jon Hanifin with about 12 participants. Like me almost all of them have been attracted by this disease in the following decades; we have met often and became good friends. Many of them will be quoted in this book.

J. Ring, *Atopic Dermatitis: Eczema*, DOI 10.1007/978-3-319-22243-1_1

You cannot study atopic dermatitis without questioning the phenomenon of allergy. In the meantime, the disease—most likely due to the rapid increase in prevalence—has attracted much more followers also in clinical research. Even if 50 years ago the majority believed that allergy does not play an important role in this disease, but dry skin and psychology are the major factors, it became clear that this "atopic" disease cannot be studied without basic knowledge of allergy.

Thus, in the first edition of my allergy book "Angewandte Allergologie" (Allergy in Practice) 1982, I included a voluminous chapter on atopic eczema. In 1991 the first edition of the "Handbook of Atopic Eczema" (Ruzicka et al. 1991) appeared, in 2006 the second edition (Ring et al. 2006). In 1993 I was asked by the Ministry of Health of the Federal Republic of Germany to write an expertise regarding the "health care and prevention in children with atopic eczema," which was finally published as a book in 1998 and gave the start signal to develop an educational program "Eczema School for Parents and Children" (Ring 1998; Gieler et al. 2001).

In 2002 the booklet for lay people "Eczema—Causes and Treatments" appeared, written together with Dr. Annette von Zumbusch (Ring and von Zumbusch 2002). Meanwhile other valuable books have been published (Bieber and Leung 2002; Williams 2000; Schneider et al. 2011).

Why do we need another book on atopic dermatitis?

The state of the art has shown a tremendous increase in knowledge in molecular genetics and experimental dermatology and allergology during the last years. New concepts allow the vision of new therapeutic strategies.

Beside this progress, there is the urgent need of many affected individuals and physicians dealing with this disease; it is not enough just to write a prescription! These patients are "exhausting," and they need intense information about and introduction into causes and individual provocation factors. There is neither a "miracle" injection, "miracle" ointment, nor "miracle" pill which applied once will solve the problem forever.

On the other hand, there is no reason to become desperate; I fight against the so often used term "incurable" disease. It is true that there is a genetic predisposition with regard to barrier disturbance and hypersensitivity of the skin that gives rise to the formation of eczema, and which at the moment cannot be changed. However, the eczema itself can be treated very well and many patients are symptom-free over decades. They "grow out" of eczema.

Already today a considerable progress has been made in anti inflammatory basic dermatological and immunological therapies which unfortunately are not made available to all patients. To illustrate this in a very practical sense is one of the aims of this book.

1.2 History

1.2.1 First Descriptions

In most dermatology textbooks, historical reflections in the description of atopic eczema start with Robert Willan who in 1808 used the term "eczema" in a scientific morphological way (Schadewaldt 1980–1984; Wallach et al. 2004; Willan 1808). The term "eczema" was coined in the sixth century AD by the Greek physician Aetios from Amida who described the boiling and bubbling (eczeo = to bubble up) as it can be observed in a boiling soup (Aetios from Amida 1542). Aetios from Amida himself probably did not realize how illustratively he described the modern concept of pathophysiology of spongiosis in those times, namely, the intercellular formation of edema starting in the dermis and reaching the epidermis, flooding it with lymph until blister formation (more in Bergmann and Ring 2014).

Early descriptions can be found in the book of the Italian physician Girolamo Mercuriali (De morbis cutaneis) with a description of "lactumen" as crustose skin lesions on the scalp (Mercuriali 1601) which look like burned milk in a pan and were later called "cradle cap" or, in German, "Milchschorf." Cradle cap is often regarded to be the first manifestation of atopic dermatitis in infants.

The first documented individual patient of history may have been emperor Octavianus Augustus

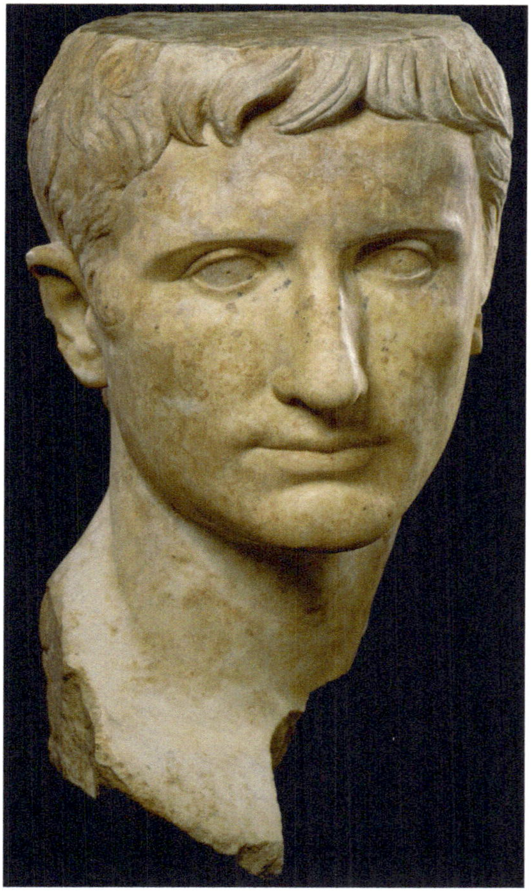

Fig. 1.1 Emperor Octavianus Augustus from the Julian-Claudian emperor family

(Fig. 1.1) from the Julian-Claudian emperor family (Mier 1975; Ring 1985) who, as we find in Suetonius "De Vita Caesarum (Suetonius 1958)," was suffering not only from "catarrhus" at the time of spring winds and episodic "tightness of the chest," but also from "tormenting itch" with lichen-like skin changes (which he used to scratch on his back with a long instrument). Also in the Julian-Claudian emperor family, a positive family history (even according to today's standards) can be found in emperor Claudius with perennial rhinoconjunctivitis and Britannicus as a horse-allergic individual (Ring 1985). The diagnosis "atopic eczema" for Octavianus Augustus seems plausible. Unfortunately, the many statues and images are of no help, since they always were idealized and did not represent individual portraits (Paul Zanker, personal communication 1983).

Table 1.1 Atopic dermatitis/eczema: names in history

Eczema	Aetios from Amida
Eczema	Willan
Constitutional prurigo	Hebra
Neurodermite diffuse	Brocq
Prurigo diathésique	Besnier
Early or late exudative eczematoid	Rost
Atopic dermatitis/atopic eczema	Wise and Sulzberger
Endogenous eczema	Korting
Neurodermitis constitutionalis sive atopica	Schnyder and Borelli
Atopic eczema dermatitis syndrome (AEDS)	Johansson et al. (EAACI task force)
Eczema	Johansson et al. (WAO consensus JACI 2004)

Literature see Ring et al. 2006
EAACI European Academy of Allergy and Clinical Immunology, *WAO* World Allergy Organization

The great rival of Robert Willan, the French Jean-Louis Alibert, described itchy and oozing skin changes in infants under the name "teigne muqueuse" where teigne, like "tinea," just meant an inflammatory skin disease (Taïeb et al. 2002).

1.2.2 Milestones and Terminology

In Table 1.1 the most important milestones of history of atopic dermatitis are listed which also reflect the wide spectrum of names used for this disease.

Erasmus Wilson described in detail an "infantile eczema," and he also included skin changes without blisters as dry eczema. Ferdinand von Hebra, the great Viennese dermatologist, described a "constitutional prurigo" which we today would call a prurigo type of atopic eczema.

The great breakthrough came with the French School and was connected with the names Vidal, Jacquet, Brocq, and Besnier. Besnier coined the term "prurigo diathésique"("dermatites multiformes prurigineuses chroniques exacerbantes et paroxystiques de prurigo de Hebra") (Besnier 1892, 1901). For a long time, the disease also was called "Prurigo Besnier."

Brocq and Jacquet coined the term "neurodermite" (Brocq 1903, 1927; Jacquet 1904), focusing on the dry lichenified skin lesions, and by enlarging the lichen simplex chronicus, Vidal gave a name for a similar, more generalized eruption. In Germany the pediatrician Czerny coined the term "diathesis" as a concept (Czerny 1905). Rost defined an "exudative state," "früh- bzw. spät-exsudatives Ekzematoid" ("early or late exudative eczematoid") (Rost 1929; Rost and Marchionini 1932). Soon in Germany, the term "neurodermitis" prevailed, while it was forgotten in France.

The discovery of transferability of allergy with serum by Prausnitz and Küstner (1921) and the observation of a familial tendency for atopic diseases with the definition of the term "atopy" by Coca and Cooke (1923) in the USA led to inclusion of allergic reactions in the description of this disease. In 1906 the Viennese pediatrician Clemens von Pirquet had created the term "allergy" (von Pirquet 1906). Today we see allergy as an environmental disease where, on the basis of a genetic predisposition, the organism reacts against environmental substances (Figs. 1.2 and 1.3). Allergy can be regarded as a specific alteration of immune reactivity towards a hypersensitivity disease (Ring 1982a).

Many dermatologists have problems in describing the morphology of this disease due to its wide spectrum and the difficulty to identify a classical primary lesion. Therefore, on national and international congresses, generally intense debates arose about this disease. In 1933 the American Marion Baldur Sulzberger—who had joined Joseph Jadassohn and Bloch in Switzerland—together with Wise defined the unifying concept of infantile and adult disease as atopic dermatitis or atopic eczema (Wise and Sulzberger 1933). For a long time this concept was neglected in Europe. Robert Degos in Paris liked the term "constitutional eczema" (Degos 1953). In the handbook chapter in the "Jadassohn-

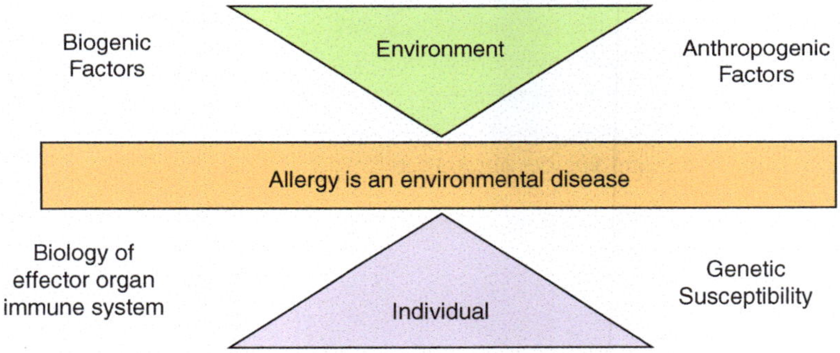

Fig. 1.2 Allergy as environmental disease (According to H. Behrendt)

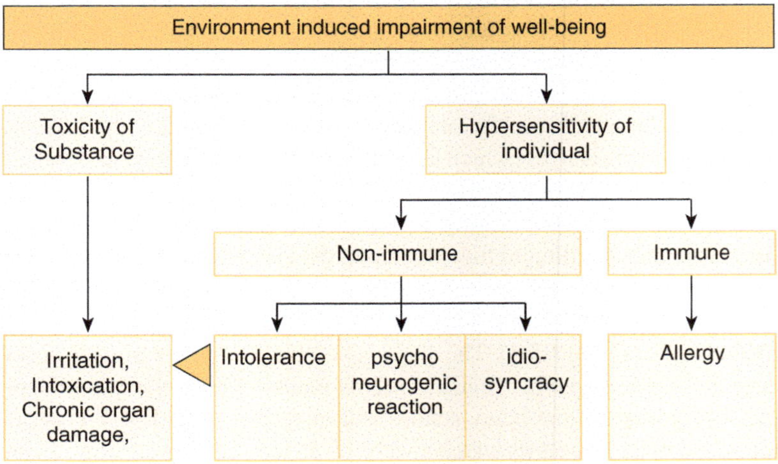

Fig. 1.3 Not every impairment of well-being through environmental factors is an allergy

Ergänzungswerk," edited by Alfred Marchionini, Urs Schnyder and Siegfried Borelli wrote on "Neurodermitis diffusa constitutionalis sive atopica" (Borelli and Schnyder 1962; Schnyder and Borelli 1962). Korting wrote his thesis on "endogenous" eczema where he focused on the abnormal reactivity patterns in the autonomic ("vegetative") nervous system not only affecting the skin, but also provoking cardiovascular and even pupillary reactions with an increased cholinergic and decreased adrenergic reactivity (Korting 1954).

Hans-Jürgen Bandmann was an allergist and dermatologist and a supporter of the term "Neurodermitis" (Bandmann 1962). The transatlantic differences were overcome by the pioneers Georg Rajka in Oslo and Jon Hanifin in Portland/Oregon who, at an international symposium organized by Georg Rajka focusing on atopic dermatitis, developed a consensus on diagnostic criteria which are used until today (Hanifin and Rajka 1980). These symposia became the platform of researchers and clinicians all over the world interested in atopic dermatitis and a place for free discussions and exchange of information. It was there where the "Scoring System for Atopic Dermatitis (SCORAD)" was born, allowing an objective determination of various severity grades of this chronic disease (Kunz et al. 1997; Stalder et al. 1993).

In 1983, Brunello Wüthrich—in analogy to respiratory atopy—proposed an "extrinsic" versus an "intrinsic" variant of this disease (IgE associated versus non-IgE associated) (Wüthrich 1983, 1989). Around the millennium, this conflict culminated in an intense nomenclature debate both in the European Academy of Allergology and Clinical Immunology (EAACI) (Johansson et al. 2001) and finally in a task force of the World Allergy Organization (WAO) (Johansson et al. 2004). Today the debate on terminology is not led quite so emotionally by many dermatologists, allergists, or patients. On the other hand, terminology is not a matter of sophisticated debate, rather pathophysiological concepts are hidden in names, and these concepts lead to quite different management approaches both in diagnostics and therapy.

Therefore it makes sense to understand what researchers, patients, or physicians mean when they talk about atopic dermatitis or atopic eczema.

1.2.3 Summary

The disease "atopic dermatitis" (atopic eczema) most likely is not new; the term "eczema" was coined around 600 AD. First descriptions of the disease can be found in the nineteenth century under various names, and only around 1900 the term "neurodermitis" was clearly differentiated from other types of eczema. In 1933, Wise and Sulzberger proposed the name "atopic dermatitis" or "atopic eczema."

1.3 The Term "Atopy"

In a book on this disease, it cannot be avoided to briefly also touch the history of allergy and the term "atopy" (Table 1.2).

The term "atopy" has provoked a variety of interpretations during the 90 years following its birth. Atopic diseases, according to the classification of Coombs and Gell, range among type I (immediate-type) reactions (Fig. 1.4) (quoted in Bergmann and Ring 2014). In 1923, Coca and Cooke coined the term "atopy" to describe an "inherited" hypersensitivity against environmental allergens which manifests as asthma or "hay fever" (Coca and Cooke 1923). Different from other physicians who are not so critical, they knew their limits in philology and asked the Greek philologist Perry from Columbia University in New York to propose a term for this condition. Perry proposed "atopy," meaning "not on the right place, out of order" (Ring 1983).

Two years later, Coca and Grove proposed the term "atopic reagins" for the substances in serum with which the hypersensitivity of the immediate type can be transferred according to Prausnitz' and Küstner's experiments (Coca and Grove 1925). They added this characteristic to the term of atopy. Translated into today's language this means that IgE antibodies are an important part of atopy.

Table 1.2 Milestones in the history of allergy (quoted in Ring et al. 2006)

Pollen: skin and provocation tests	Blackley	1873
Mast cell	Ehrlich	1877
Neurodermite diffuse	Brocq	1891
Prurigo diathésique	Besneir	1892
Patch test for contact allergy	Joseph Jadassohn	1895
Anaphylaxis	Richet and Portier	1902
Allergy	von Pirquet	1906
Histamine effects mimic anaphylaxis	Dale and Laidlaw	1910
Immunotherapy ("prophylactic inoculation")	Noon and Freeman	1911
Transfer of hypersensitivity with serum	Prausnitz and Küstner	1921
Atopy	Coca and Cooke	1923
Reagins in atopy	Coca and Groove	1925
Allergic diathesis	Kämmerer	1928
Bronchial hyperreactivity	Tiffeneau	1945
Shock fragment	Hansen	1941
Cortisone	Hench and Kendall	1949
Autonomic nervous dysregulation	Korting	1954
Genetic basis	Schnyder	1960
Types of pathogenic immune reactions	Coombs and Gell	1963
Immunoglobulin E	Ishizaka K and T	1966
	Johansson	1967
House dust mite	Vorhoorst and Spieksma	1967
Beta blockade in asthma	Szentivanyi	1968
Fc-epsilon receptor	Metzger	1977
Th1-Th2 concept	Mossman	1987
Interleukin 4	Coffman	1988
Filaggrin mutation in eczema	McLean and Irvine	2006

Literature see Ring 2005

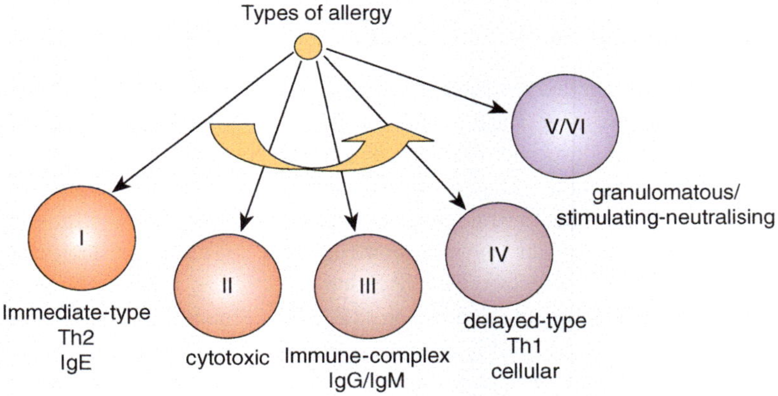

Fig. 1.4 Types of allergic reactions in the classification of Coombs and Cell (Modified by Ring)

In 1933, Wise and Sulzberger also included the skin manifestations in this spectrum and called it "atopic dermatitis" or "atopic eczema."

In 1943, Coca modified his definition towards "atopy comprising a group of allergic diseases with a common hereditary influence and characterized by atopic reagins" (Coca 1943).

1.3.1 The Role of Immunoglobulin E

After the discovery of immunoglobulin E (IgE) as a carrier of the immediate-type hypersensitivity by the groups of Ishizaka (Ishizaka and Ishizaka 1967) and Johansson (Johansson 1967), atopy was identical with IgE-mediated disease for many authors (Juhlin et al. 1969; Ohman and Johansson 1974).

However, it soon became apparent that this was too simple. There are individuals with IgE-mediated diseases without family background like IgE-mediated penicillin anaphylaxis or insect venom anaphylaxis (Ring 2005).

In the 1980s, it was J. Pepys who stressed the concept that all human beings or all organisms under certain conditions can form IgE antibodies against protein allergens either after heavy exposure or when they have the "atopic background" (Pepys 1975) in abnormal concentrations.

1.3.2 Definition of Subpopulations

The normal relation between atopy and IgE antibodies can also be used to define subpopulations of allergic diseases, e.g., "atopic" asthma with IgE association versus "non-atopic" asthma without detection of IgE sensitization.

According to clinical experience, the disease itself does not differ as "asthma bronchiale" or "noninfectious rhinoconjunctivitis," even if patients do not show IgE-mediated hypersensitivity reactions. Therefore the term "intrinsic" or "non-IgE associated" became popular in respiratory atopy and was also used for atopic dermatitis by Wüthrich (1983).

1.3.3 Definition of EAACI and WAO

The new considerations of subpopulations "atopic" versus "non-atopic," based on the detection of IgE antibodies, were not problematic in respiratory diseases; however, in the description of the skin condition, absurd terms like "non-atopic atopic eczema" appeared. While this was never a serious nomenclature in dermatology textbooks, in international debates these discussions took place, and the necessity was felt to come up with a new atopy definition. This was then started with a task force of the European Academy of Allergy and Clinical Immunology (EAACI) and later of the World Allergy Organization (WAO) with the following definition:

"Atopy is a personal or familial tendency, commonly starting in childhood and adolescence, to become sensitized and produce IgE antibodies after normal exposure against allergens, commonly proteins. In consequence, these persons develop typical symptoms like asthma, rhinoconjunctivitis or eczema" (Johansson et al. 2004).

According to this definition, all patients with asthma, rhinoconjunctivitis, or eczema without detectable IgE antibodies would not suffer from an "atopic" disease. In consequence, this terminology then would lead to an "atopic" versus a "non-atopic" "atopic dermatitis." Therefore it became necessary to come up with a new name for the skin manifestations of atopy. The EAACI Nomenclature Task Force proposed "atopic eczema dermatitis syndrome AEDS" which aroused intense criticism and was not accepted, not the least for lack of logic since the adjective "atopic" again was used for the definition of the atopic disease and furthermore because of the association with the immunodeficiency syndrome AIDS.

Therefore the task force of the WAO found consensus by defining the term "eczema" anew in a way that dermatitis is the headline, and the term "eczema" defines the disease which before was called "atopic dermatitis" or "atopic eczema." So the adjective "atopic" would only be used when IgE antibodies could be detected (Johansson et al. 2004, Table 1.1). In consequence, there would be an "atopic" versus a "non-atopic" eczema, similar to Wüthrich's extrinsic versus intrinsic variant of atopic dermatitis.

The future will show whether these definitions will be adopted by practicing allergists and dermatologists (Bos 2002; Wüthrich 1999a).

The root of the problem in terminology can be found in the endeavor to define a clinical symptomatology and a pathophysiological mechanism with one term.

Early definitions started with the clinical symptomatology of disease and later included the detection of IgE antibodies.

The WAO definition starts from the laboratory determination of IgE and only later includes the typical clinical symptoms.

1.3.4 Our Definition of Atopy

Our definition from the *Handbook of Atopic Eczema* starts with the clinical symptomatology:

> Atopy is a familial tendency to develop certain diseases (rhinoconjunctivitis, asthma bronchiale, eczema) on the basis of hypersensitivity of skin and mucous membranes against environmental agents, associated with increased IgE production and/or altered nonspecific reactivity (Ring 1991a). Today I would like to add "… plus epithelial barrier dysfunction."

Therefore atopy is on the one hand a subgroup of IgE-mediated diseases, and on the other hand it is more (Fig. 1.5).

With this definition it is possible to describe intermediate states which can be found in the type of a "Gauss distribution" of atopic diseases which can be observed when comparing the two dimensions of "increased IgE production" with "altered nonspecific reactivity" (Fig. 1.6). Where both parameters overlap, there is no doubt of an atopic disease. Towards both sides of the curves, however, the situation becomes increasingly unprecise with entities such as "latent atopy" (only detection of positive skin tests or IgE antibodies in serum without clinical symptoms) or so-called "intrinsic" variants of atopic diseases (Ring 1982a, 2005).

This dilemma only will be solved when the term "intrinsic" or "non-atopic" will not only be negatively defined by exclusion, but by a positive detection of a characteristic marker.

In my experience, the atopy definition from our textbook seems to be most useful for clinical practice.

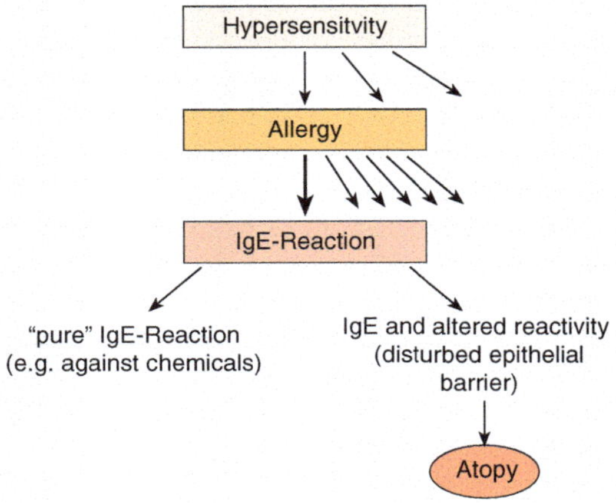

Fig. 1.5 Atopy as subgroup of IgE-mediated allergic reactions

1.3.5 Summary

The term "Atopy" has been coined in 1923 by Coca and Cooke and since then has changed its meaning several times. The problem is the lack of a clear-cut biomarker. If one uses immunoglobulin E as marker, there are clear-cut IgE-associated diseases which do not belong to "atopy" as, e.g., insect venom anaphylaxis. On the other hand, there are atopic diseases like asthma, rhinoconjunctivitis, or eczema without IgE involvement. Therefore the definition given by the task force of the World Allergy Organization (WAO) which is based on the laboratory detection of IgE may be

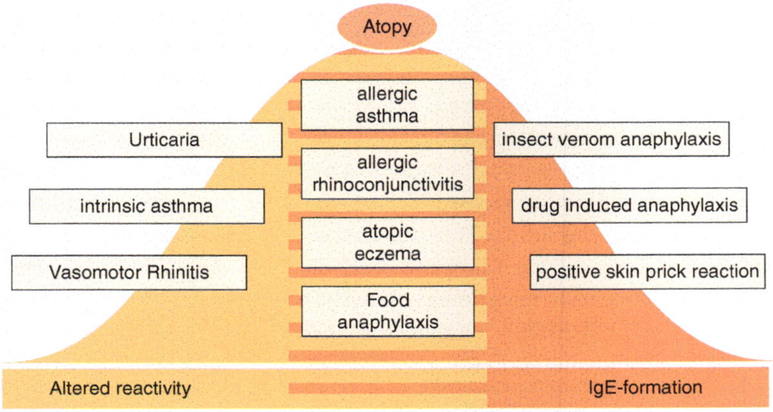

Fig. 1.6 "Gauss" distribution of atopic reactivity

difficult in clinical practice. It excludes the clinically identical disease conditions where IgE association cannot be found ("intrinsic"). The author—together with others—believes that not only the tendency to IgE formation, but also nonspecific alterations of the epithelial barrier represent a basic feature of "atopy."

1.4 Epidemiology of Atopic Eczema

There is no doubt that atopic eczema has increased in prevalence since the 1960s of the twentieth century dramatically in the general population (Kuehr 1999; Marsh et al. 1981; Ring 1991b; Ring et al. 2001a; Schäfer et al. 2003a, b, Schultz Larsen 1993; Schultz Larsen and Holm 1985; Schultz Larsen et al. 1986; Wahn and Wichmann 2000; Williams 2000). Significant differences exist in reported prevalence all over the world which only can be partly explained by methodological differences.

Some studies just describe an increase in incidence in the patients of a clinical department or office, others use population-based studies with questionnaires, and others require the diagnosis of a physician (dermatologist?). Other population-based studies with actual dermatologic examination have been performed (Schäfer et al. 1996). Most of these studies describe examinations in childhood; there are only few data regarding the prevalence of atopic eczema in adults (Worm et al. 2006; Möhrenschlager et al. in prep). Clinical examinations usually only represent a point prevalence, while questionnaires can detect cumulative prevalence rates over a lifetime.

According to general estimations, approx. 3 % of adults and 12 % of preschool children are affected, with consistently changing numbers between 1 and 25 % in the general population (Ring et al. 2012).

1.4.1 Prevalence of Atopic Eczema in Childhood

Atopic eczema is the most common noncontagious chronic inflammatory skin disease in childhood with a dramatic increase in prevalence in the last decades.

Early investigations from various countries in the years between 1939 and 1964 indicate a prevalence of 1.3–3.1 % in various populations (Ring 1991b; Wüthrich 2001). Studies between 1980 and 2005 show dramatically increased numbers ranging between 26 % for questionnaire-based and 32 % for actual investigations with dermatological inspections (Ring et al. 2012). The highest numbers were detected in the International Study of Allergy and Asthma in Childhood (ISAAC) (Asher et al. 2006; ISAAC 1998): in 90 centers, 256,410 children at the age of 6–7 years and 151 centers with 458,623 children at the age of 13–14 years were examined in 56 countries (Figs. 1.7 and 1.8). In these studies there was a worldwide variation with rather low figures in Albania and Iran and exceeding 20 % in the UK. Generally the prevalence of atopic eczema seems to be higher in Australia and Northern Europe compared to Asia and Eastern Europe.

Studies from Germany have been reported in the so-called KiGGS study (Kindergesundheits-Survey) (Schlaud et al. 2007) (Fig. 1.9). Contrary to hay fever and asthma (von Mutius et al. 1994a, b, 1998), atopic eczema showed a higher prevalence in Eastern Germany compared to West Germany (Table 1.3) (Schäfer 1996).

Only few studies followed the prevalence rates over longer time periods with a consisting identical methodology: most of them show marked increases in prevalence (Fig. 1.10) (Schäfer et al. 1996). Most of these studies have been performed in Europe. Some of these studies now show a plateau formation or even slight decreases in prevalence in some European countries.

1.4.2 Causes for Increase

The causes for the increasing prevalence of this disease are still largely unknown. However, there are hypothetical concepts trying to give an explanation (Tables 1.4 and 1.5). The most popular is the "hygiene hypothesis" (Strachan 1989, 1997).

Apart from the genetic predisposition with an immunological and an epithelial basis, environmental factors play a role in modulating allergy development in an enhancing or protective

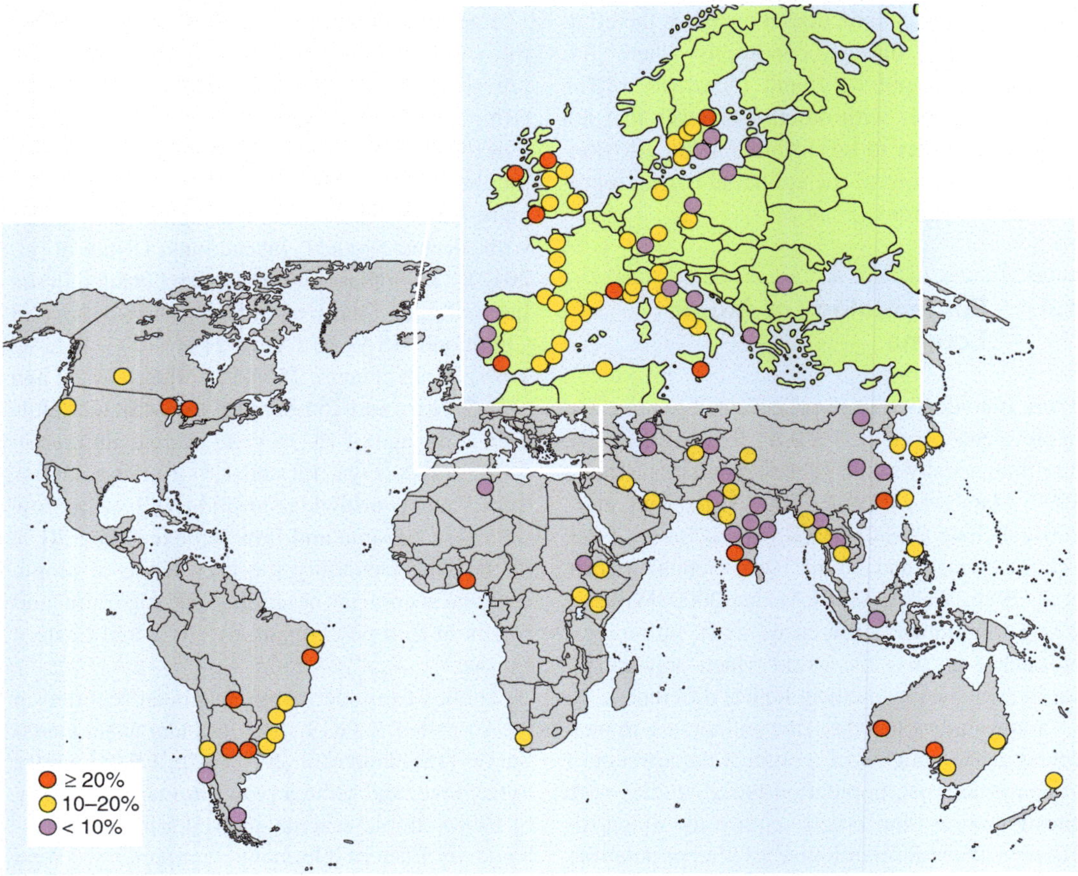

Fig. 1.7 ISAAC study: prevalence of allergic rhinitis worldwide in 13–14-year-old children (ISAAC 1998)

manner (Behrendt et al. 1999; Wichmann et al. 1995). Allergen exposure may not be regarded as the only causal factor (Arshad 2003). A variety of additional substances or factors from the environment can modulate allergy development, in the sense of an enhancement like traffic exhaust with diesel particles, tobacco smoke, volatile organic compounds [VOCs], or in a protective way, like infections in early childhood, microbial contacts, and nutrition (Behrendt et al. 1999; Behrendt and Ring 2011; Cramer et al. 2007; Ege et al. 2008a, b) (Fig. 1.11). Climate change with an increasing tendency towards global warming may additionally contribute to a further increase in allergy prevalence (IPCC 2007, Behrendt and Ring 2011).

Defective training of the immune system by improved hygiene, less infection, and less parasite infestation (IgE antibodies in evolution provided the defense against large intruders) has been summarized under the term "jungle" or "hygiene" hypothesis (Behrendt et al. 1993; Björksten 1999; Herz et al. 2000; Krämer et al. 1999a; Ring and Behrendt 1993; Strachan 1989). Though these hypothetical concepts may be interesting for scientific investigations, they are no real basis for practical recommendations. General headlines like "dirt is allergy protective" or "natural infection is healthier than vaccination" have no scientific basis.

The triad of atopic diseases shows large overlaps between eczema, asthma, and rhinoconjunctivitis (Schäfer et al. 1993, 1997c) (Fig. 1.12).

1.4.3 Own Investigations

At the Dermatology Department of the Ludwig-Maximilians-Universität (LMU) in Munich,

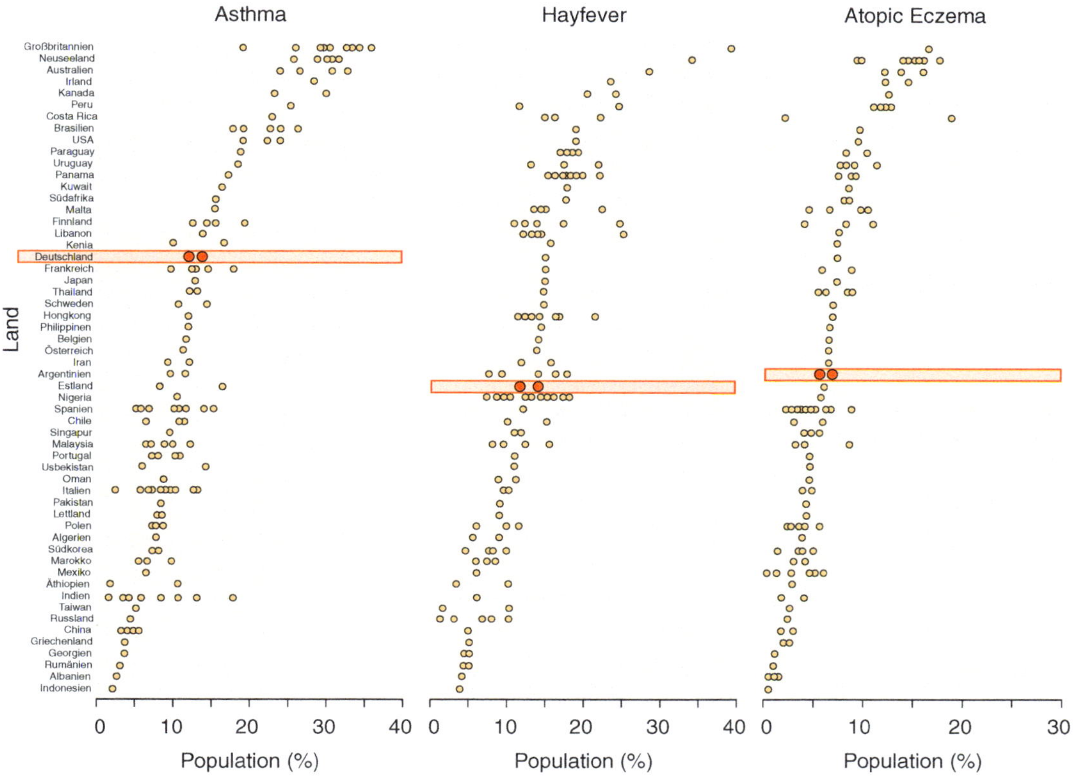

Fig. 1.8 Symptom prevalence of allergic diseases including atopic eczema in the ISAAC study in 14-year-old children (ISAAC 1998)

later at the Department of Dermatology and Allergy at the University Hospital Eppendorf in Hamburg, and then at the Department of Dermatology and Allergology at the Technische Universität, Munich, together with the Medical Institute for Environmental Hygiene (now Institut für Umweltmedizinische Forschung IUF) at the Heinrich-Heine-Universität in Düsseldorf, since 1988 we have studied over 40,000 children of the age of 5–6 years during the preschool medical examination; these investigations have been performed in various states of the Federal Republic of Germany (Bavaria, North Rhine Westphalia, Saxony, Saxony-Anhalt, Hamburg, Schleswig-Holstein) (Krämer et al. 2002; Schäfer et al. 1996; Überla et al. 1988). We found large differences between the different states in Germany, but especially between East and West Germany (Table 1.3), there was a clear-cut increase in the prevalence of hay fever with markedly increasing prevalence rates in East German children during 10 years from 1991 until 2000.

The rate of atopic eczema was high already, in some parts even significantly higher than in West German children in 1991 (Krämer et al. 2015).

1.4.4 Eczema Over Lifetime

One of the most common misconceptions when dealing with atopic dermatitis is the note that it starts "at birth." This is what mothers often say to me; only when I precisely ask "was the baby born with eczema?," she answers "of course not!" This is a crucial question since there are skin diseases occurring at birth or in the immediately following days which, however, almost never represent atopic dermatitis. This disease starts later, classically after 3 months, sometimes maybe already after 4–8 weeks. Since the differential diagnosis in neonates is difficult, the term "infantile

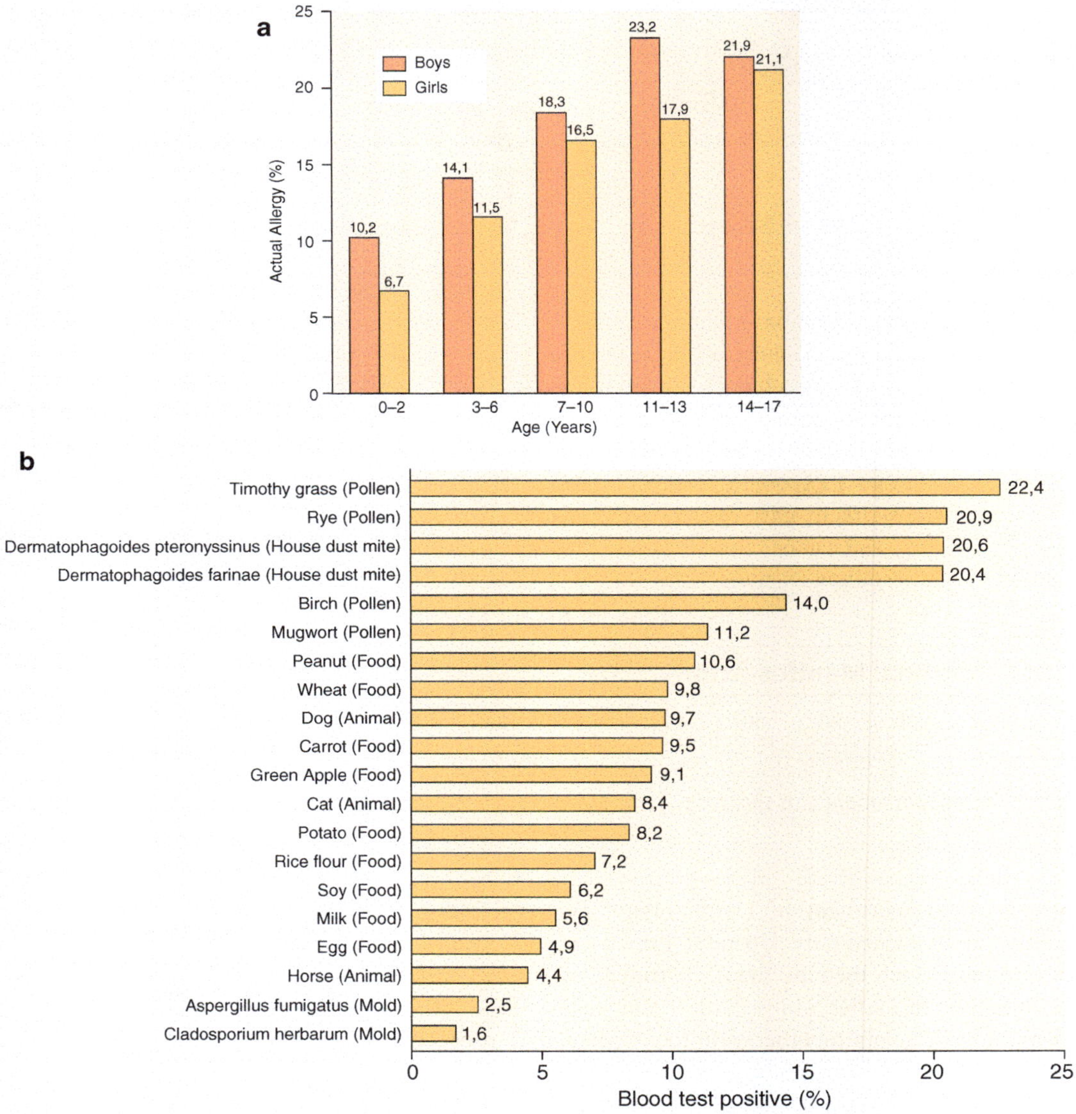

Fig. 1.9 Results of the KiGGS study (health survey of children and adolescents) of the Robert Koch Institute from the year 2003 to 2006 in 17,641 children and adolescents at 167 locations (representative sample). (**a**) Physician diagnosed atopic disease: atopic eczema, hay fever, allergic asthma. (**b**) Prevalence of sensitization against 20 common allergens (sIgE in serum), sensitization totally 41 %, aeroallergens 37 %, food allergens 20 % (According to Schlaud et al. (2007))

eczema" (eczema infantum) is not bad. Apart from genodermatoses and infectious disease, it is mostly seborrheic dermatitis making problems in the differential diagnosis (see Sect. 2.4).

Probably 80 % of atopic dermatitis starts before the second year of life, yet there is an increasing number of patients showing or developing atopic dermatitis in adulthood.

With regard to the developing immune response over lifetime, the "miracle of tolerance" during pregnancy stands at the beginning, in the neonatal period Th2 predominates, and during childhood the immune system is stimulated and trained to become mature. In puberty hormonal influences play a role (see Sect. 3.6).

During adulthood, our immune system lives from memory. The first organ to really go into senescence is the thymus which already begins to turn into fatty tissue around the 17th year of life. During senescence, the immune system suffers a loss of regulation and a tendency to facilitate autoimmune phenomena.

1.4.5 Atopic Eczema in Adulthood

Several studies have been performed to determine the prevalence of atopic dermatitis in adulthood (Williams and Wüthrich 2000).

Table 1.3 Prevalence of atopic dermatitis in East and West Germany ($n = 1404$ children) (Schäfer and Ring 2000)

Area in West Germany	Prevalence (%)	Area in East Germany	Prevalence (%)
Essen	3.4	Osterburg	7.1
Duisburg North	4.1	Gardelegen	8.4
Borken	4.9	Halle/Saale	11.2
Duisburg South	6.2	Salzwedel	11.7
		Magdeburg	13.8

In 1980, Vickers published a prospective study on 2000 children from the pediatric dermatology department in Leeds with a follow-up of up to 21 years: in around 90 % of the children, eczema disappeared, and they stayed in remission when they had reached the age of ten (Vickers 1980). However, there were critical comments to this study, since it was only one observer who designed the study and examined the children, and also the definition of "remission" was not clear. Furthermore—and this is the most crucial critical issue—he also included "eczema infantum" which at first might have been seborrheic dermatitis (see above). Other studies showed a significantly worse prognosis with remission rates of only 10–70 % (Rystedt 1986). A retrospective study in Australia in 2600 outpatients comprised 519 patients with atopic eczema; 47 % had observed the new occurrence of atopic dermatitis at the age over 20 years (adult onset, 158 women, 85 men) (Bannister and Freeman 2000). The peak of the age group was between 40 and 50 years, but also over 70 years, and 10 % of newly occurring eczema were found.

The largest study was performed in Berlin as a cross-sectional study involving 13,300 subjects randomly selected at the age from birth to 99 years and in the years 1999 and 2000. This study

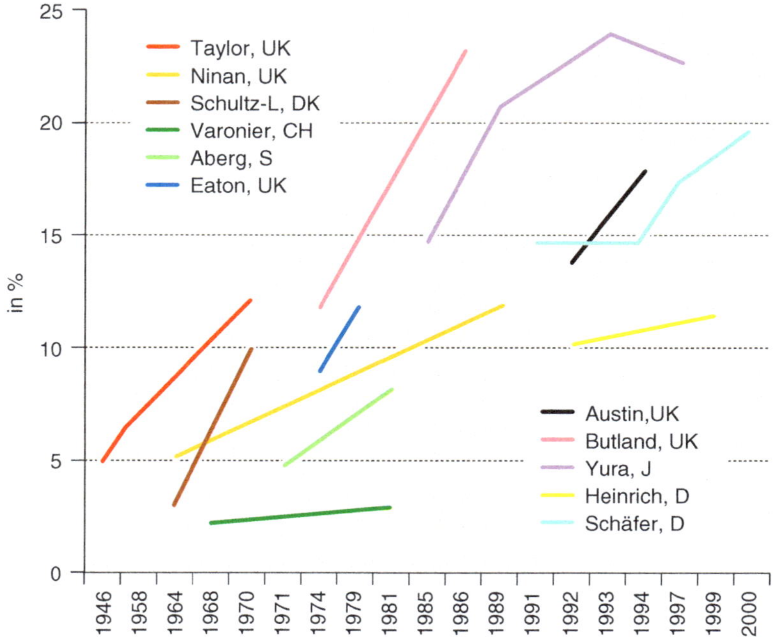

Fig. 1.10 Increasing prevalence of atopic eczema in various studies in the second half of the twentieth century (From Ring et al. (2006))

Table 1.4 Hypothetical concepts trying to explain the increase in allergy prevalence

Increased awareness and improved diagnostics
Psychosocial influences
Allergen exposure
Lack of adequate stimulation of the immune system ("jungle" or "hygiene" hypothesis)
Iatrogenic (medication)
Environmental pollution
Climate change

Table 1.5 Prevalence of atopic dermatitis in German children in the years 1990–2000 (Ring et al. 2012)

	Atopic dermatitis (%)
5–8-year-old children	
Mecklenburg Pomerania (1994)	9.9
Brandenburg (1994)	7.0
Saxony (1995/6)	17.5
Saxony/Saxony-Anhalt (1990–1995)	14.3
Saxony-Anhalt (1992–1993)	10.0
North Rhine Westphalia (1985–1989)	6.8
North Rhine Westphalia (Duisburg 1990–1995)	9.2
North Rhine Westphalia (Münster 1994–1995)	14.7
Bavaria (1988–1989)	13.4
Bavaria Augsburg (1996)	13.1
Bavaria Munich (1996)	15.9
8–15-year-old children	
Mecklenburg Pomerania (1994–1995)	5.9
Berlin (1992–1993)	10
Saxony (1995–1996)	16.6
North Rhine Westphalia (Münster 1994–1995)	10.6
North Rhine Westphalia (Bielefeld 1996–1997)	7.2
Bavaria (1989)	13.3
Bavaria (1995–1996)	17.5

used telephone interviews and—if there was evidence of skin lesions—a dermatologic investigation. From 1739 answered questionnaires, there was a cumulative 1-year prevalence of atopic dermatitis of 8.4 % and a point prevalence of actually existing skin lesions of 1.6 % (Worm et al. 2006).

It is interesting that in the adult onset of persisting eczema, females are generally more frequently affected than males.

A similar study regarding airway allergy in a follow-up of the SAPALDIA population in Switzerland, a self-supported prevalence of allergic rhinitis in subjects over 60 years, showed 13.0 % for men and 15.4 % for women; atopic sensitization had a prevalence of 26.2 % in men over 60 years compared to 18.1 % in women (Wüthrich et al. 2013).

Own investigations: between autumn 1991 and spring 1992, an environmental epidemiological trial was performed in Hamburg as the "Projekt Bille-Siedlung" with a total of 739 persons living in a certain area possibly heavily polluted by chemicals from an industrial factory. In this study we found a point prevalence of 3.4 % for atopic eczema in the whole population; in children aged below 14 years, the prevalence was 10.2 %, whereas adults showed 2.3 % prevalence (Schäfer et al. 1997a).

We found indirectly similar rates in the first epidemiological trials in Bavaria in the years of 1988–1991, where 988 five- to six-year-old preschool children were investigated; 8.3 % suffered from atopic eczema, while the respective mothers and fathers of these children only showed prevalence rates of 4.2, respectively, 2.1 % (Überla et al. 1988). This clearly showed that in the comparison of generations, the children suffered twice as often from atopic eczema than their parents. We could observe similar findings for hay fever and asthma.

When discussing adult atopic eczema, one has to distinguish between:

- Persistent atopic eczema since childhood
- Newly developing atopic eczema in adulthood ("late onset")

A study in Berlin investigating the population with telephone interviews and questionnaires even showed a 10 % prevalence of atopic eczema in adulthood (Worm et al. 2006).

It can be concluded that newly developing atopic eczema in adulthood or even elderly individuals has been disregarded in the literature until now (Sandstrom and Faergemann 2004). Often these conditions may be misdiagnosed as "generalized eczema of unknown origin."

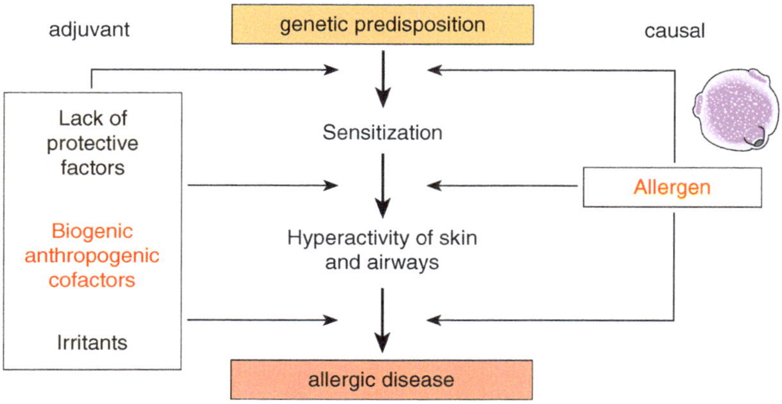

Fig. 1.11 Determinants of allergic inflammation (From Behrendt et al. (1999))

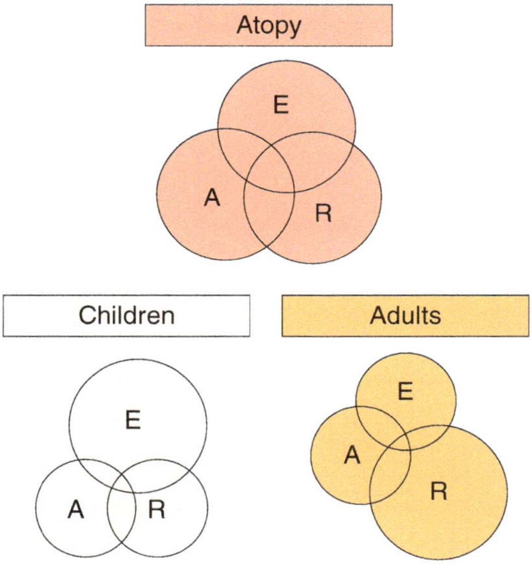

Fig. 1.12 Overlap of the three atopic diseases according to age groups in the Venn diagram. *E* atopic eczema, *R* rhinoconjunctivitis, *A* asthma

The clinical symptomatology of eczema in adulthood or in the elderly may differ a little bit from the classical early-onset childhood atopic dermatitis. A study from Turkey in 63 out of 376 patients with atopic dermatitis who had developed eczema only in adulthood showed that 22 % did not fulfill the UK working party's diagnostic criteria and that 11 % had non-flexural involvement, 6 % nummular, 3 % prurigo-like, and 1.6 % follicular patterns (Ozkaya 2005). Another study from Greece comparing adult and childhood atopic dermatitis found that the head and neck and hands are more commonly involved in adults, and in elderly patients eczematous erythroderma may be common (Katsarou and Armenaka 2011). A study from Poland observed skin manifestations predominantly on the extensor sides of the upper extremities, the neck, and the face with significant lichenification (Bozek et al. 2012). In patients with low IgE, they found significant immune reactivity against staphylococcal enterotoxin superantigens.

In two thirds of the patients, there was concomitant respiratory atopy, like allergic rhinitis or allergic asthma.

Significantly more females were affected in the adults compared to males.

The majority of the patients suffer from mild to moderate atopic dermatitis; however, in the elderly, eczematous erythroderma may be a feature of atopic dermatitis.

1.5 Clinical Course and Prognosis

The general public, but also many physicians, believe that atopic eczema is a disease which mostly disappears during childhood ("the child will grow out of it"); however, this unfortunately only holds true for a small part of the affected individuals (Fig. 1.13).

In studies following the long-term clinical course, variable rates of cure have been observed between 37 % (Kissling) and 84 % in a study by Vickers (1980, 1989).

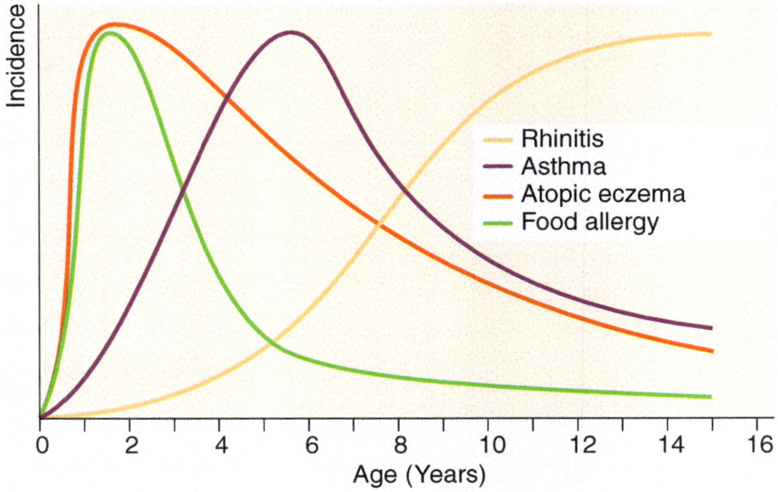

Fig. 1.13 Schematic representation of manifestation of allergic diseases over life during childhood until the 15th year of life (Acc. to T. Foucard, in Ring 2005)

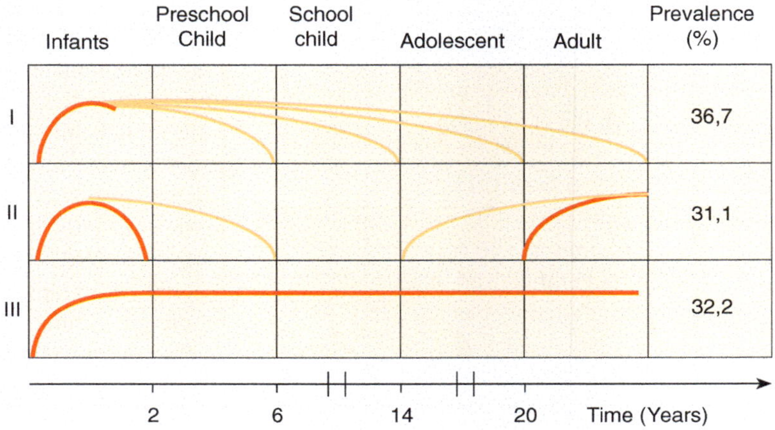

Fig. 1.14 Long-term observation and follow-up of the course of atopic eczema manifesting in early childhood over 20 years (From Kissling and Wüthrich (1993))

A very differentiated study by Kissling and Wüthrich showed that principally 3 types of clinical course of atopic eczema can be distinguished (Fig. 1.14):

- In one third of patients, eczema will disappear in early childhood.
- In another third of patients, eczema is lost until puberty, however, will appear later again.
- One last third of patients will be affected from childhood into adulthood continuously by atopic eczema (Kissling and Wüthrich 1993).

The prognostic factors are only poorly known. High IgE levels in serum, concomitant existence of atopic respiratory disease, as well as strong psychosomatic involvement seem to be risk factors for a longer persistence of eczema.

Development of asthma: the more severe the atopic eczema in infants, the higher the risk of asthma development in childhood. In a study by Gustafsson et al. with 94 children with atopic eczema, 30 % of children with mild eczema developed asthma and 25 % allergic rhinitis, while children with severe atopic eczema developed asthma after 8 years in 70 % and hay fever in 90 % (see Ring et al. 2006).

1.5.1 Intrinsic Versus Extrinsic Eczema

Intrinsic variant: for many physicians the detection of IgE-mediated sensitization is the crucial diagnostic step in the diagnosis of atopic eczema (see Sect. 4.3). However, there is no doubt that there are typical cases of atopic eczema without detectable IgE levels or specific IgE sensitization in the blood or in skin prick test. This so-called intrinsic variant (Krämer et al. 2001; Möhrenschlager et al. 2005, 2006a, b; Novak and Bieber 2003; Schmid-Grendelmeier et al. 2001; Wüthrich 1983) is not very well investigated. It might be that IgE antibodies are present, but not detectable because they are directed against allergens which are so far unknown, e.g., microbial allergens from *S. aureus* on the skin (Novak et al. 2003). Another hypothesis is that these sensitizations only develop during a lifetime. There are few studies regarding the exact prevalence of these two subvariants of atopic eczema (Wüthrich and Schmid-Grendelmeier 2003).

The intrinsic variant is more common in children than in adults as generally estimated in a study in the city of Augsburg (MIRIAM) (Krämer et al. 1996). We found significant differences with regard to gender: the intrinsic atopic eczema was significantly more prevalent in girls than in boys (Fig. 1.15) (Möhrenschlager et al. 2006b). In East-West comparison of the large study comprising children just starting school (Schulanfängerstudie West-Ost, SAWO), the intrinsic variant was more common in East German children than in the West (Krämer et al. 1999b, 2002). Taïeb observed that children with milder manifestations less often showed IgE-mediated reactions which were generally present in severe atopic eczema (Taïeb 1999).

Many authors tried to improve the definition of the subpopulation of "intrinsic atopic eczema," but this was found to be difficult. Generally, it seems that intrinsic eczema begins later in life, shows a milder severity and less skin barrier disturbance—which is very surprising! Among the atopy stigmata, intrinsic eczema often shows Dennie-Morgan folds, but rarely ichthyosis vulgaris or palmar hyperlinearity. It may be speculated that intrinsic eczema is triggered not so much by protein allergens and Th2 responses, but maybe other antigens play a role (Tokura 2010).

Surprisingly also activation of all T-cell subpopulations including Th2 has been found in a study comparing extrinsic and intrinsic atopic dermatitis in adult patients. In intrinsic atopic dermatitis, there was a higher activation of all inflammatory cells including Th2, but particularly Th17 and Th22 cells (Suarez-Farinas et al. 2013).

Gene expression studies using microarrays and protein-protein interaction (PPI) mapping from skin biopsies of extrinsic atopic dermatitis patients showed the following gene classes to be specially activated:

- Extracellular matrix and cell adhesion-related genes
- ATP- and GTP-binding genes
- Immune response genes
- Proteolytic enzyme genes
- Structural genes (Lü et al. 2009).

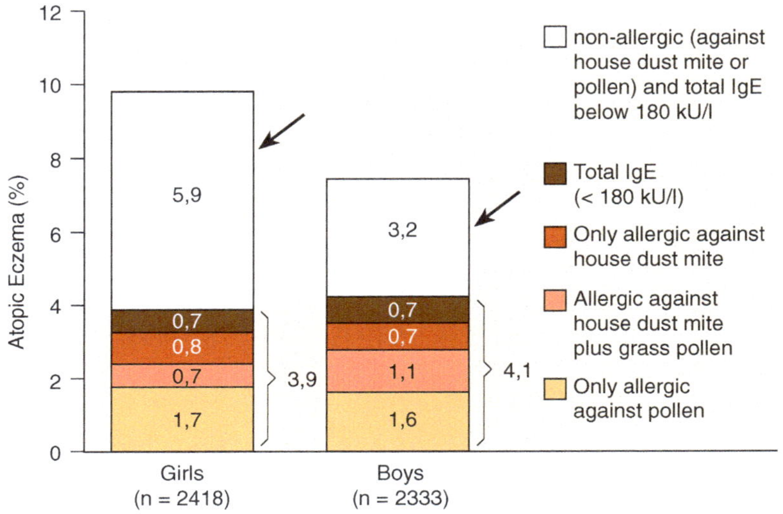

Fig. 1.15 Intrinsic atopic eczema in childhood is more prevalent in girls than in boys (investigation in 7.229 six-year-old children in Germany 1991–2000 (According to Möhrenschlager et al. (2006b))

Thomas Bieber therefore postulated that atopic eczema always starts as an "intrinsic" condition, possibly on the basis of a disturbed skin barrier function (see Sect. 3.2) and that the IgE-mediated sensitizations only develop later in life (Bieber 2008; Fölster-Holst et al. 2006a; Novembre et al. 2001). He believes that intrinsic atopic eczema in adult males is an absolute rarity.

Table 1.6 Prevalence of atopic diseases in various villages of different development on the island of Karkar in Papua New Guinea (Herbert 2009)

Center of island (original state) (Karmok)	0
Between center and shore (Did)	2.4
Shore villages (already Western influence)	
Kurum	8.1
Gaubin	7.7
Kavailo	6.7

1.5.2 Gender Differences

In adults, obviously the female gender is more commonly affected with estimated numbers between female to male 2:1 (Schnyder and Klunker 1957; Schnyder 1960). Some authors also report increased incidences in girls compared to boys (Schäfer et al. 1996). In early childhood, however, boys seem to be more often affected.

It remains a matter of speculation whether here genetic influences play a role. When regarding the differences between childhood and adult age, also hormonal influences should be considered, such as allergy-protective effects of androgenic hormones. Similar observations have been made in other allergic diseases such as urticaria and certain forms of anaphylaxis (Chen et al. 2008, see Sect. 3.6).

1.5.3 Risk and Protective Factors

1.5.3.1 Socioeconomic Status

The influence of socioeconomic status upon the development of atopic diseases has been investigated by several authors (Diepgen 2001). Usually there was a positive linear correlation between the parameters "socioeconomic status" and "prevalence of hay fever or allergic asthma" or "atopic sensitization" (Krämer et al. 1997). Also with regard to atopic eczema, there was a significant association with a higher socioeconomic status in affected adults.

A study from Hannover investigated 4219 children just starting school and found a significant correlation of atopic eczema to maternal education or paternal occupational categories (Schmidt-Ott et al. 1999, 2003; Werfel et al. 2009). The reasons of this influence of socioeconomic status upon allergy development are unclear; some authors speculate about exaggerated hygiene procedures in these families (see below).

"Western lifestyle": It would be wrong to conclude from these data that atopic eczema is a disease of the "rich" only (Williams et al. 1995). Experiences in sub-Saharan Africa Oceania and from inner-city slums in US American metropoles observe a high incidence of atopic diseases and also of atopic eczema in children investigated (George 1989; Ferié et al. 2006; Schmid-Grendelmeier et al. 2003; Waite et al. 1980).

Western lifestyle seems to favor allergy-enhancing factors. A recently published study from a very remote island in Papua New Guinea showed that in the center of the island of Karkar where people still live in a very original way (no electricity, no houses, etc.), there are no allergies, while in villages closer to the sea, allergies are known, and in villages at the seashore with more Western influence, prevalence rates of 6–8 % can be observed (Table 1.6) (Herbert et al. 2009). Also the number of children seems to influence the rate of atopy (Olesen et al. 1996; Purvis et al. 2005; Strachan 1989).

A conservative lifestyle (like, e.g., on a farm or in anthroposophical families) seems to protect against allergy development in children (Alm et al. 1999; Gassner-Bachmann and Wüthrich 2000; Braun-Fahrländer et al. 2004; von Mutius et al. 2000).

1.5.3.2 Psychosomatic Influence

The strong psychosomatic influence in clinical manifestation and course of this disease is reflected in the name of the disease in German-speaking countries, "Neurodermitis," although the term originally derives from the French dermatology (see above).

Table 1.7 Life events in the family and atopic dermatitis: results of the LISA birth cohort study (Bockelbrink et al. 2006)

Life event	Odds ratio (OR)	Confidence interval (CI)
Severe disease of a family member	0.29	0.1–0.7
Separation/divorce of parents	3.59	1.6–1.7

There is no doubt that psychologic factors are able to influence considerably the clinical course of eczema, both in a positive and in a negative way (Alexander 1971; Bosse and Gieler 1987; Buske-Kirschbaum et al. 2001; Gieler et al. 1990; Richter and Dahme 1987; Richter and Ahrens 1990).

A more recent investigation studied the occurrence of eczema in early childhood and found interesting associations: in families where another family member was affected from a severe disease (cancer or traumatic accident), the incidence of atopic eczema was significantly rarer, while in families with parental disharmony (continuous quarreling, separation, divorce), the eczema rate was significantly elevated (Table 1.7) (Bockelbrink et al. 2006; Schmitt et al. 2010).

Psychosomatic factors do not only influence the course of an existing eczema, but might also be of relevance in the early initiation and triggering of first symptoms.

1.5.3.3 Pregnancy

A study from Denmark reported that prolonged gestation periods go along with an increased risk of atopic eczema in children (over 40 weeks compared to 39–40 weeks; OR 1.32, CI 1.06–1.63) (Olesen et al. 1997).

1.5.3.4 Hygiene, Infectious Disease and Vaccinations

The general aspects of the so-called hygiene or jungle hypothesis (see above) are discussed elsewhere. The question as to a possible benefit or risk of vaccination is controversially discussed.

Measles

In a large study from Denmark, 9744 children at the age of 3–15 years were investigated for the influence of measles. The majority of children (93.3 %) had received measles vaccination. 5 % had suffered from a measles infection. In children who were vaccinated against measles, mumps and rubella, there was an increased eczema incidence (OR 1.64; CI 1.24–2.16). On the other hand, the risk of atopic eczema was even higher in the group of those children who had suffered measles infections (OR 1.91; CI 1.04–3.51) (Olesen et al. 2003). Discordant results have been reported with regard to a measles infection leading to either an increase or decrease of incidence of atopic eczema (Williams 2000).

Pertussis

In our own investigations comparing East and West German preschool children, we found that vaccination against *Bordetella pertussis*, which was obligatory in the 1980s in the former East German Democratic Republic GDR, while it was only accepted by approx. 75 % of West German parents, was a decisive factor. We found a significant protective effect against the development of atopic respiratory diseases, especially bronchial asthma (Ring et al. 2004); after adjusting the East-West differences for the factor "pertussis vaccination," the East-West differences observed earlier in respiratory airway disease disappeared. There was no influence of pertussis vaccination with regard to atopic eczema.

Smallpox (Variola Vera)

Until 30 years ago, the vaccination against smallpox with vaccinia antigen was considered a contraindication in individuals with atopic eczema because of the dramatic condition of "eczema vaccinatum" which represented a generalized blistering disease with possible life-threatening consequences. Therefore it was impossible for many European young people to travel to the USA where smallpox vaccination was mandatory. In the late 1970s of the twentieth century, the veterinary virologist A. Mayr, together with Helmut Stickl, the director of the Bavarian Vaccination Institute (Bayerische Landesimpfanstalt), developed a new vaccine against smallpox using an attenuated virus (modified virus Ankara MVA) which could be applied subcutaneously, while the classical smallpox vaccination had to be applied by scarification to the epidermis (Mayr et al. 1978; Stickl et al. 1974) and dated back to 1807, when Bavaria was the first country in Europe to install an official vaccination program against smallpox.

Immunogenicity of this MVA vaccine was excellently measured by humoral and cellular immune responses against smallpox antigen. The safety was dramatically better. Among approx. 100,000 persons vaccinated with MVA only, few severe side effects were observed (Stickl et al. 1974). With the declaration of the official eradication of smallpox at the end of the 1980s (in 1987), smallpox vaccination was no longer necessary or recommended.

After September 2001, concerns of bioterrorism using still available smallpox strains (in high safety labs in the USA and Russia) gave rise to study the risk of smallpox vaccination for high-risk population groups (soldiers, medical personnel, especially dermatologists). In a prospective study in various volunteers with or without atopic diseases including atopic eczema, the MVA vaccine was found effective and safe in in vitro measurements (Sonnenburg et al. in press; Darsow et al. in press).

1.5.3.5 Vaccination Recommendations

Considering the actual controversial data and in the light of rather high risk of certain infectious diseases, it makes sense to recommend the common vaccinations also for persons with risk of atopy (Werfel et al. 2009; Grüber 2012).

1.5.4 Nutrition (See Also Chap. 6)

When discussing the influence of nutrition, one has to differentiate between effects upon initiation of development on the one hand and triggering of exacerbations of eczema on the other.

1.5.4.1 Breastfeeding

Most studies are available with regard to the effect of breastfeeding (Kramer et al. 2001). A meta-analysis showed a significant preventive effect (Gdalevich et al. 2001). However, it should not be left unconsidered that there are studies which do not show this effect or even show a higher risk of atopic eczema in breastfed infants.

1.5.4.2 Maternal Nutrition and Baby Formula

Alterations of maternal diet during pregnancy or lactation have no significant effect on eczema prevalence as has been shown in a recent Cochrane review (Kramer and Kakuma 2003).

From the results of the German Infant Nutritional Intervention Study (GINI), it became obvious that there was a significant preventive effect of certain hypoallergenic formulas (von Berg et al. 2003, 2008) on the development of atopic eczema.

1.5.4.3 Polyunsaturated Fatty Acids: Pre- and Probiotics

The role of polyunsaturated fatty acids (PUFA) has been studied in Australia where positive effects in the prevention of atopic eczema by addition of PUFA have been found (Dunstan et al. 2004).

Already in early East-West European studies, the role of intestinal microflora has been stressed (Björksten et al. 2001). Recent interesting results show a preventive effect of prebiotics (oligosaccharides) (Grüber 2012). The preventive effect of probiotics (e.g., Lactobacillus GG) has been studied mainly in Finland (Isolauri et al. 2000; Kalliomäki et al. 2001) and, however, has not been reproduced by other groups in a significant way.

1.5.5 Skin Care

There are few prospective studies to the effect of skin care which represents one of the basic therapeutic and preventive approaches in atopic eczema. At present there are studies showing a beneficial effect of the use of emollients in infants with regard to prevention of atopic eczema (*neu*!).

1.5.5.1 Peanut Oil

A study from England supported the hypothesis that peanut allergy is enhanced by applying peanut oil contained in bath oils in young children (Lack et al. 2003); however, there is no quantitative measurement of the specific skin care procedures with regard to the amount of peanut oil applied. Furthermore, one must know that in refined peanut oil there are no measurable concentrations of peanut protein and even less of peanut allergen which makes this hypothesis rather unlikely with regard to practical relevance (Möhrenschlager and Ring 2007).

The hygiene hypothesis supports the concept that too much or too intensive procedures in baby care may contribute to eczema development by changing the cutaneous microbiome. However, the fact that pathogenic microbes like *Staphylococcus aureus* are colonizing atopic skin and probably can act as triggers of eczema also has to be considered (see Sect. 5.3).

1.5.6 Life Style

1.5.6.1 Living on a Farm

The clear-cut protective effect for children growing up on a farm with regard to development of atopic diseases (Braun-Fahrländer et al. 2002, 2004; Ege et al. 2008a, b; Gassner-Bachmann and Wüthrich 2000; von Mutius et al. 2000; von Ehrenstein et al. 2000) is true for respiratory allergies and especially when the mother had been working on the farm or in the stable during pregnancy or the children had been drinking fresh warm milk directly from the cow. For atopic eczema, there is a study showing an effect with regard to the diversity of foods introduced during the first year of life, especially yogurt showing a preventive effect with regard to development of atopic eczema (Roduit et al. 2012).

1.5.6.2 Pet Keeping

The most marked change in allergy prevention recommendation has been made during the last years with regard to pet keeping. While 20 years ago it was generally agreed that avoidance of a pet with furs or feathers is an absolute requirement for individuals at risk for atopy, there have been new studies showing no such risk or, on the contrary, even a protective effect for dogs, while cats are still regarded as a risk factor for the development of atopic diseases and atopic eczema (Muche-Borowski et al. 2010). These studies were commented in lay newspapers with the headline "Snuffy the Dog found not guilty" (*Freispruch für Schnuffi*). It has to be mentioned that these data are still controversial and that in families genetically predisposed for atopy, pet keeping is significantly rarer; it may be possible that there is an effect of "reversed causality."

1.5.6.3 Environmental Pollutants

There is no doubt that exposure to air pollutants can influence the development of atopic diseases (Behrendt et al. 1999; Saxon and Diaz-Sanchez 2005).

1.5.6.4 Environmental Tobacco Smoke

In the indoor air, it is mainly exposure to tobacco smoke which is of relevance. In own large epidemiological trials, MIRIAM (Multicenter International Study On Risk Assessment of Indoor and Outdoor Pollution on Allergy and Eczema Morbidity), we could show that exposure to tobacco smoke (measured as cotinine in the urine of the children) was highly significantly associated with the development of atopic eczema, especially in families where one parent already was suffering from an atopic disease (Krämer et al. 2004) (Fig. 1.16). This study supported earlier reports where we found that "smoking during pregnancy" was enhancing the atopy risk of children significantly (Schäfer et al. 1997b, 1999).

1.5.6.5 Nitrogen Oxides

In the indoor air also nitrogen oxides are present, especially when gas is used for cooking or heating water; this could be shown in studies in East German children with a significantly elevated prevalence of atopic eczema associated with the use of gas indoors (Krämer et al. 1999c, 2002).

1.5.6.6 Traffic Exhaust

In the outdoor air, traffic exhaust seems to be the most important risk factor (Terada et al. 1999). Children growing up near a heavy-traffic road show significantly elevated incidence rates of atopic eczema (Fig. 1.17) (Krämer et al. 1999c). Similarly, exposure to truck traffic showed the

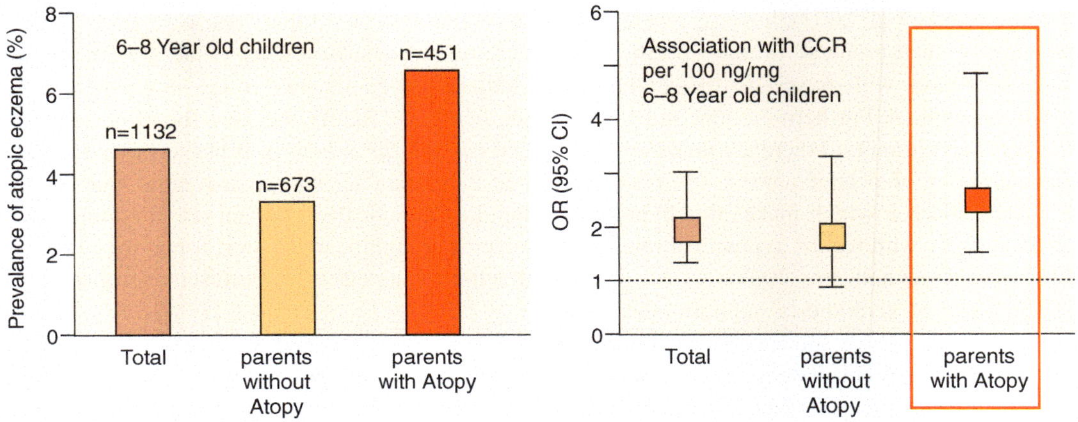

Fig. 1.16 Atopic eczema and tobacco smoke exposure measured as cotinine-creatinine ratio (CCR) in the urine (MIRIAM study Augsburg 1996–1998). OR: odds ratio, 95 %. CI: 95 % confidence interval (According to Krämer et al. (2004))

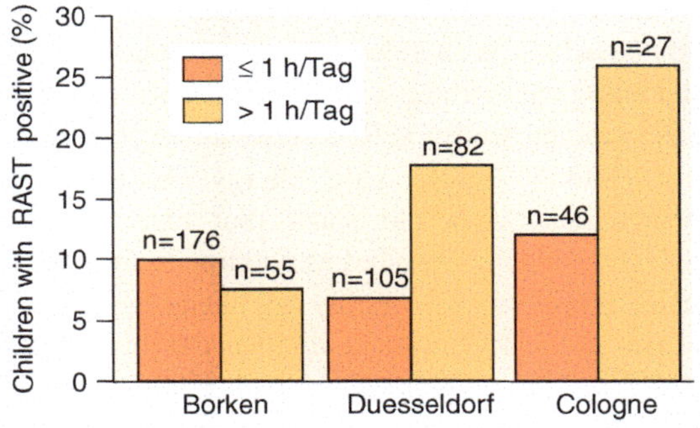

Fig. 1.17 The prevalence of allergic sensitization depends on daily traffic exhaust exposure. Investigations in 5–6-year-old children in May 1988 (Krämer et al. (1999c))

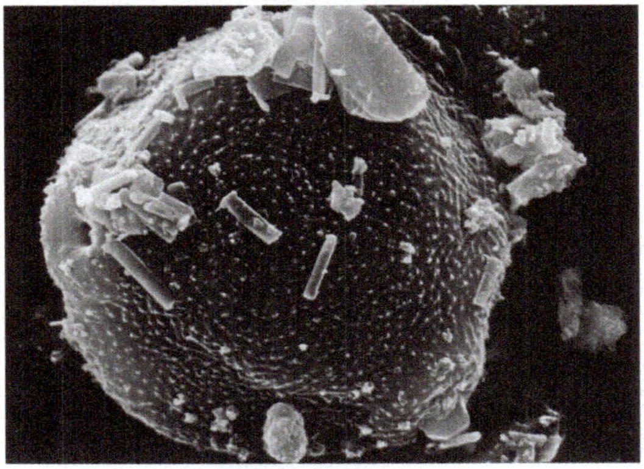

Fig. 1.18 Birch pollen grain loaded with pollution particles in the atmosphere of a West German big city (With friendly permission of H. Behrendt)

same effects (Behrens et al. 2004; Weiland et al. 1999). Experimental investigations by Behrendt et al. (1993) showed that pollutants in the outdoor air can lead to changes in the pollen surface and in the liberation of pollen grain constituents (Fig. 1.18) of possible relevance for allergy development.

A detailed study in the city of Munich showed a significant and dose-dependent increase in the prevalence of atopic diseases, also atopic eczema, in clear association to exposure to fine dust particles (Morgenstern et al. 2008). In animal experiments, allergic inflammation was enhanced over many days by pre-exposure to fine or ultrafine particles before allergen application (Alessandrini et al. 2006; Terada et al. 1999). This effect was most likely due to oxygen radical formation by fine and ultrafine particles, since antioxidant treatment could diminish inflammatory changes in mice lungs (Alessandrini et al. 2006).

1.5.6.7 Prognostic Factors

In a study from Switzerland, the following factors were correlated with a bad prognosis for children with atopic eczema (Wüthrich 1999b):

- Early onset (before the 6th month of life)
- Severe manifestation of eczema

- Single child
- High IgE concentration in serum
- Concomitant manifestation of respiratory atopy

1.5.7 Summary

Atopic eczema is one of the most common inflammatory skin diseases, and in childhood it is the most common noncontagious inflammatory skin disease with a prevalence of 10–20 %. The prevalence has increased dramatically in the last decades and seems to have reached a plateau in some countries. In 80 %, atopic eczema starts in early childhood (under 2 years), and in recent years an increase of prevalence in adults can be observed.

Only one third of the children with atopic eczema are losing the disease before puberty; in two thirds of the children affected, it can be estimated that eczema stays or reoccurs in adulthood. Risk factors from epidemiologic studies are higher socioeconomic status (as measured as educational level of parents), psychosomatic influences, alterations in the course of pregnancy, allergen exposure (especially pet keeping), and pollutant exposure (especially tobacco smoke in indoor and traffic exposure in outdoor air).

The attractive "jungle" or "hygiene" hypothesis for other atopic diseases where stimulation of the immune system in early childhood seems to have a protective effect on the development of atopic diseases seems to be predominantly true for respiratory atopy and only to a lesser extent or not at all for atopic eczema.

1.6 Socioeconomic Burden of Atopic Eczema

It is obvious that a disease like atopic eczema affects the life of affected individuals, but also their families and their environment in a dramatic way. In a time where financial aspects are becoming increasingly important, it is good to stress this "individual and socioeconomic" burden in a quantitative way.

The individual burden for a patient with atopic eczema consists in:

- Dysesthesia, especially intense itch sensation
- Loss of function (e.g., when hands or feet are affected) with occupational impairment
- Social stigmatization and disfigurement
- Sleep loss and intense pruritus lead to impairment of daily life achievements (Leistungsminderung) at school or at work (Lewis-Jones et al. 2001, Lewis-Jones 2006)

1.6.1 Quality of Life

The individual affection does not only manifest itself as diminishment of quality of life as can be measured by instruments such as the Quality Of Life (QOL) and the Dermatology Life Quality Index (DLQI) (Finlay 1996a, b, 1997; Finlay and Khan 1994; Augustin et al. 1999a, b, 2000). In Germany the DIELH (Deutsches Instrument zur Erfassung der Lebensqualität bei Hautkrankheiten) (Schäfer et al. 2001) has been developed together with other instruments to assess the quality of life in children.

Compared to other severe diseases, it is of interest that impairment of quality of life through atopic eczema is in the same or even higher range of diseases like cancer, diabetes mellitus, or myocardial infarction. It also affects the life of the caregivers (Lewis-Jones 2006; Ho et al. 2010).

1.6.2 Financial Costs

In addition to the impairment in quality of life, rather high financial costs have to be considered not only for drugs and medical aids, but also for a variety of other aspects of daily life which are necessary for affected individuals (Augustin et al. 2000; Gieler et al. 1999; Schmitt et al. 2009c). These direct and indirect costs can be measured and estimated to be about 3 to 5×10^9 euros per year in Germany (Ring et al. 2010; Ehlken et al. 2005).

In spite of these alarming figures, eczema is not regarded as one of the major health problems by relevant authorities such as insurances or health politics officials in many countries (Ring et al. 2012).

1.6.3 Personal Burden

The personal burden of an individual affected by atopic eczema manifests itself differently during lifetime.

Infants only learn to scratch between the 3rd and 6th month of life; earlier they only can express their dysesthesia by a whimpering noise which often is not understood as itch. The lack of scratch marks cannot be regarded as a sign of absence of itch!

Psychologic consequences for lifetime are often underestimated, when a young human being never knows the feeling of normal skin, but only a hypersensitive, rough, and destroyed skin surface with intense itch (Borelli 1950). The lack of understanding of many adults expressing itself in admonitions like "Stop scratching yourself once and for all!" leads to additional isolation. Emotional changes can trigger itch crises; this can change the emotional life of a human being. Anger can lead to scratch attacks. In families sometimes this is used as "weapon" by the child which makes educational procedures difficult.

In kindergarten or at the latest in school, stigmatization is a major factor for eczema children; even in our modern and rational society, archaic reflexes of 3000 years ago are still prevalent which associate any skin disease with contagion, and there are reflexes like "Put the contagious leppers out of town!." In Munich the first skin patients were treated at the Gasteig outside of the city walls, on the right side of the river Isar (Borelli 1995).

Sleep loss and intense itch lead to diminished concentration and achievements in school, but also to conflicts with teachers. Maybe this is one of the reasons often "hyperactive" syndromes are diagnosed, when eczema children just cannot remain seated because of the intense pruritus.

Attention deficit and hyperactivity disorder ADHD and eczema show interesting overlaps: in a large study it has been shown that sleep loss is a major factor for the development of ADHD, and sleep loss due to intense itch occurring in early childhood in eczema children may also lead to a higher prevalence of ADHD in atopic eczema (Romanos et al. 2010; Schmitt et al. 2009c).

Special dietary requirements—sometimes not indicated—in the case of concomitant food allergy, together with the requirement for time-consuming skin care procedures or selection of certain textiles for clothing, make life additionally difficult for eczema children.

In adolescence, young people are suffering tremendously by the stigmatization when their skin is not "smooth and pure," as can be seen in TV advertising around the clock, and their skin shows red patches, scales, or eyelid edema or halo formation. Social stigmatization leads to isolation and makes friendships or partnerships more difficult.

When the genital area is involved, which often occurs in the lichenified manifestation, problems in sexual life are obvious. Few people and physicians can openly discuss these very important problems of many eczema patients.

1.6.4 Financial Burden

1.6.4.1 International Figures

The financial burden of eczema is difficult to measure; there are different estimates from different countries. The direct costs of atopic eczema in childhood have been estimated to 47 m GBP per year in the UK and in the Netherlands to 71 m euros per year. Indirect costs have been estimated to between 0.9 and 3.8×10^9 USD per year in the USA (Ellis et al. 2002). A study from Australia showed similar figures with 1140 AUD in mild eczema up to 6999 AUD for patients with severe eczema (Kemp 1999).

1.6.4.2 Studies in Germany

The costs for atopic eczema have been studied in Germany by different authors. Yearly total costs for patients to be paid by insurances have been estimated to 1600 euros. In addition, there are costs to be paid by the patient himself/herself, as well as indirect costs adding up to a total of 6200 euros per year (Table 1.8) (Ring et al. 2012).

These costs can be explained by about 70 % direct costs, 20 % for drugs, 35 % for outpatient treatment, 12 % for inpatient treatment, and 3 % for rehabilitation. In addition, 30 % indirect costs for invalidity (8 %) or absence from work (22 %) (Ring et al. 2012) have to be considered.

Table 1.8 Average costs (per patient and year) of disease for patients with atopic dermatitis (Ring et al. White book, Allergy in Germany, 2010)

Sum of direct costs (doctor and medications)	2229.46 euros
Indirect costs (for living, clothes, diets, etc.)	4257.90 euros
Total	**6487.36** euros
Other skin diseases compared	
Psoriasis	6169.86 euros
Chronic urticaria	4321.74 euros
Acne	1342.55 euros

1.6.5 Summary

Atopic eczema not only is characterized by individual suffering, but also affects families and society with a considerable socioeconomic burden. Direct and indirect costs in Germany have been estimated to reach 3 to 5×10^9 euros per year, 70 % for direct costs, drugs, outpatient and inpatient treatment, and rehabilitation. 30 % can be estimated as "indirect" costs for daily life expenses regarding nutrition, clothing, and others.

2 Clinical Symptoms of Atopic Eczema

Describing the clinical symptomatology of this skin disease is more difficult than in other dermatoses. Maybe this is why the big masters of morphology in dermatology preferred other skin diseases like psoriasis, bullous diseases, or lichen planus with clear-cut primary lesions and well-described secondary skin changes.

Atopic dermatitis often represents as a "diffuse" skin condition. The definition of the whole disease seems to be as unprecise as the borders of affected skin areas. Sometimes the term "involved" skin is questionable, especially when the dermatohistopathological investigations used show signs of inflammation also in clinically "uninvolved" skin areas (Kunz and Ring 2000).

The susceptibility for environmental influences, especially on the psychosocial level, underlines the strong variability of this dermatosis. Itch crisis can elicit attacks of rage. Rage can elicit attacks of itch and scratching. In addition, this disease manifests itself differently in different age groups and different body regions.

For logic didactic reasons, this chapter will describe the clinical symptomatology of atopic dermatitis in the following order:

- Actual symptoms of disease
- Minimal manifestations
- Stigmata of atopic constitution
- Possible complications

However, it is clear that these four phases often exist simultaneously and are variable over time even with regard to stigmata.

2.1 Actual Symptoms of Disease

2.1.1 Primary Lesion "Itch"

Normally dermatologists in the description of a skin disease start with the "primary lesion." There is no consensus with regard to the primary lesion of atopic eczema; it is described as erythema, papule, and seropapule. Some authors, starting with Jacquet (1904) and the French School, stress the symptom "pruritus." According to good tradition the author says, together with Saint John the Evangelist or Johann Wolfgang von Goethe (Faust): "In the beginning there was the itch!" (Rajka 1980, 1989; Ring 1982a).

Rarely it is possible to observe the acute development of an eczematous skin lesion in atopic dermatitis directly; however, sometimes—e.g., with your own children or under provocation tests in the hospital—it is possible. From this experience it can be concluded that human beings, who never before have shown any signs of eczematous skin changes, triggered by some environmental or psychologic factors suddenly develop itch and start scratching on apparently normal skin. Only hours later the typical clinical manifestations of atopic dermatitis develop. These phenomena are especially common in the areas mostly affected such as the elbow, knee flexures, or eyelids. It is a pity that there is little scientific documentation with regard to these early manifestations in the individual initial phase. Many colleagues, parents, and patients have made this experience.

J. Ring, *Atopic Dermatitis: Eczema*, DOI 10.1007/978-3-319-22243-1_2

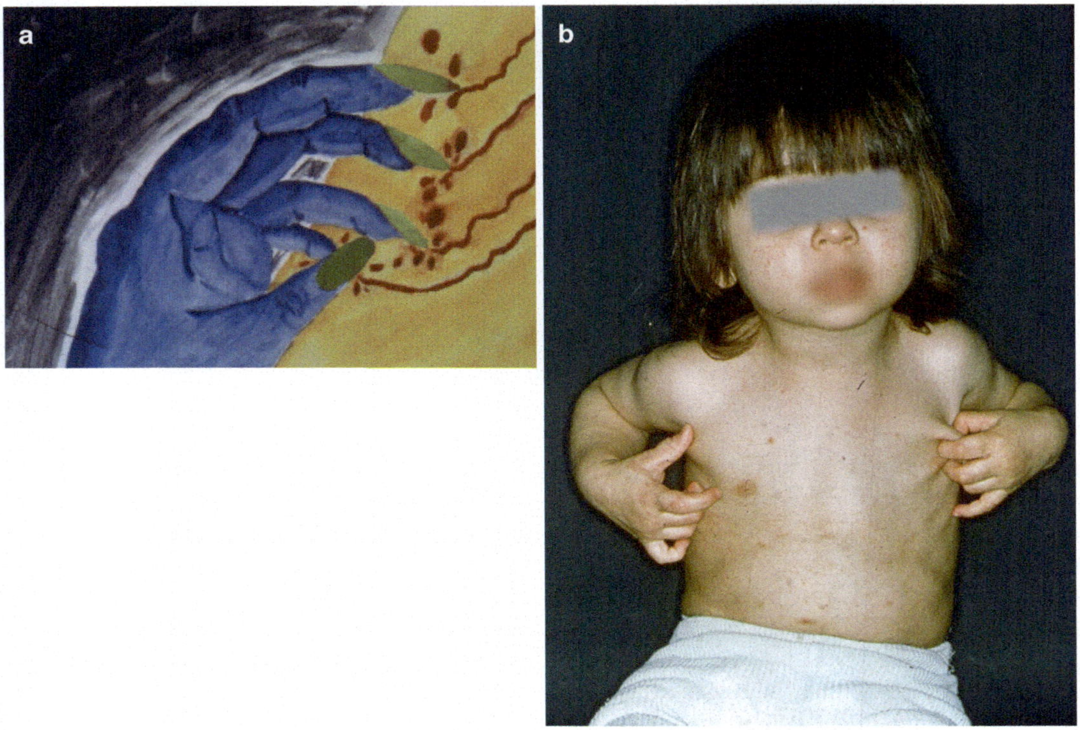

Fig. 2.1 (**a**) Itch sensation painted by a 9-year-old girl suffering from atopic dermatitis. (**b**) The primary lesion "itch" leads via scratch effects to the typical skin changes of atopic dermatitis

Itch as "dermatose invisible" is the primary lesion of atopic dermatitis which, via the scratch reaction, then gives rise to the characteristic morphologic skin changes (Fig. 2.1). Besides, it is possible that primarily skin changes occur which go along with increased itch. The borders are fluent. A typical atopic eczema without itch is extremely rare, if not inexistent. Since the French School at the beginning of the twentieth century, the central importance of itch for atopic dermatitis has been stressed by many authors (Borelli and Schnyder 1962; Braun-Falco and Ring 1984; Breit 1997; Engman et al. 1936; Haxthausen 1957; Kimura and Miyazawa 1989; Koblenzer 1999; Rajka 1989; Ring et al. 2006; Talbot 1918).

Itch is the most agonizing symptom of manifest disease and often is perceived as "incurable." It leads to sleep loss, nightly scratch attacks with bloody bedding, a feeling of "powerlessness," because it cannot be stopped voluntarily. Unfortunately this symptom is not yet taken seriously by many physicians and the society, contrary to the other main subjective symptom "pain." Regarding the latter, everybody is full of compassion (Ständer et al. 2010). I personally know patients who wanted to commit suicide because of severe itch, a fact also observed by other authors (Dieris-Hirche et al. 2009).

The old sentence "It is not the rash which itches, but the itch that rashes" (Engman et al. 1936) illustrates the situation. Early attempts of treatment 80 years ago quite brutally used procedures like fixation of children in bed or applying plaster to their extremities, so that scratching became impossible. Lesions in unreachable skin areas were indeed healing faster. Pathophysiologically this indicates that by scratching proinflammatory substances may be released (see Chap. 3).

Today the treatment of itch is the focus in the management of atopic dermatitis, and the prevention of direct scratch effects by mechanical procedures such as wet wraps with tube bandages plays a central role (see Chap. 5).

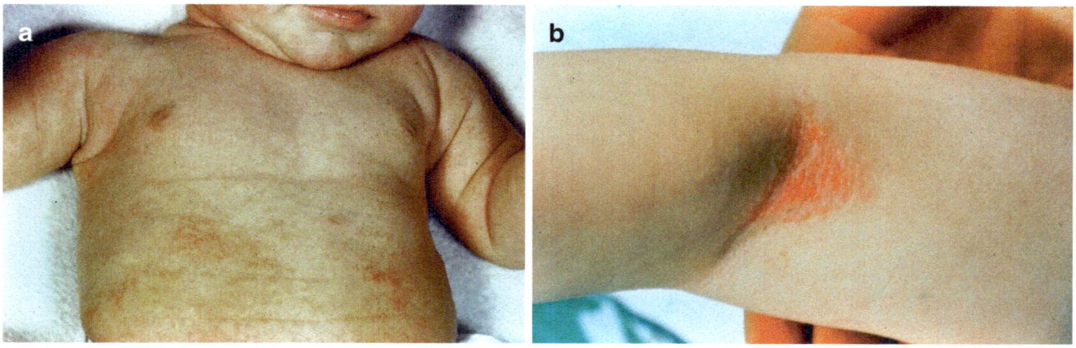

Fig. 2.2 Infiltrated erythema. (**a**) On the trunk in an infant. (**b**) In the elbow in a 1-year-old child

2.1.2 Infiltrated Erythema

Mild cases or the beginning of an exacerbation become manifest in flat, mildly infiltrated, erythematous patches with only little epidermal involvement which in the course can be excoriated and change to oozing crusting areas (Fig. 2.2).

In the severity scoring of the SCORAD (see Sect. 2.8.2, page 64), these criteria "erythema," "edema and papule," but also "lichenification" are enlisted.

It is important to stress that there are these manifestations since they are not clearly mentioned in many textbooks.

2.1.3 Erosive, Excoriated Erythema

Especially in childhood, often patchy or punctate erosive or excoriated erythematous skin changes with mild scaling are observed, going along with intense itch (Fig. 2.3).

Histologically these lesions are characterized by spongiotic changes in the epidermis. This form often has been called "eczematoid type" in the restricted sense. This may have contributed to dissatisfaction with the name "eczema" for the whole disease and may be a reason for the terminology and preference of the unprecise term "dermatitis."

In the broader definition of eczema (see Sect. 2.8.2), it becomes clear that in the local and timely course, the polymorphy of symptoms in eczema also includes other morphologies like lichenification, prurigo-type excoriated papules, etc.

Maybe strongly oozing and crusty skin changes in childhood represent signs of superinfection with, e.g., *Staphylococcus aureus* (see Sect. 2.6).

This morphology also can be observed in circumscribed skin lesions with nummular variants (see Page 37). Whether nummular eczema in childhood represents an own identity is still to be discussed. In the opinion of the author, this nummular variant is a subtype of atopic eczema in childhood.

2.1.4 Lichenification

The more chronic the skin changes, the more it shows a tendency to lichenification. This means a coarsening of the skin signs with thickening of the skin and livid red color "purple." These skin changes occur predominantly in the flexures of the big joints (elbow, knee flexure), but also as large plaques on the dorsum of the hands and feet. They also represent most likely the consequence of long-lasting scratch effects (Fig. 2.4).

The entity of lichen simplex chronicus (Vidal) or "circumscribed neurodermatitis" can be regarded as a subgroup of localized variants of atopic eczema; however, this is a matter of discussion.

Lichenification can be provoked by scratching as could be shown in classic experiments with the use of a scratch machine with a pressure of 75 g on the skin. After 60–90 h lichenification could be provoked (Goldblum and Piper 1954).

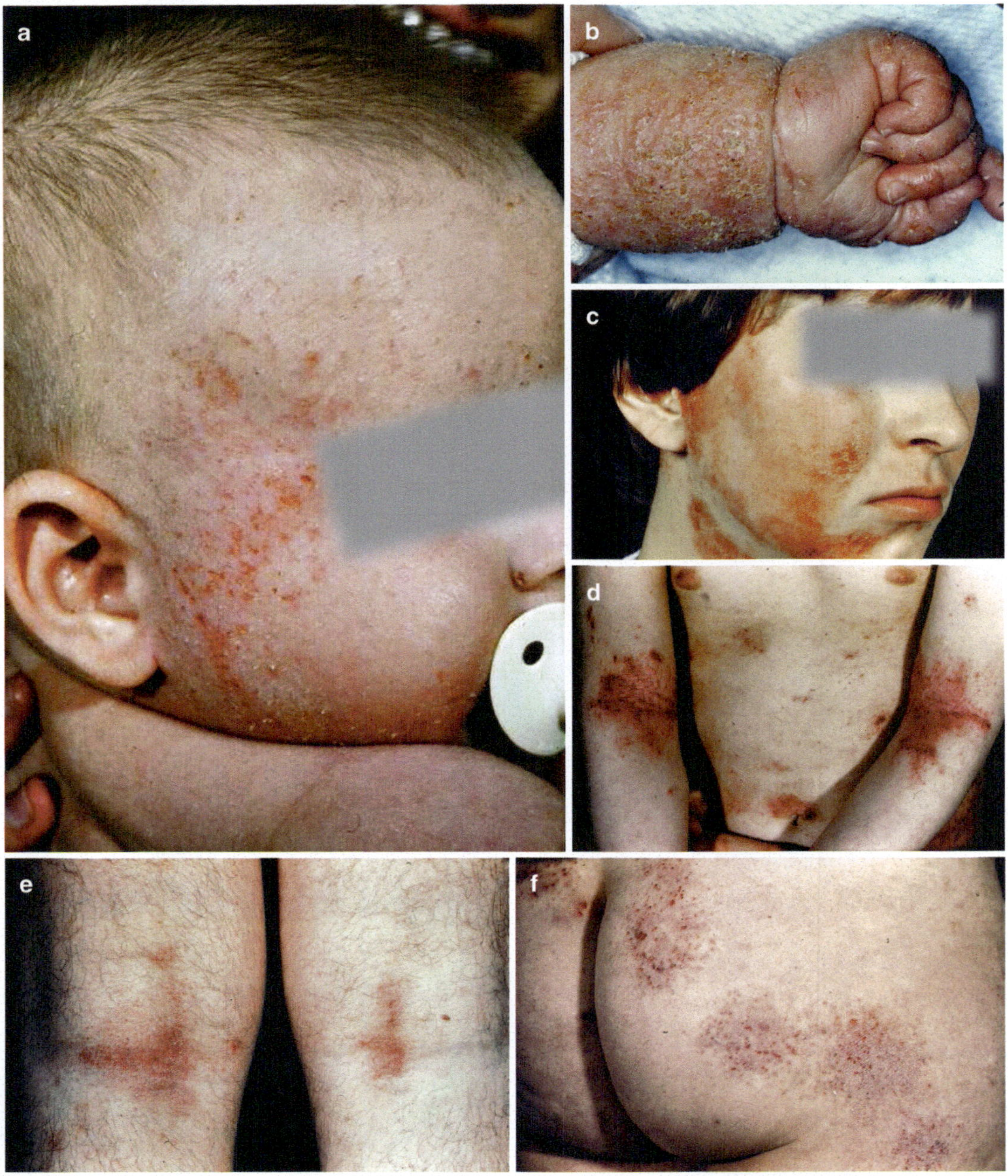

Fig. 2.3 Erosive excoriated eczematous skin changes in atopic dermatitis. (**a**) Facial eczema in an infant. (**b**) Scaling hand and forearm eczema in an infant. (**c**) Diffuse erythematous excoriations in the face. (**d**) Marked erythematous flexural eczema in the elbow. (**e**) Punctate erosive and excoriated skin changes in the knee joints. (**f**) Diffuse, partly nummular appearing erythemata with punctate erosions on the buttocks. (**g**) Massive facial eczema in an infant. (**h**) Facial eczema in an infant. (**i**) Facial eczema in a small child

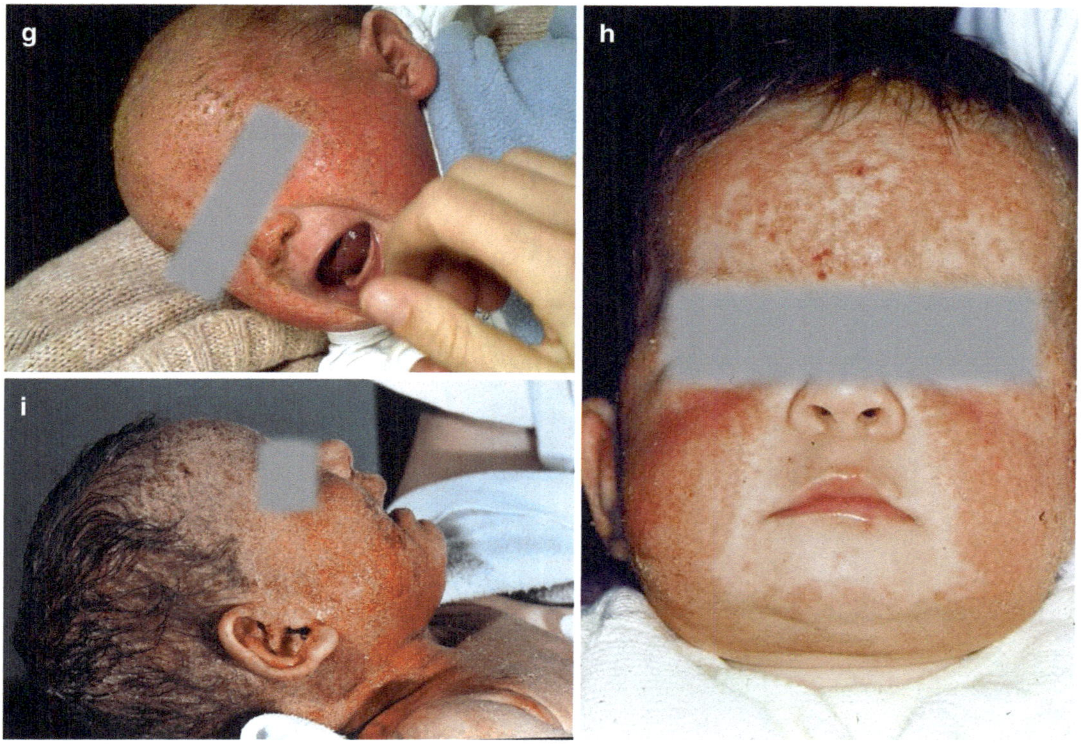

Fig. 2.3 (continued)

2.1.5 Prurigo Type of Atopic Eczema

When the follicular affection in chronic courses is prominent especially in adults, a variant can be observed which shows the clinical symptoms of prurigo; it is relatively marked by strongly itching papules or nodules with a diameter of 0.5–3 mm and central excoriation and crusting. This variant most likely gave rise to the term "prurigo Besnier" and can be found commonly in the severe manifestations in adults (Fig. 2.5).

2.2 Minimal Manifestations

Atopic eczema can change in course and localization and also in morphology over a lifetime. There are certain localizations where so-called minimal manifestations are typical: they can occur alone or sometimes in combination with other skin changes (Herzberg 1973). The affection of very small skin areas can lead to severe impairment of quality of life.

2.2.1 Minimal Manifestations in the Head Area

2.2.1.1 Lid Eczema

Sometimes only the eyelids are affected, especially in cases where aeroallergens play a causal role, sometimes also in food-induced reactions. The more chronic the course, the more difficult the treatment. Already very little contact elicits itch. Through the itch-scratch cycle, a vicious cycle develops with continuous deterioration (Fig. 2.6).

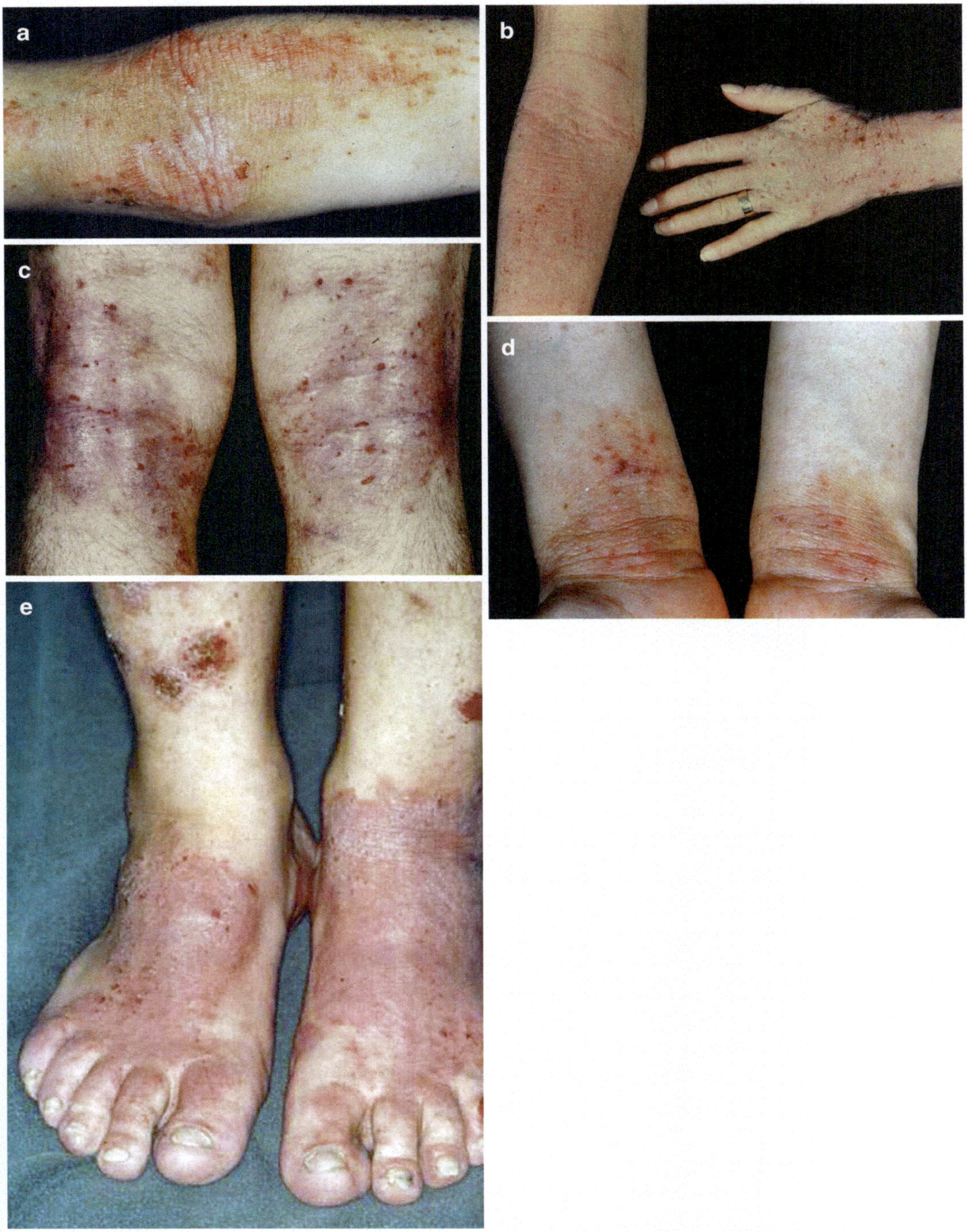

Fig. 2.4 Lichenification in chronic atopic dermatitis. (**a**) Lichenified flexural eczema in the elbow. (**b**) Lichenified eczema on the wrist. (**c**) Lichenified eczema in the knee joints. (**d**) Lichenified skin areas on the wrists. (**e**) Massive lichenification on the dorsum of the feet in an adult patient with atopic dermatitis

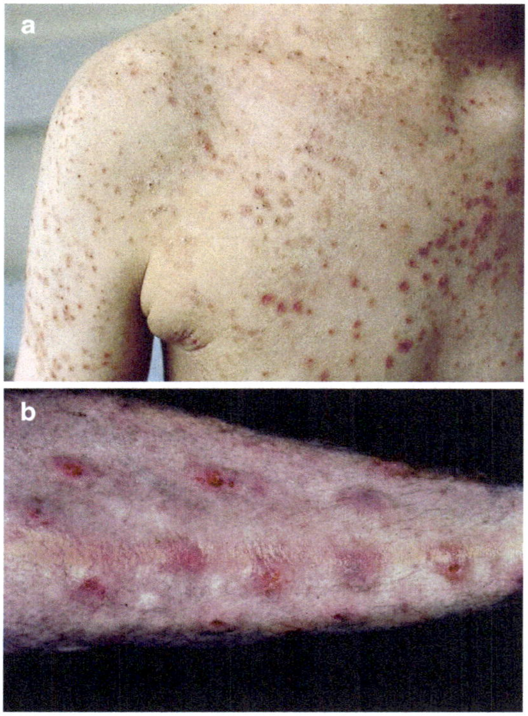

Fig. 2.5 Prurigo type of atopic dermatitis. (**a**) Centrally excoriated and crusted and papules and nodules in a 17-year-old girl with severe atopic dermatitis. (**b**) Extremely itchy excoriated papules on the trunk

2.2.1.2 Cheilitis Sicca and Perlèche

Dry lips—sometimes also with a median fissure of the lower lip—are characteristic signs of atopic eczema (Fig. 2.7), going along with fissures at the lateral angles of the mouth (perlèche) and often superinfection Angulus infectiosus (*Candida albicans*) (Temime and Oddoze 1970).

Sometimes, in the area surrounding the red part of the lip, there is an irritative eczema caused by increased lip licking (lip lick eczema) (Fig. 2.8), in infants sometimes also called suck eczema with a perioral inflammatory reaction.

2.2.1.3 Infranasal Erosion

In persons with concomitant respiratory allergy such as rhinoconjunctivitis and chronic nasal secretion or itch, sometimes erythema and fissures on the nasal entrance develop.

2.2.1.4 Infra-auricular Fissures

Infra-auricular fissures are very common at the region where the earlobe starts, which can sometimes be superinfected. It might be interesting how dressing habits—as, e.g., the rapid pulling of a T-shirt over the head of the child—can contribute to these infra-auricular fissures (Fig. 2.9).

2.2.1.5 Retroauricular Intertrigo

Similarly, signs of oozing intertrigo can be found behind the ear (Fig. 2.10).

2.2.1.6 Excoriations in the Scalp

Sometimes extremely itching skin lesions with nodules and crusts and excoriated areas can be found in the scalp as a single manifestation of atopic eczema; severe cases sometimes have been called "neurotic excoriation."

2.2.2 Minimal Manifestations on the Trunk and Extremities

2.2.2.1 Finger and Toe Eczema

Dry finger and toe changes (pulpitis sicca) can be observed especially in winter and in small children which have been described by Möller as "atopic winter feet" (Möller 1972) and sometimes were misdiagnosed as fungal infection. These changes also can look similar to dyshidrosis lamellosa sicca (Fig. 2.11).

2.2.2.2 Involvement of Nails

Strong eczematous changes on the fingers and toes can affect nail growth by matrix involvement with development of horizontal lines (Fig. 2.12a). Sometimes also paronychia develops in atopic eczema with or without superinfection (Fig. 2.12b).

Atopic dermatitis manifestations also can affect the eponychium, leading to spontaneous loss of eponychium as "epoonychitis sicca" (Ring 2005).

Inspection of nails can reveal much about scratching habits (e.g., subungual crusts or shiny nails when the skin is rubbed) (Fig. 2.13).

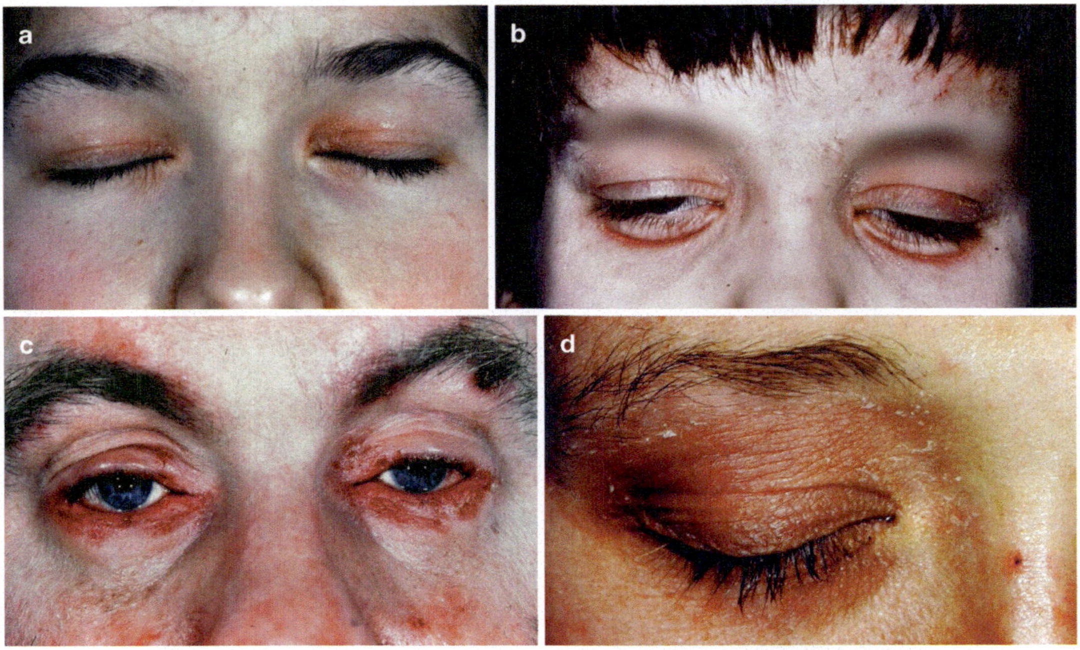

Fig. 2.6 Lid eczema in atopic dermatitis. (**a**) Upper lid eczema. (**b**) Lid eczema with edematous swelling. (**c**) Massive lid eczema of the lower lids. (**d**) Massive upper lid eczema

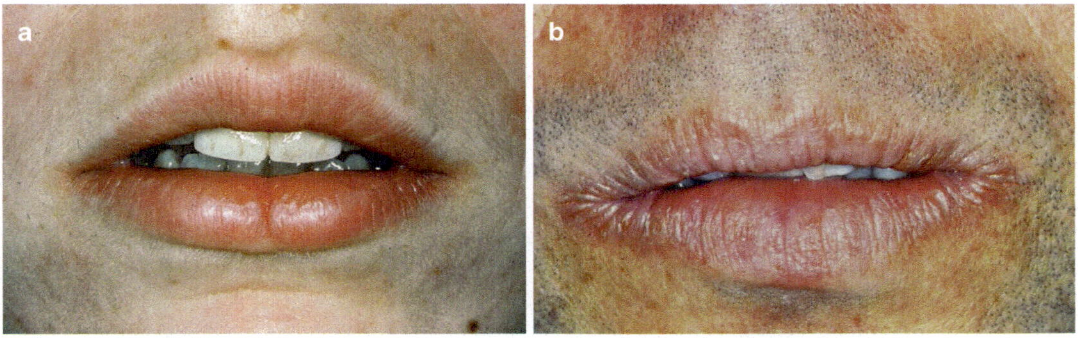

Fig. 2.7 Dry lips. (**a**) Cheilitis sicca with median lower lip fissure. (**b**) Cheilitis sicca in an adult patient with atopic dermatitis

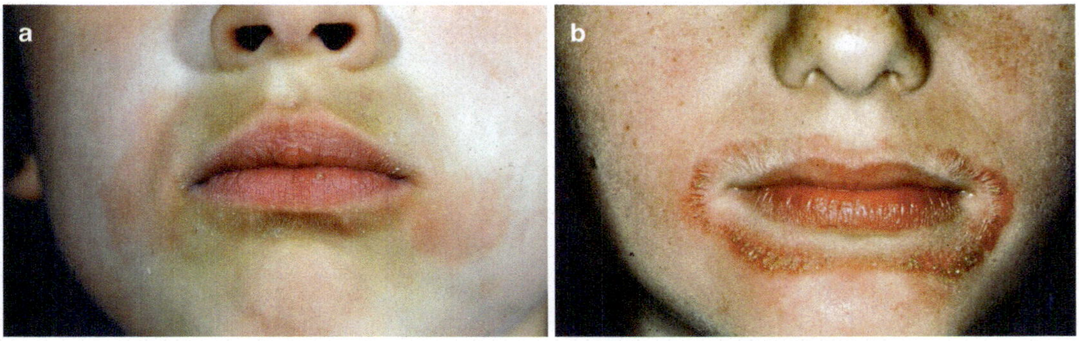

Fig. 2.8 Lip sucking eczema. (**a**) Lip sucking eczema with hyperpigmentation. (**b**) sharply marginated perioral lip eczema and cheilitis sicca

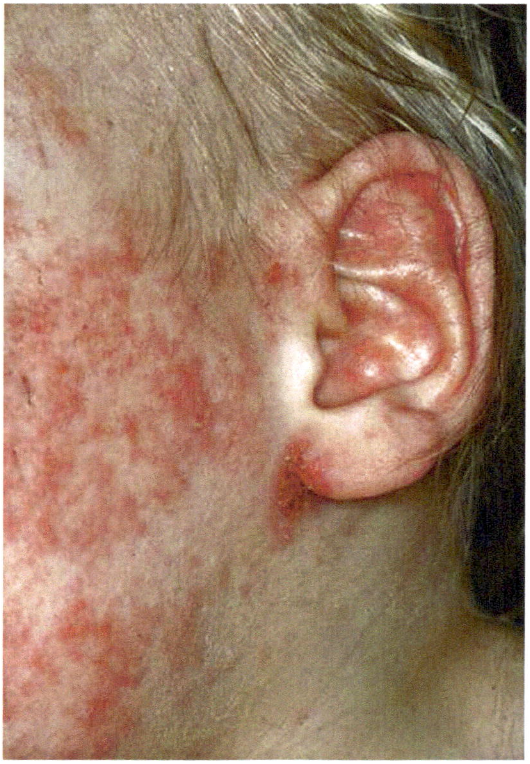

Fig. 2.9 Infra-auricular fissure in atopic dermatitis

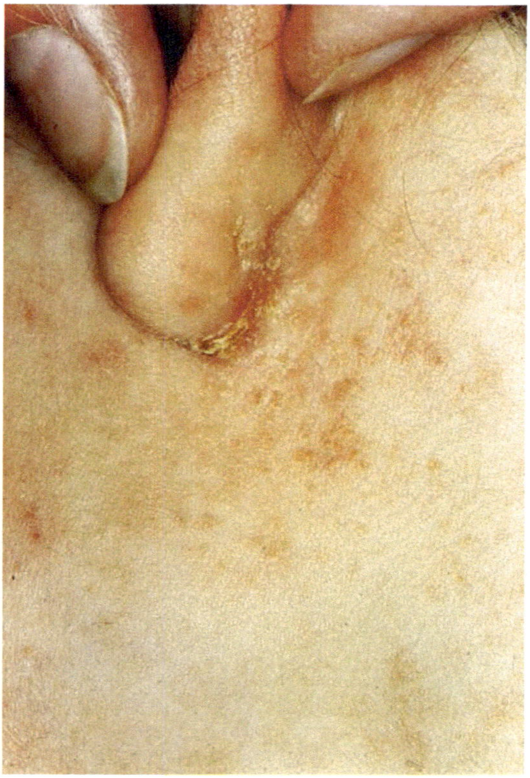

Fig. 2.10 Retroauricular fissure in atopic dermatitis

2.2.2.3 Juvenile Plantar Dermatosis

A painful variant of atopic dermatitis can be observed on the soles and lateral parts of the feet with erythema, hyperkeratosis, and fissures which is not due to contact allergy against shoe or textile material (Mackie and Husain 1976; Verbow 1989).

2.2.2.4 Eczema of the Mamilla

Mamillar eczema in atopics is a very chronic and localized variant (Fig. 2.14). It has to be evaluated in differential diagnosis in order to be distinguished from M. Paget or scabies.

2.2.2.5 Localized Genital Eczema

Similarly there are cases with exclusive affection of the genital regions as vulvar or scrotal eczema with severely lichenified variants in adults and strong psychosomatic involvement (Fig. 2.15).

2.2.2.6 Pityriasis Alba

The occurrence of whitish mildly scaling and relatively marked patches especially in light exposed skin areas during summertime is called pityriasis alba and leads to suffering in many patients (Watkins 1961), especially in colored skin (Mazenga, personal communication 2005). Most likely it is due to minimal inflammation with superficial whitish scaling (Fig. 2.16).

2.2.3 Variants and Special Forms

2.2.3.1 Dermatitis Papulosa Juvenilis

This special variant of atopic eczema goes along with development of fine papular skin changes, sometimes hypopigmented and often at the extensor sides of extremities in childhood (Bork and Hoede 1978; Fölster-Holst et al. 1996). This mani-

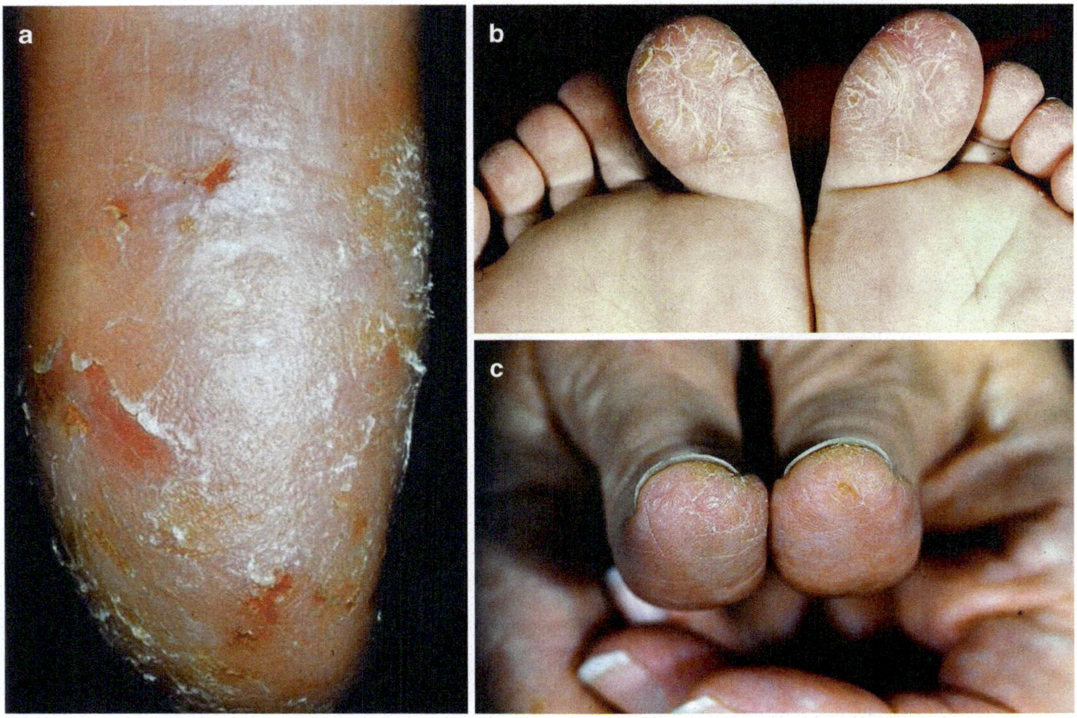

Fig. 2.11 Finger and toe eczema. (**a**) Dry finger tip eczema. (**b**) Pulpitis sicca in atopic foot dermatitis ("atopic winter feet"). (**c**) Painful eczema of the thumbs

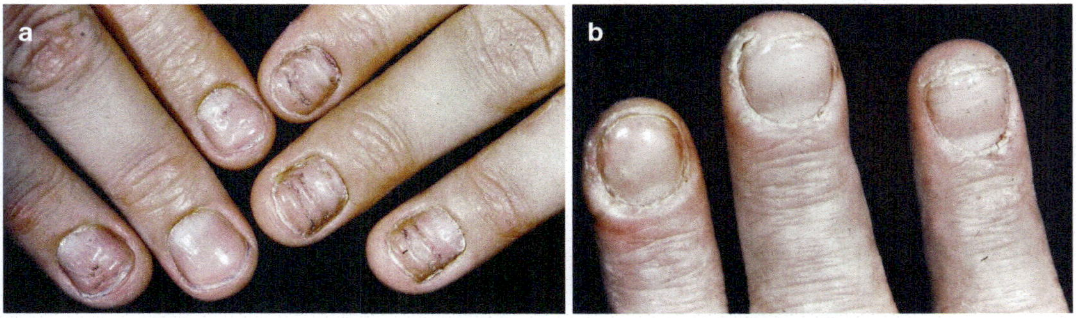

Fig. 2.12 Nail involvement in atopic dermatitis. (**a**) Eczema nails with strong horizontal grooves representing disturbance of nail growth in the matrix. (**b**) Paronychia in atopic dermatitis

festation can be found under different names (summertime pityriasis of the elbow and knee, dermatite du Tobogan, sandbox dermatitis, frictional lichenoid eruption, recurrent papillary eruption of childhood) (Dupré et al. 1974). Often the skin changes occur predominantly in spring and summer and are associated with pollen exposure. Also mechanic components like friction and sensitivity to UV light have been discussed in the pathophysiology.

2.2.3.2 Follicular Variant of Atopic Dermatitis (Patchy Pityriasiform Lichenoid Eczema)

Kitamura, Takahashi, and Sasagawa described a skin condition in Japan as plaque-type lichenoid squamous dry skin changes in children with follicular involvement and occurring predominantly on the extensor sides, sometimes similar to

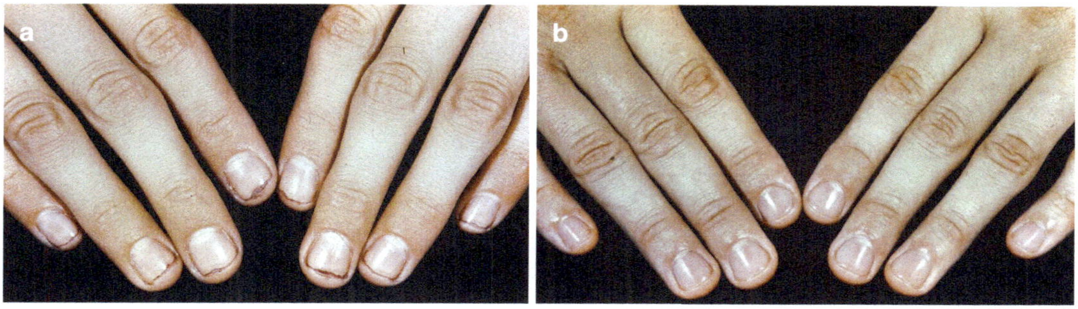

Fig. 2.13 Inspection of the nails allows information on the type of scratching. (**a**) Blood under the nail means heavy excoriation. (**b**) Shimmering nails can be derived from superficial abrasion

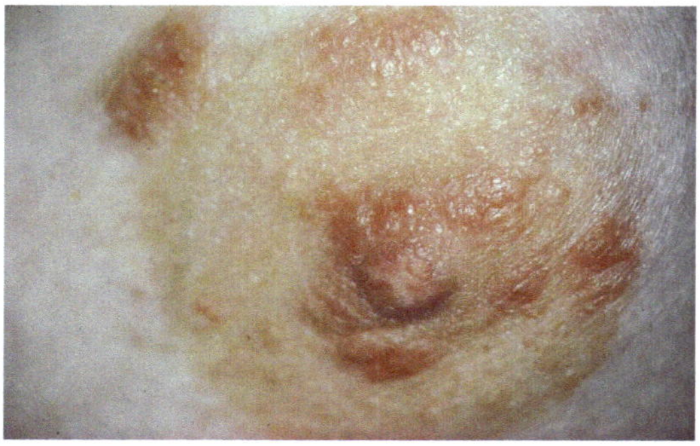

Fig. 2.14 Mamillar eczema in atopic dermatitis (when it is one-sided, scabies or Morbus Paget always have to be considered)

"goose pimples." This variant also seems to occur more often in the winter and shows improvement in the summer (Fig. 2.17) (Kitamura et al. 1950; Sasagawa 1967; Wüthrich and Schnyder 1981).

In the differential diagnosis, follicular dermatoses like lichen nitidus, Gianotti-Crosti syndrome, or follicular hyperkeratosis in certain forms of ichthyosis have to be considered.

2.2.3.3 Nummular Variant of Atopic Eczema

Especially in childhood, nummular eczema can occur with sharply demarcated nummular erythematous skin changes with scaling and excoriation and oozing aspect. Especially the lower extremities, but also the arms and trunk, can be involved. While in adults nummular eczema seems to be an own entity, it is the opinion of the author that nummular eczema in childhood represents a subvariant of atopic dermatitis (Fig. 2.18).

2.2.3.4 Special Considerations in Infants

Atopic eczema most commonly develops at the end of the first trimenon and then occurs in the face and extensor surfaces; commonly the so-called cradle cap is the first manifestation (Fig. 2.19). In the diaper area there are various differential diagnoses to atopic eczema. Interestingly, the diaper area itself is often uninvolved ("diaper sign") (see Sect. 2.4).

2.2.4 Special Localizations

2.2.4.1 Face

In many patients, atopic dermatitis only affects the face (Fig. 2.20).

2.2.4.2 Neck

Apart from the face, also the neck region is affected in many patients which can be regarded as a "big flexure" (Fig. 2.21). In chronic eczema, the clinical manifestation of a "dirty neck" develops as a postinflammatory hyperpigmentation, sometimes without real symptoms (Colver et al. 1987) (Fig. 2.22).

2.2.4.3 Hand Eczema

Often the hands and feet show the main manifestation of atopic eczema, with or without concomitant contact allergy. Here scaling eczematous skin changes and dry chronic skin lesions with lichenification, but also, when the palms and soles are involved, dyshidrosis and erosive crusty skin changes can be observed, leading to hyper-

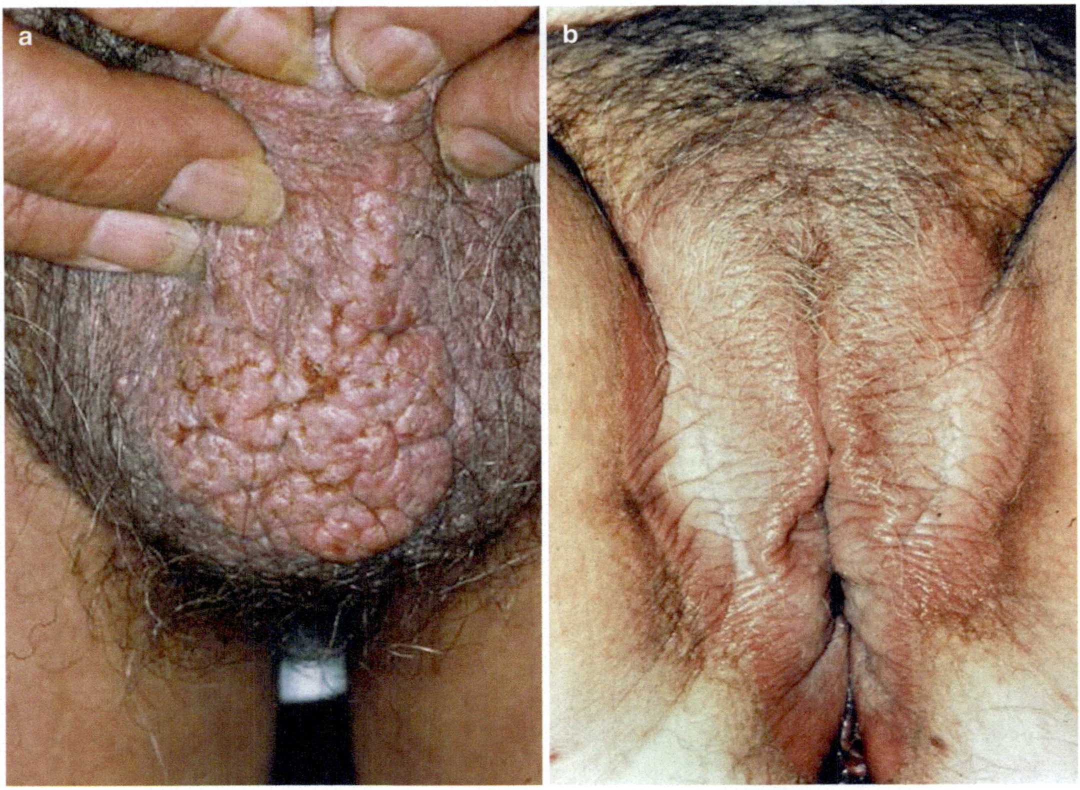

Fig. 2.15 Atopic dermatitis in the genital area. (**a**) Chronic scrotal eczema. (**b**) Chronic vulvar eczema

Fig. 2.16 Pityriasis alba in atopic dermatitis

keratotic fissuring manifestations (Fig. 2.23). Often the nails are also affected (Fig. 2.24).

Hand eczema represents a special problem as one of the most common occupational skin diseases and is pathogenetically classified between irritant, contact allergic, and atopic dermatitis. Furthermore, sometimes the differential diagnosis to psoriasis of the palms and soles may be difficult. In a retrospective study, the most frequent subdiagnoses of chronic hand eczema were allergic contact dermatitis, allergic plus irritative contact dermatitis, irritant contact dermatitis, atopic hand eczema, atopic plus irritant hand eczema, vesicular hand eczema (dyshidrotic = pompholyx) and hyperkeratotic eczema (Diepgen et al. 2009).

2.2.4.4 Erythroderma

Atopic dermatitis also can manifest as erythroderma with involvement of the whole integument in the sense of an exfoliative dermatitis with redness and scaling. Erythroderma by definition is a clinical condition which often cannot be attributed to a single disease at first glance. Several diseases can lead to erythroderma:

- Allergic contact dermatitis
- Psoriasis

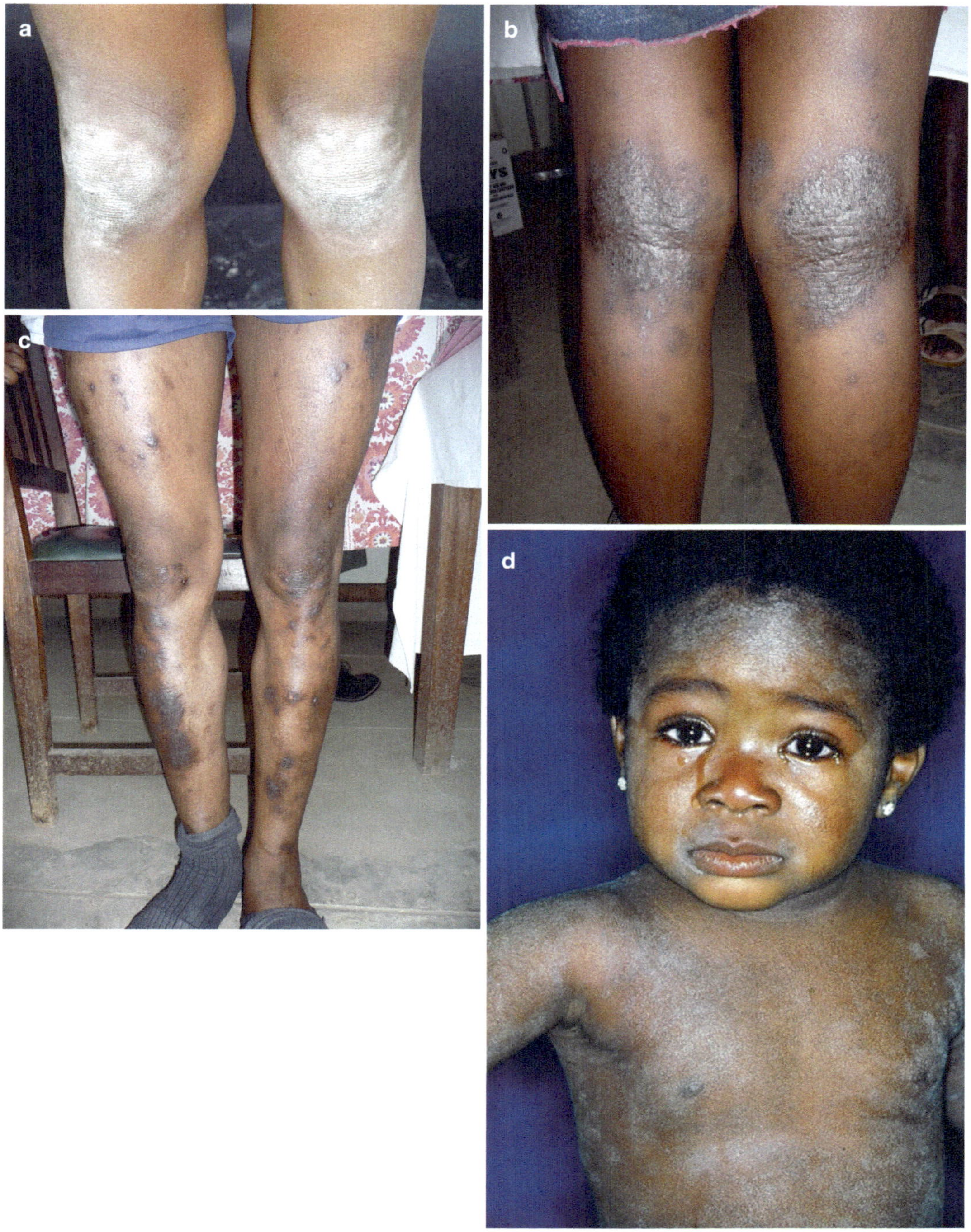

Fig. 2.17 Patchy pityriasiform lichenoid eczema as special variant of atopic dermatitis appearing on the extensor sides of the joints. These skin changes are particularly common in dark skin. (**a**) Lichenoid papules and plaques on the extensor side of the knee. (**b**) Atopic dermatitis of the knee joints in an African patient from Tanzania. (**c**) Atopic dermatitis (nummular pattern) on both legs in an African patient from Tanzania (With friendly permission of P. Schmid-Grendelmeier). (**d**) Facial eczema in an African child

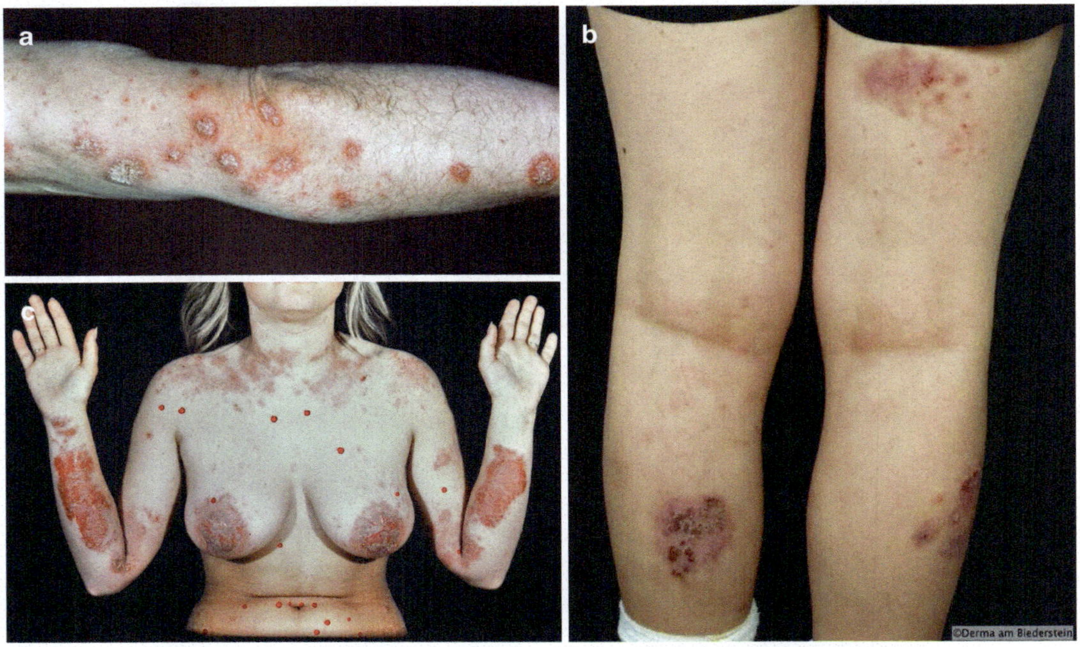

Fig. 2.18 Nummular variant of atopic dermatitis. (**a**) Scaling nummular lesions in atopic eczema. (**b**) Nummular eczema of the legs in atopic dermatitis. (**c**) Sharply marginated massive atopic eczema with nummular distribution

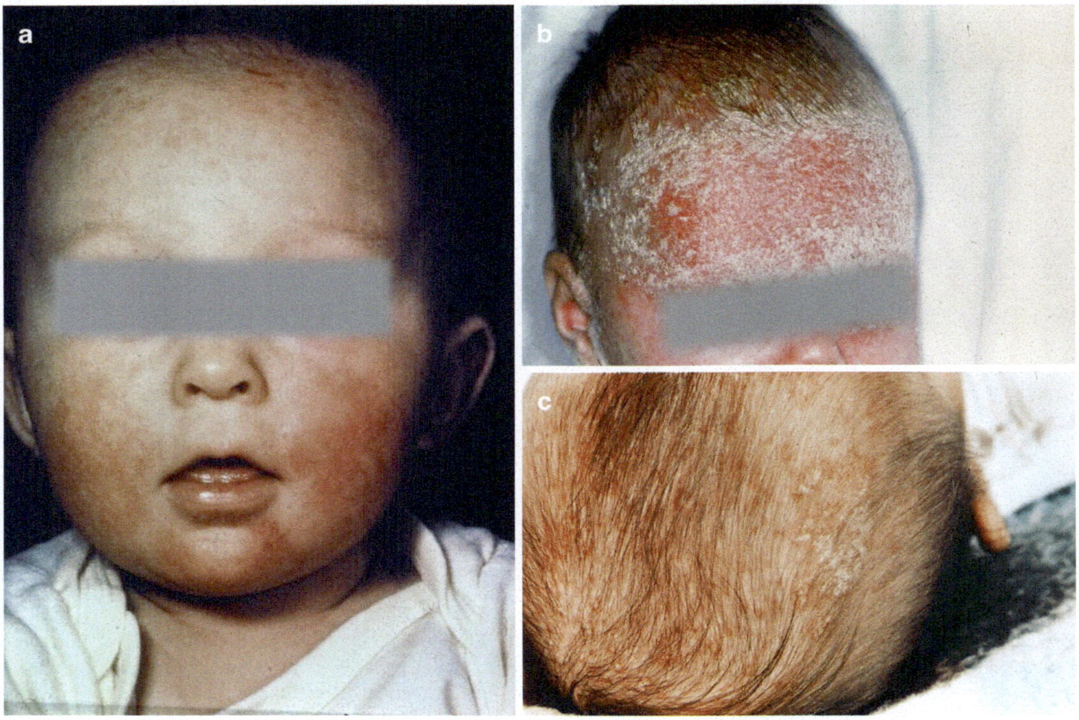

Fig. 2.19 Atopic dermatitis in infants. (**a**) Facial eczema in infants. (**b**) Cradle cap ("Crusta lactea" reminding of crusted milk in a pan). (**c**) Cradle cap on the scalp

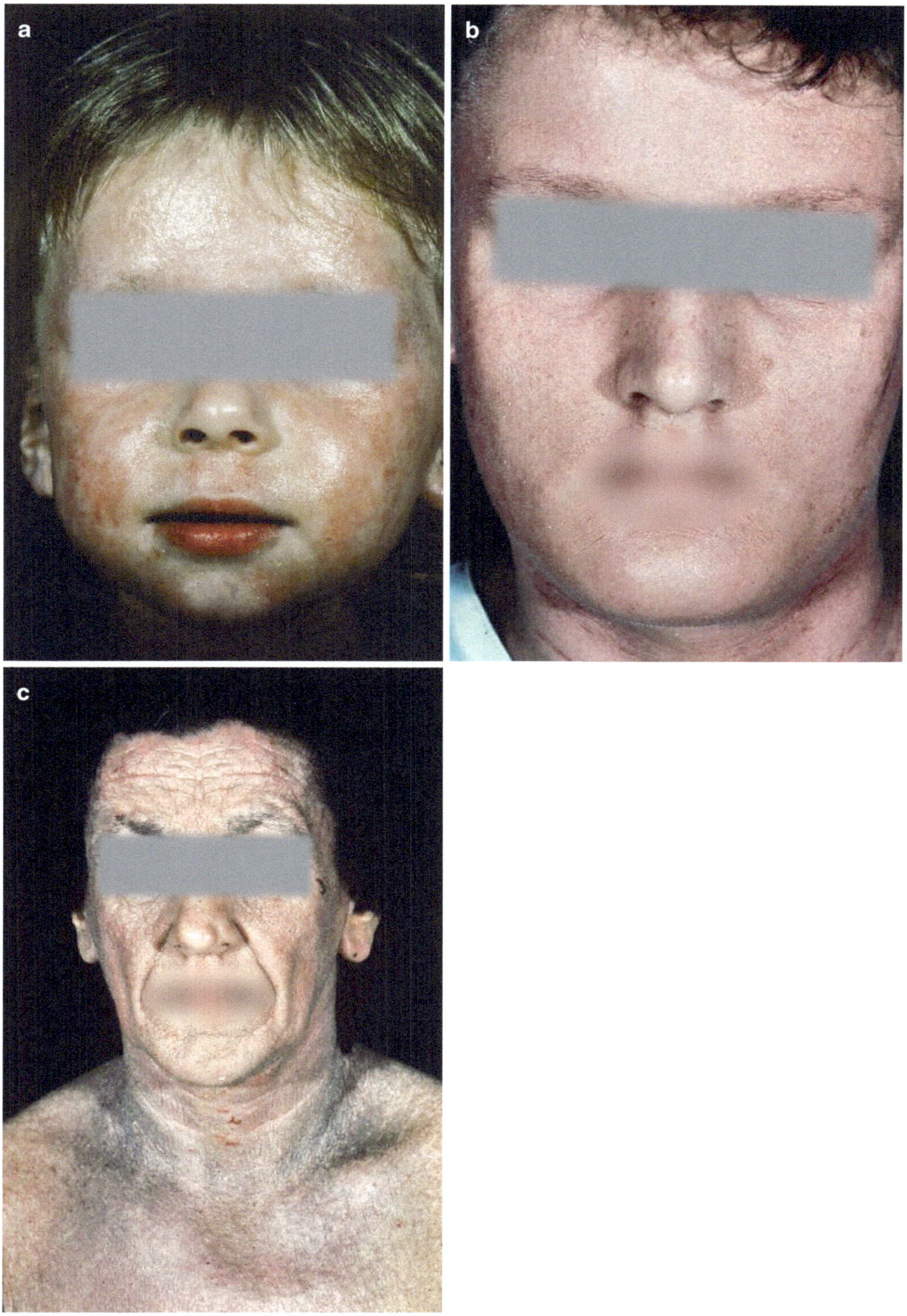

Fig. 2.20 Atopic dermatitis in the face. (**a**) in childhood. (**b**) In adulthood. (**c**) Massive atopic dermatitis of the face with lichenification

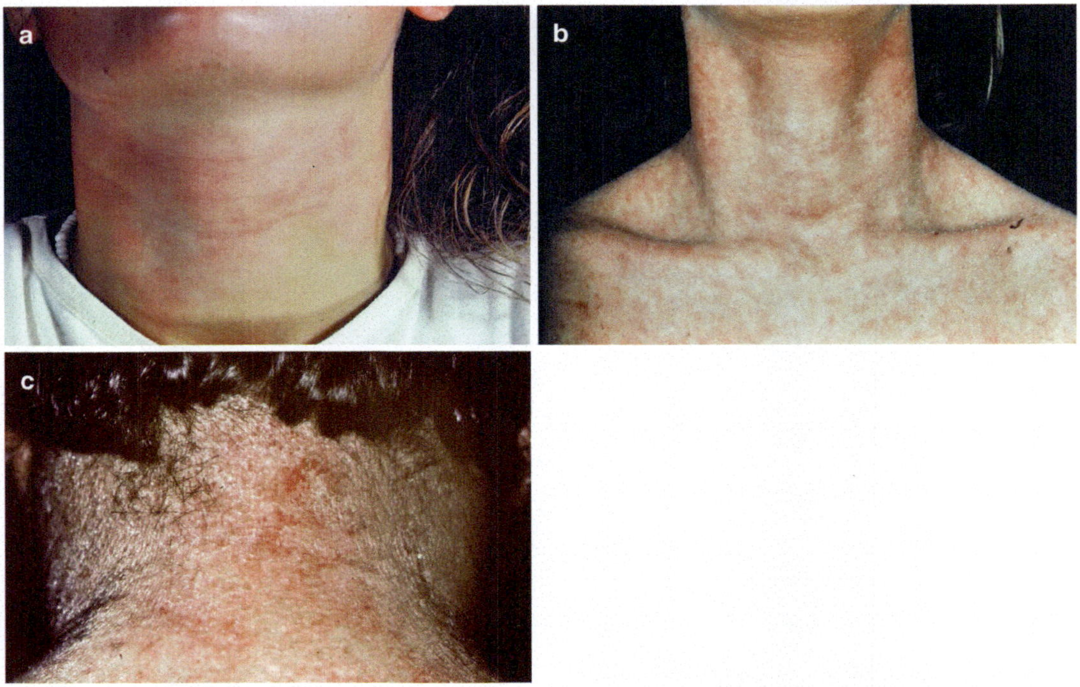

Fig. 2.21 Atopic dermatitis of the neck. (**a**) Atopic dermatitis of the neck region. (**b**) Scaling atopic dermatitis of the neck. (**c**) Atopic dermatitis of the neck with lichenification

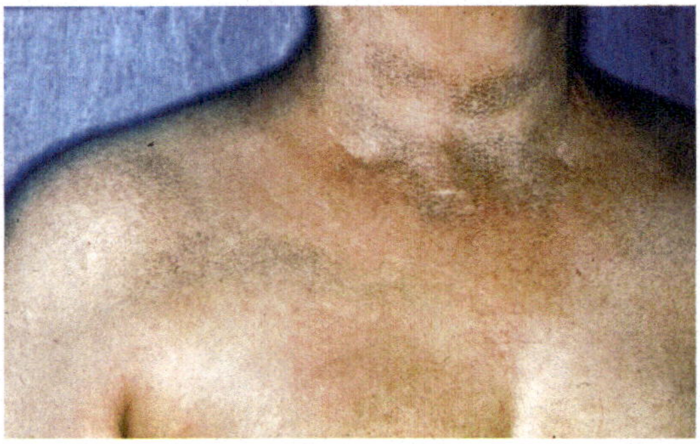

Fig. 2.22 "Dirty neck" following postinflammatory hyperpigmentation in atopic dermatitis

- Pityriasis rubra pilaris
- Cutaneous T-cell lymphoma (Sezary syndrome)
- Idiopathic melano-erythrodermia cachectica
- Exanthematous drug eruption

2.2.5 Summary

Contrary to other dermatoses, atopic dermatitis does not show a clear-cut morphology. The primary lesion can best be described as itch which then via scratching leads to the formation of skin changes. Several variants with "infiltrated erosive erythema," "chronic lichenification," or "prurigo type" of atopic dermatitis can be observed. Exudative eczematous skin changes can be found predominantly during childhood or when superinfection occurs. Minimal manifestations comprise infra-auricular fissures, cheilitis sicca, infranasal erosion, eyelid eczema, finger or toe eczema, and pityriasis alba.

2.3 Stigmata of Atopy

Contrary to actual signs and symptoms of disease and minimal manifestations, the so-called stigmata represent characteristics of the organ skin, not necessarily going along with feeling sick nor being sequels of the disease. Rather they can be regarded as constitutional signs of an "atopic diathesis"; thus, they can give the experienced physician valuable information without additional laboratory diagnostics or history analysis with regard to the existence of atopy in the individual.

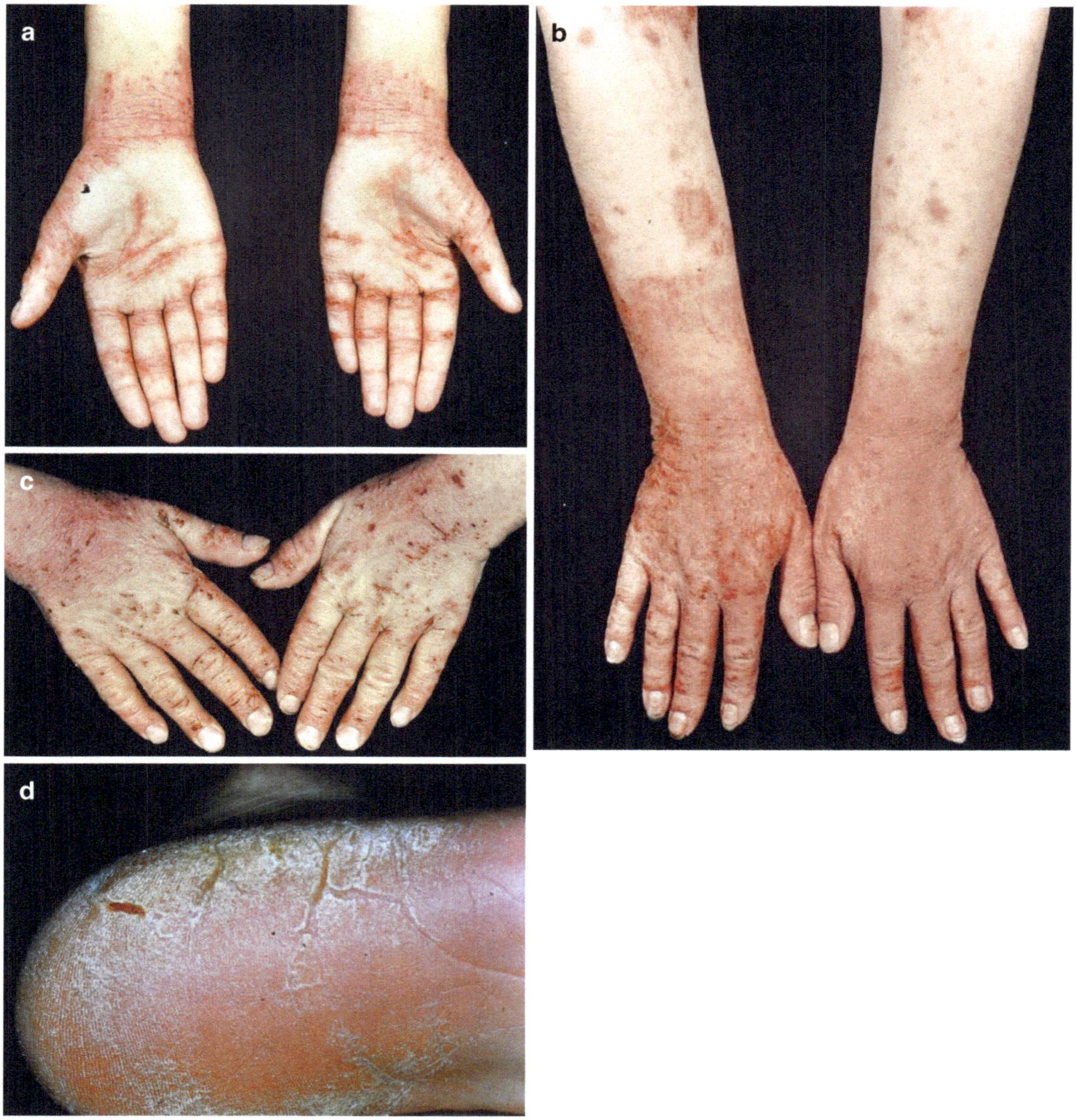

Fig. 2.23 Hand and foot eczema in atopic dermatitis. (**a**) Hand eczema with palmar involvement. (**b**) Dorsum of the hands with strong excoriations. (**c**) Dry atopic dermatitis of the dorsum of the hands. (**d**) Foot eczema with deep fissures

Table 2.1 shows the most common stigmata which also have been quantitatively evaluated in epidemiologic studies.

2.3.1 Dry Skin (Xerosis)

Dry skin is a major characteristic of atopic dermatitis, also called sebostasis or xerosis; it is visible as rough skin, sometimes slightly scaling (Fig. 2.25). The term "dry" skin can be questioned pathophysiologically since, in investigations with regard to the percentage of water in the skin, no real decrease has been found, but an increased transepidermal water loss (TEWL) due to disturbed skin barrier function. Furthermore, mild signs of inflammation have been found in "dry skin of atopic dermatitis" in uninvolved areas (Uehara 1985).

The term sebostasis indicates a diminished sebum secretion which is controversial. The lipid

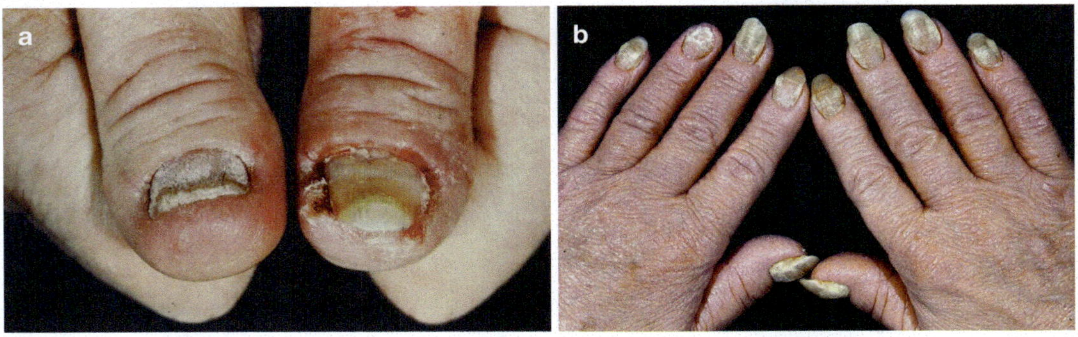

Fig. 2.24 Nail changes in hand eczema. (**a**) Eczema nails. (**b**) Nail dystrophy in eczema

Table 2.1 Stigmata of atopic dermatitis/eczema

Dry skin (sebostasis, xerosis)
Hyperlinearity of palms and soles ("ichthyosis hands or feet")
Linear grooves of fingertips
Atopy fold of the eyelid (Dennie-Morgan)
Scattering of lateral eyebrow (Hertoghe)
Low temporal hairline
Facial pallor with periorbital halo
White dermographism
Delayed blanch reaction after acetylcholine

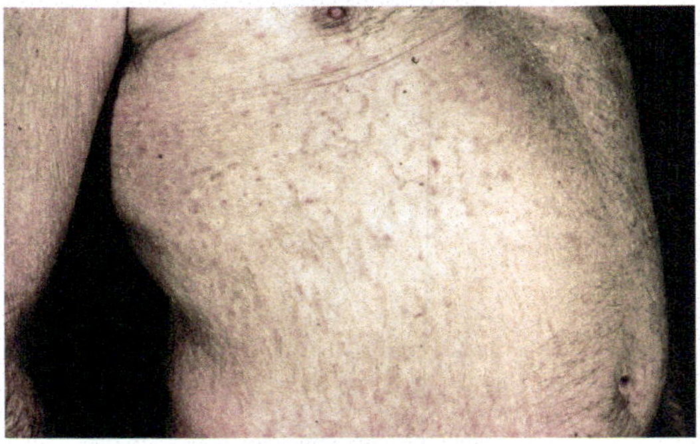

Fig. 2.25 Dry skin, eczema craquelée

content of the epidermis has been investigated by several groups and found to be altered especially with regard to different patterns of ceramides (see Chap. 3).

Finally a major characteristic is roughness which can be recognized by the patient and physician and feels like "dryness." It is not clear whether this "dry" aspect actually corresponds to the deficiency of the epidermal protein filaggrin (see Chap. 3) found in many patients with atopic eczema.

2.3.2 Ichthyosis Hands and Feet (Hyperlinearity of Palms and Soles)

This stigma is well known in patients with the autosomal dominant disease ichthyosis vulgaris. Marked linear furs or lines can be seen, partly in a bizarre or linear configuration mostly on the palms, but in infants commonly also on the soles (Fig. 2.26).

This sign, first described by Leutgeb et al. (Leutgeb et al. 1972), was regarded for a long time as proof for concomitantly occurring ichthyosis vulgaris and can now better be explained by the filaggrin deficiency in heterozygous states in many atopic dermatitis patients. Only in a small part of eczema patients the typical signs of ichthyosis vulgaris can be seen in histopathology or by electron microscopy, namely, abnormal keratohyalin granules (Fartasch et al. 1989).

A subgroup of ichthyosis hands or feet can be seen in linear grooves often horizontal to the papillary lines on the fingertips (Fig. 2.27).

2.3.3 Infraorbital Fold (Atopy Fold, Dennie-Morgan)

This sign has first been described in a letter by Dr. Morgan as "definite wrinkle just beneath the margin of the lower lid of both eyes," who mentioned it to Dr. Dennie (Morgan 1948) as a sign of atopy. The fold can be single or double. Mostly it is present on both lower eyelids, sometimes, however, only unilaterally. The exact defi-

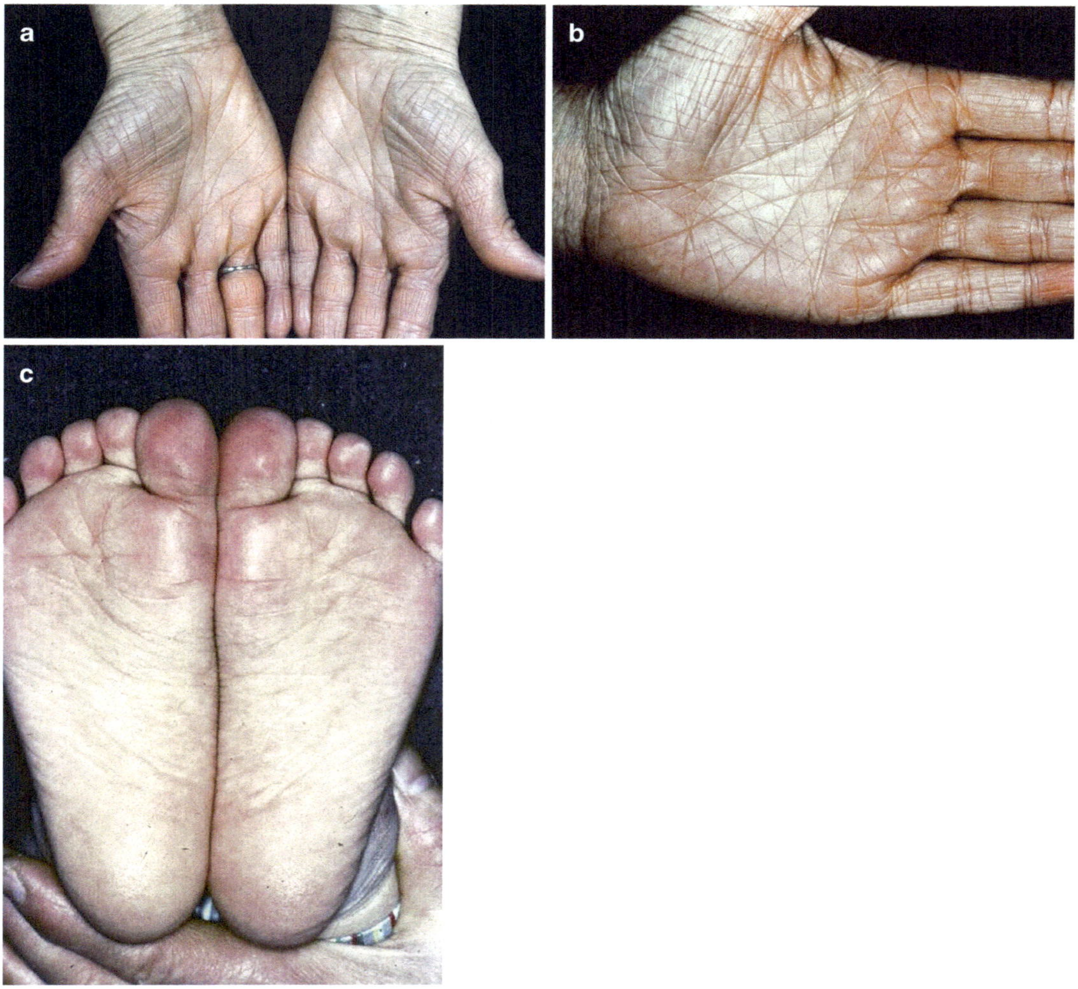

Fig. 2.26 Hyperlinearity of palms and soles (ichthyotsis hands/feet). (**a**) Massive skin changes in the palms. (**b**) Hyperlinearity of hand. (**c**) Ichthyosis feet

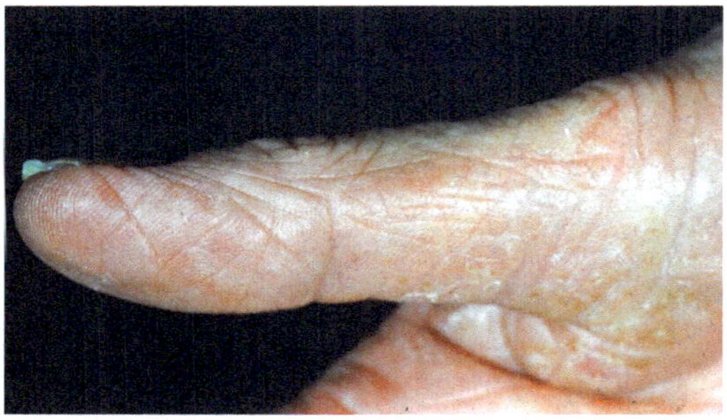

Fig. 2.27 Linear grooves on the finger tips

nition implies a clear-cut double fold beginning mostly at the inner (medial) canthus and reaching laterally at least beyond the center of the pupil. The atopy fold must not be confounded with the physiological sulcus palpebralis inferior (Przybilla et al. 1991; Uehara 1981) (Fig. 2.28). Many authors regard the Dennie-Morgan fold as a sequel of lid eczema due to increased rubbing and scratching. However, clear-cut clinical observations have shown that this stigma can be present many years before the first occurrence of atopic dermatitis, mostly starting in other body areas like the elbows or knee joints and without lid eczema.

The atopy fold is also present in respiratory atopic diseases. In Asian patients, the infraorbital fold seems to be a less suitable marker.

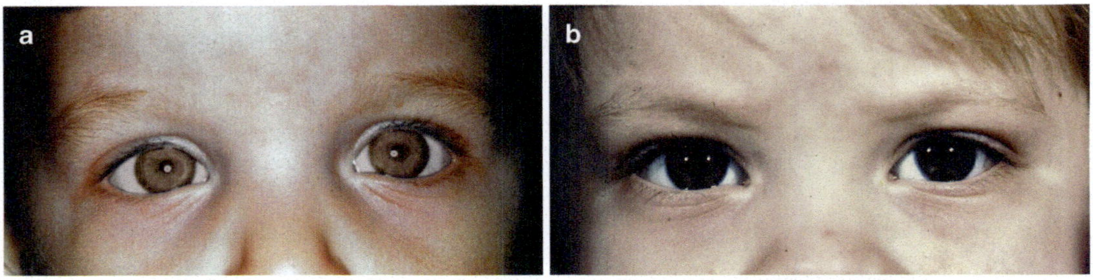

Fig. 2.28 Dennie-Morgan fold (atopy fold). (**a**) Double fold starting on the inner cantus reaching over the middle of the pupil. (**b**) Atopy fold in a child with atopic dermatitis

2.3.4 Periorbital Halo and Facial Pallor

This sign, also called halo eyes (Fig. 2.29), can be observed in atopic eczema, but also in respiratory atopy as allergic rhinoconjunctivitis and has been called "allergic shiners"; the manifestation is a dark gray, brownish discoloration of the periorbital areas, sometimes associated with mild edema. The patients give an impression of sleeplessness ("bleary eyed"). Some of my coworkers call them "disco shadows." Once an actress came to me as a patient just because of this skin change, for the director would not give her a role in a play anymore, since she looked "worn out" ("kaputt").

Pathophysiologically swellings and congestion of postcapillary venules in the area of the nasal sinuses have been incriminated. Occasionally a secondary hyperpigmentation on the basis of existing chronic eczema has been observed; this, however, does not correspond to a stigma. Together with the common pallor of the face, this stigma can be regarded as imbalance of the autonomic nervous system with increased alpha-adrenergic and cholinergic impulses and decreased beta-adrenergic reactions (Korting 1954).

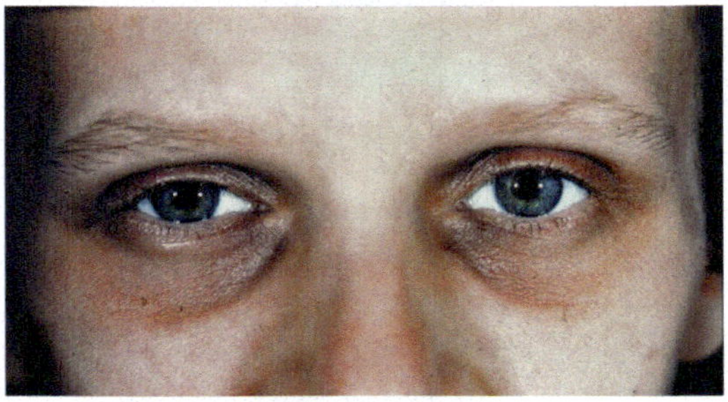

Fig. 2.29 Periorbital shadowing ("halo eyes," "disco eyes")

2.3.5 Rarefaction of Lateral Eyebrows (Hertoghe)

This sign has been first described at the beginning of the twentieth century by Hertoghe in a patient with hypothyreosis. In patients with atopic eczema, some authors see an association to increased rubbing of eyebrows, when eyebrow eczema can be diagnosed at the same time (Fig. 2.30). For a long time it was regarded as a classic stigma of altered skin independent of immune reactivity. Saurat observed a regrowth of lateral eyebrow hair after successful bone marrow transplantation in patients with Wiskott-Aldrich syndrome with massive atopic eczema and atopy stigmata (Saurat 1985). It is obvious that artificial manipulations (plucking of eyebrows) (pseudo-Hertoghe) have to be differentiated from the true stigma.

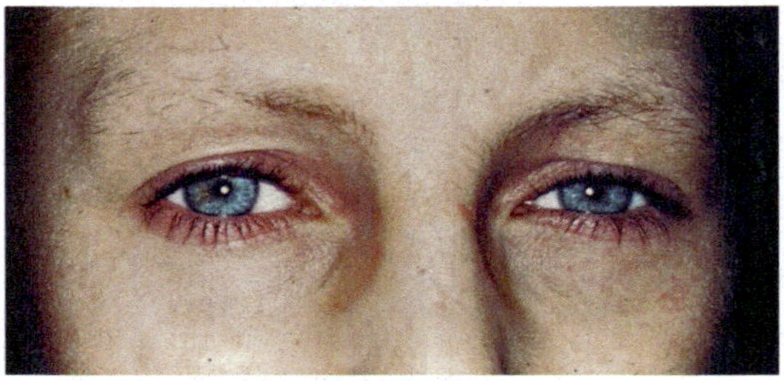

Fig. 2.30 Lateral part of eyebrows with sparse hair ("Hertoghe sign")

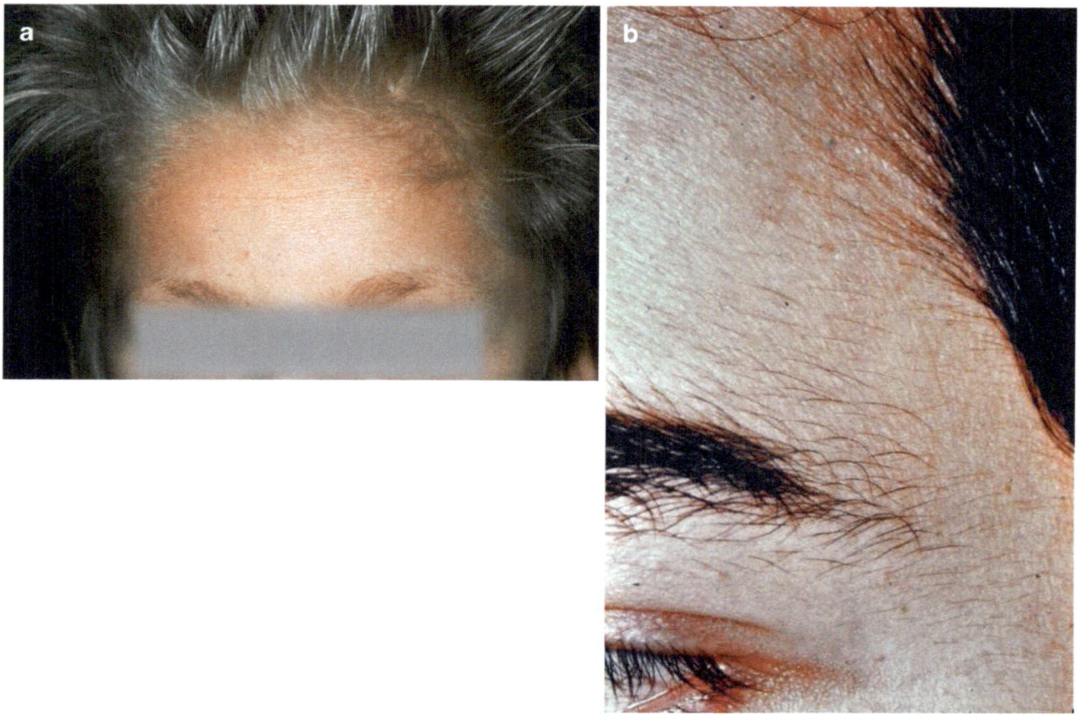

Fig. 2.31 Low temporal hairline ("fur cap"). (**a**) Reduction of the distance between temporal and hair and end of lateral eyebrows. (**b**) Low temporal hairline

2.3.6 Low Temporal Hairline, "Fur Cap Hair Growth"

This stigma describes a decreased distance between the temporal hairline and the end of the lateral eyebrows; sometimes there is no distance in between (Fig. 2.31). Quantitatively the distance between the temporal hairline and eyebrow should be more than 3 cm. The stigma can be observed in almost 90 % of patients with atopic dermatitis (Przybilla et al. 1991).

A positive Hertoghe phenomenon does not exclude a low temporal hairline sign.

2.3.7 White Dermographism

The white dermographism is one of the best-known stigmata of atopy. While in healthy individuals tangential pressure (e.g., with a spatula) leads to a redness of the skin within 30–60 s (red dermographism), in atopic individuals sometimes the skin turns white (Fig. 2.32); sometimes there is a contrasting whitening next to a central red part (red dermographism with a white edge). Pathophysiologically most likely an increased local vasoconstriction is the basis of white dermographism (Wong et al. 1984).

2.3.8 Delayed Blanch

After injection of acetylcholine (intradermal), some patients with atopic eczema develop a long-lasting white discoloration in the injection area called delayed blanch reaction or delayed white reaction (Hanifin and Lobitz 1977; Lobitz and Campbell 1953; Whitfield 1938).

White dermographism and delayed blanch can be regarded as signs of autonomic dysregulation in atopics. They are not specific for atopic dermatitis but also can be seen in respiratory atopy.

It is important not to elicit white dermographism in an involved or inflamed skin area. On

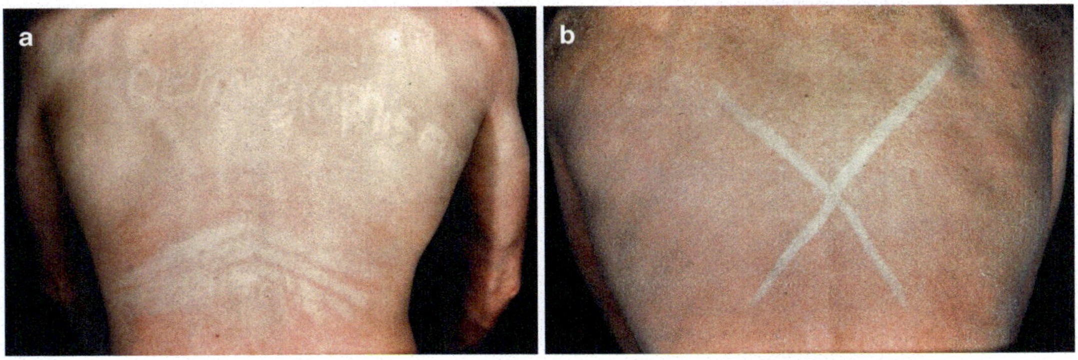

Fig. 2.32 White dermographism. (**a**) After tangential pressure the skin turns white instead of red. (**b**) Massive whitening within 30–60 s

inflamed skin, white dermographism can be elicited also in other skin conditions.

2.3.9 Role in Diagnosis

Many studies have investigated the prevalence of atopy stigmata in patients with atopic eczema and other atopic diseases as well as in healthy control persons. In an intense and quantitative measurement in patients with various atopic diseases and healthy controls, we found that all of the abovementioned stigmata were significantly more prevalent in atopics compared to non-atopic controls (Przybilla et al. 1991). The strongest association with atopic eczema (and significantly higher than in respiratory atopy) were:

- Dry skin
- Ichthyosis hands
- White dermographism
- Hertoghe phenomenon

Similar to the increased tendency to IgE production (see Sect. 1.3.1), there also may be overlaps in the manifestation of atopy on the skin with "minimal" or "latent" atopy which only become manifest in stigma or presence of stigmata without ever turning into actual clinical eczema.

2.3.10 Summary

Stigmata have to be distinguished from actual symptoms of disease. They are signs of the skin organ not necessarily connected with feeling ill which give hints to the existence of an "atopic" diathesis. They comprise dry skin (xerosis, sebostasis), hyperlinearity of the palms and soles (ichthyosis "hands" or "feet"), increased infraorbital fold (atopy fold Dennie-Morgan), facial pallor with periorbital halo, rarefaction of lateral eyebrows (Hertoghe), fur cap hair growth with low temporal hairline, as well as white dermographism and delayed blanch.

2.4 Differential Diagnoses

Even if the diagnosis of atopic dermatitis is not difficult for an experienced dermatologist or allergist, a variety of differential diagnoses have to be considered, partly depending on the age group.

The most common differential diagnoses are listed in Table 2.2 and comprise chronic inflammatory skin diseases, infectious skin diseases, immunopathologies, hereditary skin diseases, metabolic disorders, malignant skin diseases, drug reactions, as well as all other forms of dermatitis or eczema (see also Fölster-Holst et al. 2004; Rajka 1989; Ring et al. 2006).

2.4.1 Differential Diagnosis in Infants

In the first months of life, it is mainly seborrheic dermatitis or diaper dermatitis which has to be considered (Fig. 2.33). Often there is no clear-cut

Table 2.2 Differential diagnoses of atopic dermatitis

Chronic inflammatory skin diseases
Seborrheic dermatitis
Psoriasis
Lichen simplex chronicus
Allergic contact dermatitis
Irritative toxic contact dermatitis
Infectious skin diseases
Impetigo contagiosa
Candidiasis
Tinea
Scabies
Ictus insectorum (strophulus)
Immunodeficiency syndromes
Ataxia telangiectasia
Wiskott-Aldrich syndrome
Hyper IgE syndrome
Severe combined immunodeficiency (SCID)
Autoimmune diseases
Bullous pemphigoid
Pemphigus foliaceus
Dermatitis herpetiformis
Dermatomyositis
Graft-versus-host disease
Genodermatoses
Netherton syndrome
Dubowitz syndrome
Erythrokeratodermia variabilis
Metabolic diseases
Phenylketonuria
Tyrosinemia
Zinc deficiency
Side effects of drugs

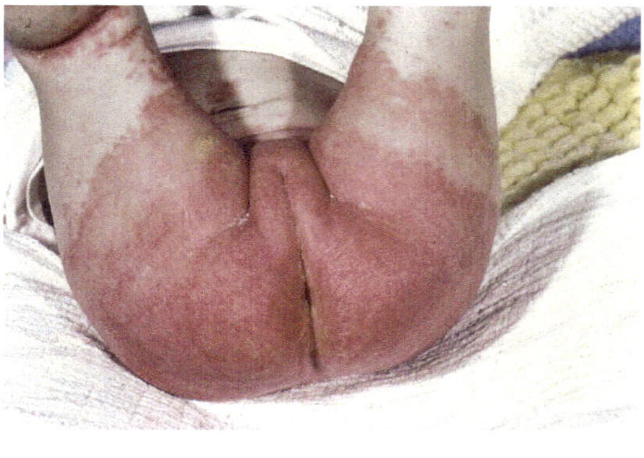

Fig. 2.33 Diaper dermatitis with marked erythema in the diaper area

diagnosis in the first months of life, and then the term "eczema infantum" (infantile eczema) is helpful (Edgren 1943).

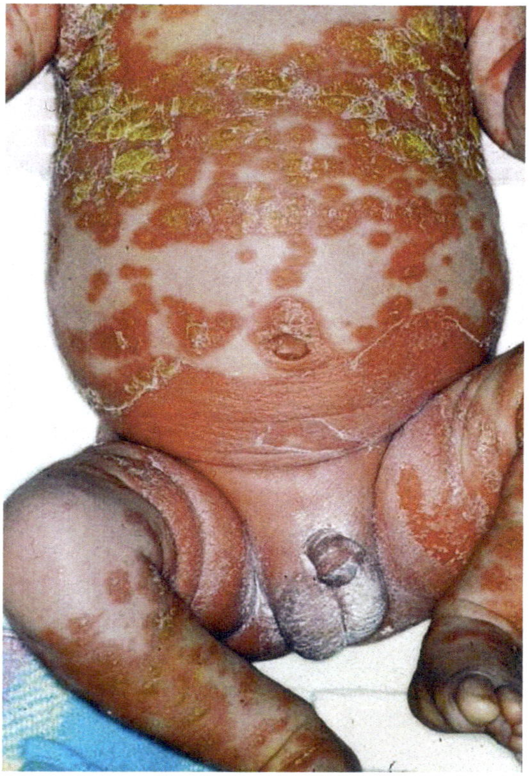

Fig. 2.34 Yellowish crusts in seborrheic dermatitis in an infant

There is a valuable rule: bipolar occurrence (especially head and scalp and genital area involved) allures seborrheic dermatitis (Fig. 2.34). Skin changes in the head and trunk with the uninvolved diaper area are typical for atopic eczema. This commonly observed "diaper phenomenon" is poorly investigated scientifically. One can speculate whether the diaper offers protection against scratching or the contents act like a wet wrap. It is surprising that in severely affected infants with atopic eczema, often only the diaper area is totally uninvolved (Fig. 2.35).

Another sign visible to everybody but not often recognized is the absence of eczema on the tip of the nose (Yamamoto sign, personal communication via Kristian Thestrup-Pedersen 2005).

2.4.2 Chronic Inflammatory Skin Diseases

In infants, but also in small children, psoriasis can be a difficult differential diagnosis, especially in

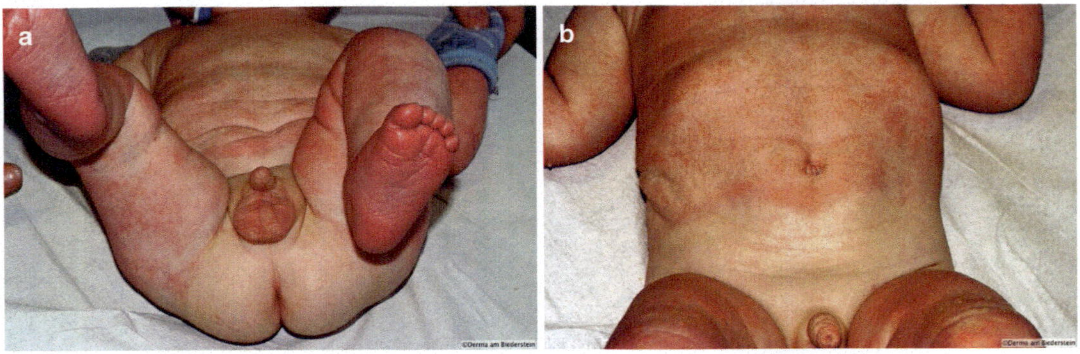

Fig. 2.35 Diaper sign in atopic dermatitis: the diaper area is surprisingly often uninvolved. (**a**) Uninvolved diaper area. (**b**) Uninvolved diaper area with strong general skin involvement

cases of so-called figurated eczema or when there is a coincidence of both diseases. Thirty years ago this was no problem; eczema and psoriasis seemed to exclude each other. Only by the epidemiological studies by Henseler and Christophers (1995), it became clear that psoriasis and atopic eczema can occur in one and the same individual, although rarely. Due to the increase in eczema prevalence, this subgroup of patients may be seen more often.

Furthermore existing eczema may trigger latent psoriasis via scratching and mechanical traumatization in the sense of a Koebner phenomenon.

A difficult differential diagnosis can be the localized involvement of palms and soles together with dyshidrosis (pompholyx). This type of hand eczema can occur in atopic eczema, but also in allergic contact dermatitis, and also in patients with tinea. According to some authors, dyshidrotic hand or foot eczema always corresponds to atopic dermatitis and should be called atopic palmoplantar eczema (Schwanitz 1992).

The co-occurrence or absence of other inflammatory diseases in atopic dermatitis is an interesting phenomenon and gives rise to new pathophysiological concepts (see Chap. 3).

Other allergic skin diseases, especially allergic contact dermatitis, have to be differentiated; allergic contact dermatitis also can occur in childhood, which is not mentioned in many textbooks (see Chap. 4). Especially when the dorsum of the feet is involved, contact allergy against shoe constituents should be considered.

In adult life, lichen simplex chronicus is a differential diagnosis in chronically lichenified areas (Fig. 2.36) or may represent a subtype of atopic dermatitis in a localized variant. Similarly irritative reactions, due to strong mechanic traumatization and individual susceptibility, have to be considered as differential diagnosis of atopic dermatitis.

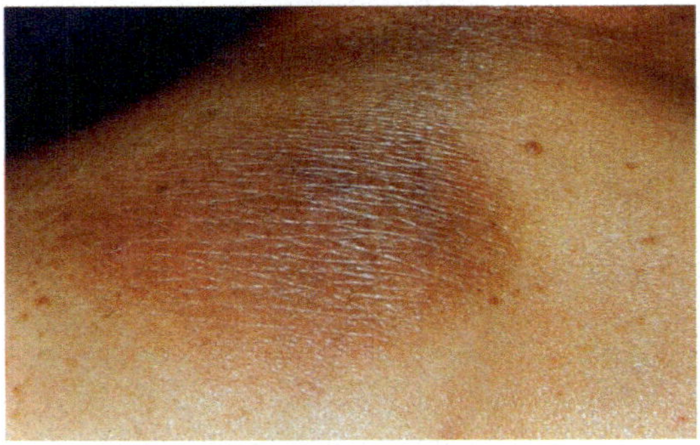

Fig. 2.36 Lichen simplex chronicus Vidal

Also systemic allergic contact dermatitis (hematogenous contact eczema) may sometimes be difficult to distinguish from a generalized flare of atopic eczema. Pathophysiologically, it is a Th1 reaction with activation of homing receptors of specific reactivated T cells producing generalized or symmetric eczematous skin lesions after parenteral or oral allergen application (Ring 1990; Ring and Merkel 2012).

2.4.3 Inflammatory Tumor Responses

An interesting variant of eczematous skin disease is an inflammatory phenomenon occurring around congenital pigmentary nevi with a mostly transitory character. This inflammatorily altered nevus is called Meyerson's nevus (Meyerson 1971).

The differential diagnosis between atopic dermatitis and cutaneous T-cell lymphoma, especially of an erythrodermic variant, also may be difficult. Total serum IgE or measurement of certain chemokines do not really differentiate; however, absence of specific IgE, extremely high CD4/CD8 ratio, and CCR10 positivity in the skin and Sezary cells in peripheral blood may be a strong indication for cutaneous T-cell lymphoma (Miyagaki and Sugaya 2011).

2.4.4 Infectious Skin Diseases

Scabies may be overlooked by the inexperienced and diagnosed as atopic eczema, since it also goes along with extreme itch. The typical mite furrows on the wrist or in the interdigital areas together with typical papules in the genital area (penile papules) are characteristic. Using the dermatoscope, the detection of scabies mites has become much more easy (typical scabies "kite").

Regarding the existing cross-reactivities between scabies mite (*Sarcoptes scabiei*) and house dust mite (*Dermatophagoides pteronyssinus* or *farinae*) as well as storage mites (Lepidoglyphus destructor), one can speculate about a primitive evolutionary defense reaction against mites via IgE antibodies in the development of atopic dermatitis.

Other infectious diseases which have to be considered include staphylococcal infection (impetigo) and herpes simplex, which can give rise to the serious complication of eczema herpeticum (see Sect. 2.6) as well as tinea.

2.4.5 Metabolic Diseases, Immunodeficiencies, or Immunopathies

A variety of metabolic diseases can become manifest in eczematous skin changes: when the orificia (perioral and perianal) are involved in infants, one has to think of zinc deficiency and acrodermatitis enteropathica. Short stature has been observed (David 1989).

In several congenital or acquired immune deficiencies, atopic eczema seems to be more prevalent than in the normal population (Saurat 1985; Saurat et al. 1985; Vieluf et al. 1989) (see also Sect. 2.5).

Immunopathies may be considered in the differential diagnosis with regard to early stages of bullous pemphigoid in the elderly or other blistering diseases like dermatitis herpetiformis Duhring or pemphigus foliaceus.

Graft-versus-host disease can show eczema-like skin changes with itch and dysesthesia and follicular papules.

Skin changes in dermatomyositis in childhood are characteristic, but can be confounded in the initial phase with facial involvement, erythema, and swelling with eczema. Sometimes lid eczema is diagnosed, although only swelling (without epidermal involvement) of the eyelids is present.

2.4.6 Malignant Diseases

Atopic dermatitis has to be differentiated from a variety of malignant skin diseases, especially T-cell lymphoma of the skin and Langerhans cell histiocytosis (histiocytosis X). In infants, Langerhans cell histiocytosis can occur preferably in the diaper area or in the neck-shoulder region and looks similar to atopic eczema with crusted papules and seborrheic squamous areas. In these cases, dermatopathology is crucial.

In adults, unexplained and not clearly attributable eczematous skin changes should give rise to the differential diagnosis of lymphoproliferative disease of the skin, the most common being mycosis fungoides as a variant of cutaneous T-cell lymphoma as well as Sezary syndrome (Rajka and Winkelmann 1984) (see Sect. 2.4.3).

Especially in the maximal variant of erythroderma which can occur in atopic eczema, the differential diagnosis of T-cell lymphoma is crucial.

A hint for malignant T-cell proliferation can be seen in the poor response to anti-inflammatory treatment of the eczematous skin changes. The simple question as to "whether this patch has been there in the same spot all the time or has disappeared and reoccurred at another skin area"

Table 2.3 Differential diagnoses of atopic eczema in infancy

	Atopic dermatitis	Seborrheic dermatitis	Scabies
Onset	2–3 months	First days of life	All ages
Gender	6 M=F	M=F	M=F
Prevalence	Common	Common	Variable
Genetic mutation	Filaggrin +	0	0
IgE	Increased	Normal	Normal/increased
Eosinophilia	Common	Rare	Common
Morphology	Typically age dependent	Diaper area, axillae, capillitium	Interdigital areas, genital area
Itch	Strong	Almost absent	Strong
Dermographism	White	Red	Red
S. aureus infection	Common	Rare	Rare
Other infections	Rare	*Malassezia furfur*	Rare
Concomitant respiratory atopy	Common	Rare	Rare
Food allergy	Common	Rare	Rare

According to Fölster-Holst et al. (2004)

is one of the most important questions in this differential diagnosis.

The most important differential diagnostic aspects of atopic dermatitis in infant and adult age are enlisted in Tables 2.3 and 2.4.

2.5 Associated Diseases

2.5.1 Hereditary Dermatoses

Some hereditary skin diseases can either directly be accompanied by atopic dermatitis or be associated with similar skin changes (Hoeger and Harper 1998) (Table 2.5).

In 50 % of the cases with phenylketonuria, eczematous skin lesions can be observed which in early childhood can be mixed with atopic eczema, but which clear under the correct diet with avoidance of phenylalanine.

2.5.2 Ichthyosis Vulgaris

The autosomal dominant and most common form of ichthyosis is closely associated to atopic dermatitis (Rabinowitz and Esterly 1994; Rajka 1989). The basic defect is a homozygous deficiency of the epidermal protein filaggrin which, when in heterozygous manifestation, gives rise to an increased risk of atopic eczema (see Sects. 3.1 and 3.2). In ichthyosis vulgaris, the second important aspect of pathophysiology in atopic dermatitis, namely, the immunodeviation toward Th2 and IgE, is missing. Ichthyosis patients only suffer from extremely dry skin.

2.5.3 Netherton Syndrome

The triad:

- Congenital ichthyosis in linear configuration (ichthyosis linearis circumflexa)
- Atopic diathesis with increased IgE and hypereosinophilia
- Hair growth disturbance (trichorrhexis invaginata or "bamboo hair") comprises the Netherton syndrome (Caputo et al. 1984)

Pathophysiologically the underlying defect is a deficiency of the gene for SPINK5 on chromosome 5q32 which encodes for the serine protease inhibitor LEKTI (lymphoepithelial Kazal type-related inhibitor) and plays a role in skin barrier function (Cork 1997).

2.5.4 Dubowitz Syndrome

Another autosomal recessive dermatosis going along with eczematous skin changes is the Dubowitz syndrome, which is character-

Table 2.4 Differential diagnosis of atopic eczema in adulthood

	Atopic dermatitis	Seborrheic dermatitis	Scabies	T-cell lymphoma	Allergic contact dermatitis
Onset	Early childhood	All ages	All ages	50–60 years	Adults
IgE	High	Normal	Normal	High	Normal
Eosinophilia	Common	Rare	Common	Rare	Rare
Morphology	Large flexures	Seborrheic areas	Wrists, interdigital and genital area	Persistent patches	Often localized
Itch	Strong	Mild	Strong	Mild	Strong
Dermographism	White	Normal	Normal	Normal	Normal
Concomitant respiratory allergy	Common	Rare	Rare	Rare	Rare
Food allergy	Common	Rare	Rare	Rare	Rare
Others			Other family members affected	T-cell receptor rearrangement	Positive patch test

Table 2.5 Hereditary dermatoses with association to atopic dermatitis

Ichthyosis vulgaris
Netherton syndrome
Dubowitz syndrome
Wiskott-Aldrich syndrome
Hyper IgE syndrome
Anhidrotic ectodermal dysphasia
Omenn syndrome
DiGeorge syndrome
Phenylketonuria

ized by dysmorphia of the face together with psychomotoric irritations (Dubowitz 1965, Möhrenschlager et al. 2007).

2.5.5 Wiskott-Aldrich Syndrome

The Wiskott-Aldrich syndrome develops through an X-chromosomal recessive defect on chromosome XpL 22 and occurs almost exclusively in boys. It goes along with eczema, thrombocytopenia, and purpura with normal megakaryocytes and increased susceptibility to infections. Eczematous skin changes with increased blue patches in male infants should make think of Wiskott-Aldrich syndrome.

Genetically a mutation of the WASP (Wiskott-Aldrich syndrome protein) has been found which plays a role in the actin formation of the cytoskeleton (Bradley et al. 2001). A decrease of IgM concentrations has been described in the Wiskott-Aldrich syndrome. Bone marrow transplantation is the life-saving therapy (Saurat 1985).

2.5.6 Hyper IgE Syndrome

An extreme elevation of serum IgE levels together with skin changes often occurring in the first years of life together with severe deep tissue infections (*Staphylococcus*, *Candida*) are typical for the hyper IgE syndrome (Buckley and Becker 1978; Ring and Landthaler 1989). In the pathology, mutations in the STAT3 gene are likely to be responsible.

A characteristic clinical sign is the delayed dentition with concomitant existence of both primary and secondary teeth.

For a long time, the differential diagnosis between severe atopic dermatitis with impetiginized and superinfected skin lesions from hyper IgE syndrome (HIES) (Job's syndrome) was difficult. Through molecular analysis and better characterization of phenotypes, it has become clear that a papulopustular eruption especially on the face and scalp in the first 8 weeks of life seems to be typical of a hyper IgE syndrome and can be distinguished from other neonatal skin lesions. Furthermore, clinical signs of nail infection and chronic candidiasis of the oral mucosa are more often seen in HIES, where the STAT3 mutation is autosomal dominant (Olaiwan et al. 2011, Boos et al. 2007, Schmincke et al. 2008).

Also anti-IgE has been found to be helpful in occasional cases with hyper IgE syndrome (Bard et al. 2008).

There is a subtype of hyper IgE syndrome characterized by mutations in the DOCK1 gene (ca. 5 % of hyper IgE syndrome patients which show more severe infections) (Boos et al. 2007).

Some other severe immunodeficiency syndromes (thymic hypoplasia DiGeorge) as well as severe combined immunodeficiency (SCID) can go along with eczematous skin changes.

2.5.7 Keratosis Follicularis (Pilaris)

There is an endless controversy whether keratosis follicularis should be regarded as a stigma or a minimal manifestation of atopic dermatitis which until now is not clear. According to our experiences it is sometimes associated with atopic eczema, but not significantly more prevalent in atopic individuals generally.

When the face is involved, so-called ulerythema ophryogenes can be a differential diagnosis to atopic eczema with involvement of the eyebrows and redness of the cheeks together with keratotic papules.

Classically keratosis follicularis involves the lateral side of the upper arms and responds well to mild keratolytic treatment.

2.5.8 Anhidrotic Congenital Ectodermal Dysplasia

This severe skin disease can also go along with an increased prevalence of atopic diseases (Vanslow et al. 1970).

2.5.9 Hair Diseases

Some forms of hair disease seem to be associated with an increased prevalence of atopic dermatitis such as the syndrome of incombable hair (cheveux incoiffables) (Braun-Falco et al. 1982; Dupré et al. 1981).

There is a controversial discussion whether there is an association of atopic eczema and alopecia areata (De Weert et al. 1984). Some authors regard the typical alopecia areata pathophysiologically as "eczema of the hair follicle."

In a study from Japan, 10–52 % of patients suffering from alopecia areata have been found to be atopic (Ring et al. Handbook 2006), and this association was particularly apparent in childhood.

2.5.10 Atopic Respiratory Diseases and Other Allergic Reactions

Per definition, atopic dermatitis is associated to a high degree with atopic respiratory diseases such as rhinoconjunctivitis and bronchial asthma, but also with other allergic, especially IgE-mediated reactions (Bergmann et al. 1994; Nowak et al. 1996; Schnyder 1960; Wise and Sulzberger 1933).

2.5.11 Bronchial Asthma and Rhinoconjunctivitis

The occurrence of atopic respiratory diseases in atopic dermatitis is common, especially in children and adolescents. Over 50 % of atopic eczema patients suffer from respiratory symptoms. The risk of allergic bronchial asthma for infants with atopic eczema is three to four times increased compared to the normal population; there is a clear-cut dependence on the severity of the skin disease (Beyer and Wahn 1999). Approximately 80 % of children with atopic eczema suffer from asthma or allergic rhinoconjunctivitis. Salop et al. found in 90 % of children an existing bronchial hyperreactivity which was unknown to patients and parents (Salob et al. 1993).

In the classic Venn diagram, the overlap of asthma, rhinoconjunctivitis, and eczema shows a focus of eczema in childhood, while rhinoconjunctivitis is more prominent in adults (Fig. 1.12, page 14) (Ring et al. 2006).

Children with atopic dermatitis without known asthma often show bronchial hyperreactivity (Corbo et al. 1989) or increased concentrations of exhalable nitric oxide (FeNO) (Eberlein et al. 2009a)

2.5.12 Protein Contact Dermatitis, Food Allergy, and Gastrointestinal Diseases

IgE-mediated reactions, such a contact urticaria or protein contact dermatitis, are more frequent in atopics. IgE-associated food allergies, especially food anaphylaxis, seem to be more common in atopic eczema patients than in normals (Brockow and Ring 2008; Eigenmann et al. 1998; Przybilla and Ring 1990; Steinke et al. 2007; Zuberbier et al. 2004).

Apart from gastrointestinal symptoms of IgE-mediated food allergy, other gastrointestinal problems like gluten-sensitive enteropathy, eosinophilic gastroenteritis, eosinophilic esophagitis, or other inflammatory bowel diseases can be increased in atopy (Bernard 1953; David 1983). Common genetic markers for M. Crohn, psoriasis, and atopic eczema have been found (Cookson and Moffatt 2002).

2.5.13 Anaphylaxis to Seminal Plasma

This rare, but life-threatening, condition affects females developing anaphylactic shock after coitus and almost exclusively occurs in atopic females, especially in patients with severe atopic dermatitis and concomitant food allergy. Only recently the eliciting allergen could be identified as prostate-specific antigen (PSA) (Weidinger et al. 2006).

2.5.14 Food Allergy and Food Anaphylaxis

In discussing the role of food hypersensitivity in atopic dermatitis, one has to consider different aspects (Jäger and Wüthrich 2001):

Food allergens can elicit exacerbations of existing eczema lesions and contribute to continuous maintenance of atopic dermatitis.

Food allergens—sometimes the same, but sometimes other or different allergens—can elicit life-threatening symptoms of anaphylaxis in eczema patients, independent of eczema or oral allergy syndrome with swelling of the lips and tongue; this preferably occurs with pollen-associated food allergens in patients also suffering from hay fever.

Finally non-IgE-associated food hypersensitivities may also occur in eczema patients and may contribute to eczema flares, especially after application of preservatives or sulfites or other food additives (Ring et al. 1989; Ring et al. 2006).

2.5.15 Drug-Induced or Insect Venom-Induced Anaphylaxis

IgE-mediated anaphylactic reaction against drugs or insect venoms can occur in patients with atopic eczema, but they do not seem to be more prevalent than in other populations (Galli 2004). Maybe the special hyperreactivity of the mucosal surfaces in the allergen contact is a prerequisite for increased occurrence in atopic individuals.

2.5.16 Ocular Diseases

Many different clinical and pathogenetic conditions can occur in the eye, sometimes difficult to diagnose. The major allergic diseases in the eye include:

- Seasonal or perennial allergic conjunctivitis
- Vernal keratoconjunctivitis which may be IgE, but also non-IgE associated
- Giant papillary conjunctivitis with no allergy history
- Superficial punctate keratitis
- Atopic keratoconjunctivitis (more prevalent in atopic dermatitis)
- Classical allergic contact dermatitis (involving the eyelid and the conjunctiva: blepharoconjunctivitis) (Ring 2005; Leonardi et al. 2012)

In a review of the literature, it was found that atopic dermatitis alone seems to be a risk factor to develop both anterior and posterior subcapsular cataracts, the latter often being associated with systemic glucocorticosteroid use. The authors speculate about a role of oxidative stress during an inflammatory reaction as a causal factor (Bair et al. 2011).

Not only allergic rhinoconjunctivitis is more often associated with atopic dermatitis, but also a variety of other ocular complications such as atopic keratoconjunctivitis, atopic cataract, and keratoconus (Friedländer 1988; Reinhard et al. 1999, Allansmith 1995).

The association of cataract and atopic eczema is well referred to in the textbooks, but may have been overestimated in earlier times (Beetham 1940) with studies showing prevalences between 0.4 and 33 % (!) (Ring et al. 2006). In our own experiences this occurs much rarer. In the slit lamp examination, one has to differentiate between anterior and posterior subcapsular cataracts; the latter ones usually are a sequel of long-term glucocorticosteroid use and thus can be more common in eczema patients.

It may be interesting to speculate whether common pathophysiologic mechanisms in the skin and the eye lens could play a role in the development of atopic cataract (Uehara et al. 1995).

Severe eye changes usually can be seen in patients with otherwise very severe clinical course of atopic eczema (Fig. 2.37).

In adult patients with lid eczema, of course, contact allergy to ophthalmic preparations in eye drops has to be considered.

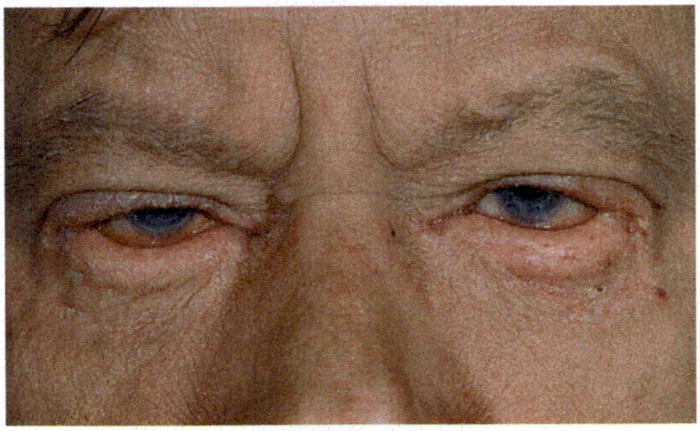

Fig. 2.37 Marked ocular changes in severe atopic dermatitis in an adult with keratoconjunctivitis and blepharitis

2.5.17 Nephrotic Syndrome

In some patients with atopic diseases, a steroid-sensitive nephrotic syndrome can occur with proteinuria, edema, and clear-cut deterioration after allergen contact (pollen, house dust mite, or food allergens).

2.5.18 Vitiligo

There is an opinion in the literature that, in patients with severe atopic eczema, concomitant vitiligo has a poorer prognosis (Ortonne et al. 1976). Whether there is a clear association between vitiligo and atopic dermatitis is not established.

2.5.19 Photosensitivity

While UV treatment and heliotherapy is benefitting many patients, ca. 10 % report about deterioration or exacerbation of skin symptoms after UV exposure.

The most common—in common parlance called sun allergy—photohypersensitivity reaction is polymorphous light dermatosis (polymorphous light eruption) (PLE) which occurs characteristically in spring after the first heavy sun exposure and ameliorates during summer. This condition seems to be more prevalent among atopics compared to the general population (Przybilla et al. 1991). The eliciting agent in this type of photohypersensitivity is unknown. The skin lesions clearly can be differentiated from eczematous skin lesions and are polymorphous in nature with regard to the manifestation in a group of various patients, but monomorphous in the individual patient with either urticarial or papular eruptions with rather little itch. This is a major differential diagnostic criterion in distinguishing PLE from sun-induced atopic eczema.

2.5.20 Ear Disease

Relapsing inflammations of the middle ear (otitis media) are more common in patients with atopic diseases, especially in patients with respiratory atopy. There has been abundant literature with regard to swelling of the eustachian tubes and also increased staphylococcal colonization and inflammation of the external auditory canal.

Rarely an association of deafness with atopic eczema has been described.

2.5.21 Neurologic Diseases

Some authors report about increased prevalence of lesions of vertebral nerves using magnetic resonance techniques in patients with atopic eczema (Toropova, personal communication 1998).

2.6 Complications of Atopic Eczema

The most common complications of atopic dermatitis regard infectious skin diseases which can give rise to very severe, partly life-threatening conditions.

2.6.1 Bacterial Infections

The skin of patients with atopic dermatitis is heavily colonized with *Staphylococcus aureus* (over 90 %) in unlesional skin, in the nose, and under the nails. Regarding the itch-scratch processes, this can lead to transfer and impetiginization of eczematous skin changes (Biedermann 2006; David and Cambridge 1986; Lacour and Hauser 1993; Leung 2002, 2003) (Fig. 2.38).

Impetiginized atopic eczema lesions are not only infected with staphylococci, but also with streptococci and other microbes (Adachi et al. 1998; Aly 1980; Aly et al. 1977; Bode et al. 1982; Zollner et al. 2000).

In a population-based cross-sectional study in over 1000 children between 0 and 6 years in Japan, it was found that the lifetime prevalence of impetigo contagiosa was significantly higher in atopic dermatitis than in control children, and mollusca contagiosa was more pronounced in boys, while there was no difference in the prevalence of herpes simplex infection (Hayashida et al. 2010).

2.6.2 Fungal Infections

Patients with atopic eczema show an increased susceptibility to fungal infections, especially *Trichophyton rubrum* and *Candida albicans*. Some authors have found immediate-type reactions against *Trichophyton rubrum* antigens (Jones et al. 1973a, b), and the pathophysiological relevance is unclear.

Malassezia furfur as saprophyte and inducer of pityriasis versicolor also is common in patients with atopic dermatitis and can be found especially when the scalp and neck areas are involved ("head and neck dermatitis") (Hjorth and Clemmenson 1983; Waersted and Hjorth 1985). IgE-mediated reactions against *Malassezia* have been detected as well as positive atopy patch test reactions with this fungus (Schmid-Grendelmeier et al. 2002; Novak et al. 2003).

2.6.3 Viral Infections

2.6.3.1 Herpes Simplex: Eczema Herpeticum

One of the most severe complications of atopic eczema is the so-called eczema herpeticum (Kaposi's varicelliform eruption), which presents as a disseminated form of infection with herpes simplex virus HSV type 1 or 2 on the basis of atopic dermatitis. It goes along with high fever and possible development of central nervous inflammation (Kaposi 1891). Often the diagnosis is made too late since doctors think of a mere exacerbation of atopic dermatitis. The infection occurs frequently by skin contact with affected persons (kissing, mother and child, etc.) (Wollenberg et al. 2003a, b).

The diagnosis is made by detection of HSV antigen in the lesion together with the clinical manifestation and the acute occurrence of vesiculopustular, commonly eroded point-like skin changes (Fig. 2.38).

The prognosis has been improved by the introduction of intravenous antiviral therapy with acyclovir or, for acyclovir-resistant infections, foscarnet or ganciclovir.

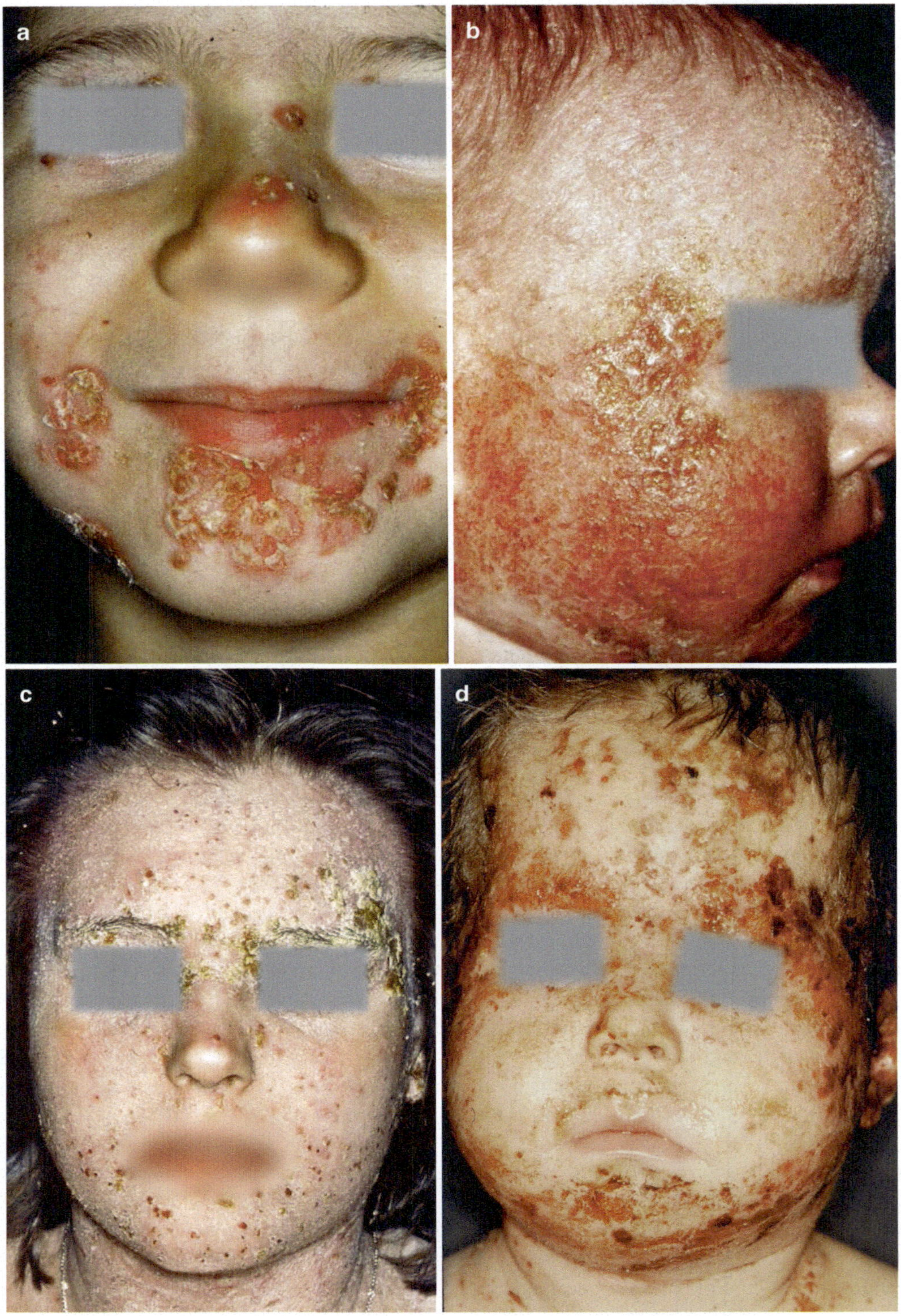

Fig. 2.38 Bacterial superinfection in atopic dermatitis. (**a**) Impetiginized eczema in the face. (**b**) Impetiginized infantile eczema. (**c**) Impetiginized atopic dermatitis with crusts and oozing. (**d**) Massive superinfected atopic dermatitis (*S. Aureus*)

2.6.3.2 Eczema Vaccinatum

When smallpox infection (Variola vera) still was a threat to mankind and vaccination programs were common, this was a major complication of vaccination. Eczema vaccinatum occurred in patients with atopic dermatitis and corresponded clinically to eczema herpeticum with severe general disease, fever, lymph node swelling, and malaise (Fig. 2.39).

Because of this complication, patients with atopic dermatitis could not be vaccinated against smallpox. In those days, these individuals were not allowed to travel to the USA. By the development of a prevaccination with a modified smallpox vaccine (modified virus Ankara) (MVA), it was possible to reduce these complications (Stickl et al. 1974) (see above).

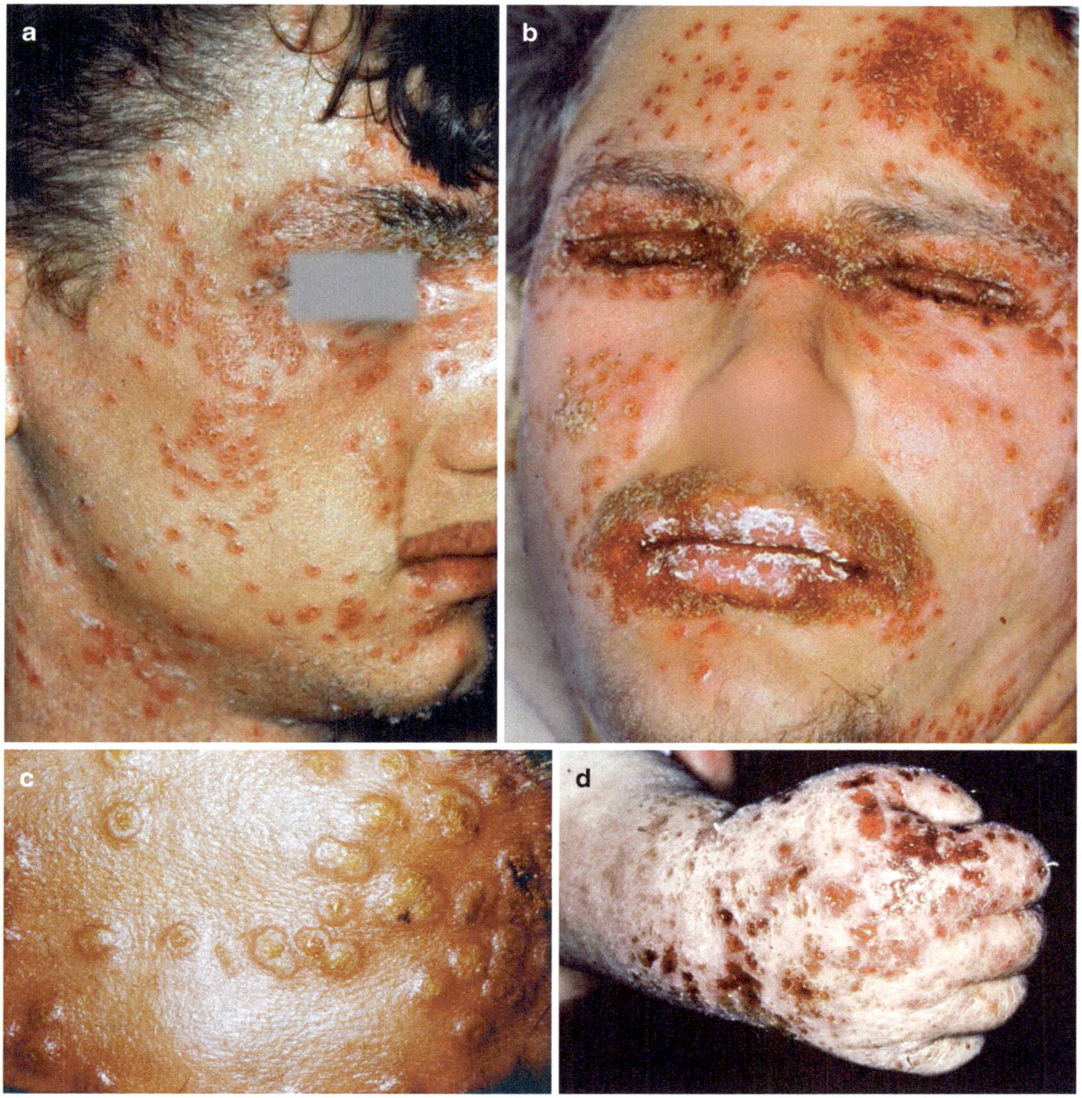

Fig. 2.39 Eczema herpeticum, a severe complication of atopic dermatitis. (**a**) Vesicular pustular skin changes. (**b**) Disseminated erosive punctate skin changes. (**c**) In the magnifying perspective the vesicular pustular character resembles varicella. (**d**) Eczema herpeticum of the hand with large erosions

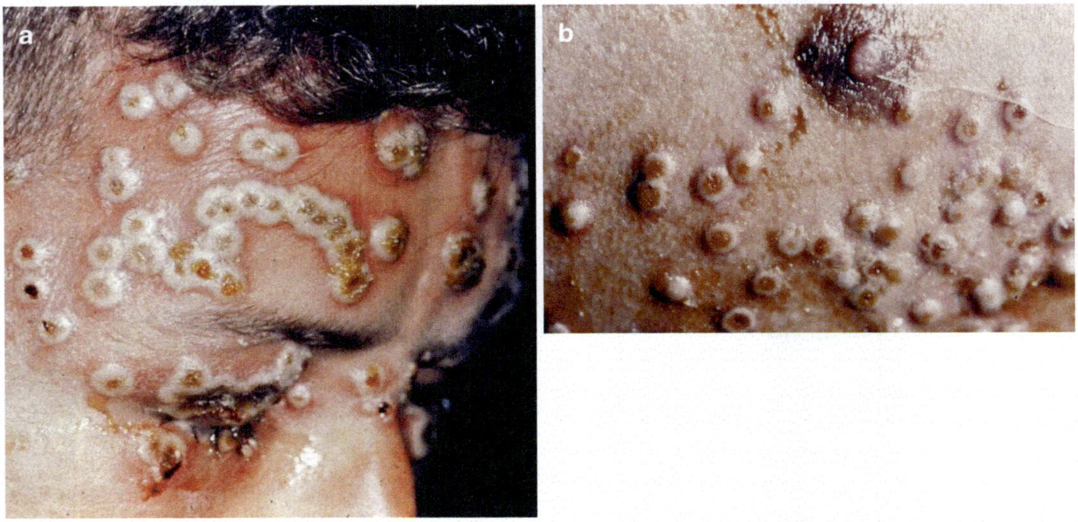

Fig. 2.40 Eczema vaccinatum. (**a**) Severe complication of smallpox vaccination in a person with atopic dermatitis. (**b**) Detail

2.6.3.3 Molluscum Contagiosum

This typical infection with the epidermotropic DNA virus of the pox group is very common in childhood and occurs in especially intense manifestation in patients with atopic dermatitis; H. Wolf spoke of "eczema molluscatum" (Wolf, personal communication 1985) (Fig. 2.40).

Also severe clinical manifestations of orf (ecthyma contagiosum) have been described in atopic eczema (Dupré et al. 1981).

2.6.3.4 Warts

Infections with human papillomavirus (HPV) seem to be more common in atopics and show a more intense severity, especially with regard to common warts (verruca vulgaris). In some patients with severe manifestations in the hand and around the nails, the term "eczema verrucatum" could be used (Fig. 2.41).

2.6.3.5 HIV Infection

The association of HIV infection and IgE-mediated diseases is controversially discussed; in the initial phase of HIV infection, atopic diseases and immunoglobulin E do not seem to play a role; however, in manifested AIDS, severe exacerbations of atopic eczema together with superinfection can be observed.

2.6.3.6 Other Viral Diseases

An increased prevalence of extracutaneous viral infections has been discussed with regard to the pathophysiological immunodeficiency of Th1 reactions. Compared to the normal population, viral infections of the upper respiratory tract seem to be increased in prevalence in atopic dermatitis (Verbow and Hart 1986).

Infections with Epstein-Barr Virus (EBV) also seem to be more frequent in atopics (both respiratory atopy and atopic eczema).

Activation of a subclinically existing cytomegalovirus infection (CMV) in patients with severe eczema has been observed.

2.7 Diseases Rarely Associated with Atopic Eczema

While literature is abundant regarding atopy-associated diseases and complications, only few epidemiological trials study the occurrence of certain diseases which, according to general experience, are less prominent in atopic individuals compared to the normal population. On the basis of the pathophysiological concept of Th1 and Th2, this should be apparent (Olesen 2006) for the following diseases:

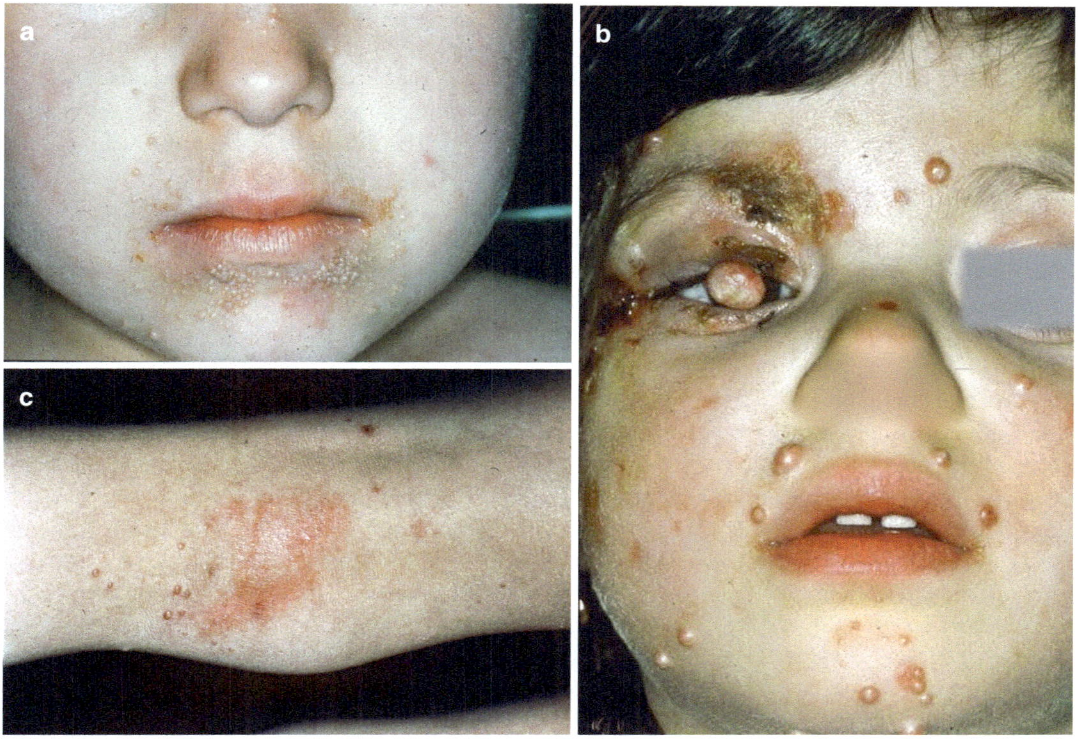

Fig. 2.41 Mollusca contagiosa. (**a**) Intensive appearance of Mollusca contagiosa in the perioral region with cheilitis sicca. (**b**) Massive Mollusca contagiosa in a child with atopic dermatitis. (**c**) Mollusca contagiosa next to flexural eczema

2.7.1 Diabetes Mellitus

Juvenile diabetes mellitus (type 1) occurs by an autoimmune Th1 reaction against the beta cells in the pancreas. It therefore was of interest whether diabetes type 1 is more common in atopics.

A study from the Netherlands found a lower prevalence of atopic diseases in 7- to 12-year-old children with insulin-dependent diabetes mellitus (IDDM) (Meerwaldt et al. 2002). Another study reported an increased prevalence of atopic diseases, especially asthma, in IDDM with controversial results regarding atopic eczema (EURODIAB).

A Danish study in 3- to 15-year-old children with IDDM found a significantly lower incidence of atopic eczema in diabetes patients in comparison to the normal population (OR 0.49, CI 0.39–0.63). When diabetes mellitus was manifest, there were no significant differences in the prevalence of atopic eczema in diabetics compared to normal persons (Olesen et al. 2001).

The increased prevalence of type 2 diabetes in middle-aged adults was also investigated: Again lower prevalence rates of atopy were found in diabetes patients.

2.7.2 Rheumatoid Arthritis

A similar situation seems to be found in rheumatoid arthritis with data showing an inverse association between atopic diseases and rheumatoid arthritis (Verhoef et al. 1998; Olesen 2006).

There was a significantly lower incidence of atopy among rheumatoid arthritis patients compared to healthy controls (OR 0.39, CI 0.19–0.81) (Hilliquin et al. 2000). On the other hand there was a significantly lower incidence of eczema among rheumatoid arthritis (2.9 % compared to healthy controls 4.9 %).

2.7.3 Melanocytic Nevi

Many doctors have seen; however, few have realized the specific phenomenon that patients with atopic eczema often show fewer melanocytic nevi than normal persons. The inspection and registration of the eczematous skin lesions is in the focus. Sometimes nevi are registered as side finding, and sometimes they give rise to further investigations because of atypia. There are few scientific investigations with regard to the incidence and prevalence of melanocytic nevi in atopy or atopic dermatitis.

In a Swedish study, Broberg et al. found in a group of patients with severe atopic eczema significantly decreased numbers of melanocytic nevi compared to non-atopic controls. They found a significant negative association between the level of serum IgE and the number of melanocytic nevi in atopic eczema (Broberg and Augustsson 2000).

In a larger Danish study, 2030 adult patients with atopic eczema were examined and compared with the General Cancer Registry in Denmark. Thereby no single case of malignant melanoma was found in the group of patients with atopic eczema, although cases should have been expected theoretically (Olesen 2006).

There are other studies showing similar findings.

However, it seems too early to generally speculate whether atopic individuals or atopic dermatitis patients have a really decreased risk to develop malignant melanoma.

2.7.4 Inflammatory Bowel Disease

Roberts et al. found a two times higher prevalence of atopy and atopic eczema in patients with ulcerative colitis (Roberts et al. 1979). Also Pugh et al. found a higher prevalence of eczema in ulcerative colitis and Crohn's disease (Pugh et al. 1979).

There was no association between atopic eczema and ulcerative colitis or M. Crohn in two studies (Mee et al. 1979; Troncone et al. 1988).

In Japan, in a large study in 47,862 adult atopic eczema patients between 18 and 62 years, Niwa found no association to Crohn's disease (OR 1.0, CE 0.45–2.2), but a clear association to ulcerative colitis with an OR of 6.5 (CI 5.1–7.3) (Mitsuyama et al. 2014).

In the survey of KiGGS (children and adolescent health survey), there was a significantly increased risk for ADHS in patients with atopic eczema (OR 1.54, CI 1.24–1.93), while there was no association to allergic rhinitis or asthma in a multivariate analysis adjusted for age, sex, SES, maternal smoking, perinatal health problems, breastfeeding, number of siblings, and family history of atopy (Romanos et al. 2012; Schmitt et al. 2009). However, in a stratified analysis taking into account sleep loss, it was found that the high association was mainly due to sleep problems, since atopic eczema without sleep disturbance was no longer showing significant associations.

So there seems to be an association between atopic eczema and ADHS, whereby atopic eczema seems to temporarily precede the occurrence of ADHS. Most likely sleep problems in early childhood due to the intense itch in atopic eczema may be causal for the later development of ADHS in these patients (Romanos et al. 2012; Schmitt et al. 2009c).

2.7.5 Cancer in General

There is abundant literature with regard to incidence of cancer and allergy; however, the literature is controversial.

Some studies have found decreased prevalences of neurologic or brain tumors (glioblastoma) (Harding et al. 2008).

In a recent large review investigating 23 publications from 1985 to 2004, Wang et al. found that atopic eczema may be associated with a decreased risk of pancreatic cancer, brain tumor, and childhood leukemia (the latter not significant) with no consistent findings with regard to skin cancer or non-Hodgkin lymphoma (Wang et al. 2008).

In 575 children with brain tumors from the UK childhood cancer study, atopic children (asthma and/or atopic eczema) showed a reduced risk for CNS tumors, while there was no significant inverse correlation for atopic eczema alone (Harding et al. 2008).

On the contrary, in a study involving 2030 adult patients with atopic eczema, comparing to the Danish Cancer Registry from 1977 to 1996, an increased risk of cancer was observed over all (OR 1.5, CI 1.2–1.9), whereby half the excess cases of cancer were nonmelanoma skin cancer diagnosed within the first 9 years of the follow-up. Others conclude that this increased rate may be due to calcinogenic potential of therapies used for severe atopic dermatitis (Olesen 2006).

In a study in 550 children 8–9 years old, those with active eczema had fewer melanocytic nevi than children without atopic disease with a median of 4 (mean 7.4) versus a median of 9 (mean 11.2) in controls (Synnerstad et al. 2008).

When the same authors studied the incidence of malignant melanoma in 6280 patients with atopic dermatitis and a mean follow-up of 36.7 years, they found 6 cases with malignant melanoma representing an OR of 0.49 (CI 0.27–1.35) which was not significant (Synnestad et al. 2008).

2.7.6 Psoriasis

The association of atopic eczema and psoriasis has been discussed and is controversial, although with regard to the Th2 hypothesis lower prevalences of atopy in psoriasis and vice versa should be expected and represent a general experience. In selected cases with concomitant simultaneous occurrence of clear-cut psoriasis and atopic eczema, interesting immunological findings could be observed with interleukin-4-producing T-cell clones only to be isolated from eczema or atopy patch test lesions and interferon gamma-, interleukin 17-, or TNF-secreting T-cell clones from psoriasis lesions (Eyerich et al. 2011) (see Chap. 3).

There are opinions that cardiovascular disease and metabolic syndrome may be occurring rarer in atopy patients; however, clear analytical studies are missing (Schäfer et al., personal communication).

2.7.7 Contact Allergy

For a long time it was postulated that contact allergy is rarer in atopic dermatitis (Marghescu 1985), and also under the light of the Th1/Th2 paradigm, this seemed to be logical. However, intense studies examining the prevalence of contact allergy in atopic dermatitis find similar rates; in our own study, we found a prevalence of positive patch tests in 41 % of atopic eczema patients compared to 40 % in the whole group of other diagnoses tested (Enders et al. 1988) (see Chap. 4).

2.7.8 Summary

While some diseases are associated significantly more often with atopic eczema as especially respiratory atopic diseases, asthma, allergic rhinoconjunctivitis, and food anaphylaxis, there are other diseases which probably occur less often in eczema patients like type I diabetes mellitus, rheumatoid arthritis, and psoriasis, but also melanocytic nevi. This area needs further research. The concomitant occurrence of psoriasis and atopic eczema seems to be possible but is rare and gives rise to interesting studies regarding mechanisms and therapeutic effects of new strategies.

For a long time, the prevalence of contact allergy was regarded to be decreased in atopic dermatitis; however, allergic contact dermatitis also occurs in atopic eczema and also in childhood. Therefore a patch test belongs to the diagnostic standard in atopic dermatitis also in childhood.

Complications of atopic eczema comprise especially infectious skin diseases, both viral (eczema herpeticum) and bacterial (*Staphylococcus aureus*, streptococci) in origin.

2.8 Atopic Eczema: Diagnostic Criteria and Severity Scoring

Many factors contribute via various mechanisms to the development and chronification of this disease, which is partly reflected in the colorful terminology. The diffuse and variable morphology with the lack of a true primary lesion and variable clinical course over lifetime makes diagnosis sometimes difficult.

2.8.1 Diagnostic Criteria

2.8.1.1 Diagnostic Criteria According to Hanifin and Rajka

Therefore it can be regarded as a breakthrough that two dermatologists, Jon Hanifin from Portland, Oregon, and Georg Rajka from Oslo, developed an internationally accepted list of diagnostic criteria based on clinical and anamnestic findings (Hanifin and Rajka 1980) (Table 2.6). In most scientific studies, these criteria are the gold standard for diagnosis of atopic dermatitis. The diagnosis of atopic dermatitis can be made when a minimum of three major and additional three minor criteria are fulfilled.

In an analysis by Diepgen et al. 1991 in 110 patients with atopic eczema and healthy controls, the following five criteria were the most common:

- Itch when sweating
- Wool incompatibility
- Dry skin
- White dermographism
- Hertoghe phenomenon

The multitude of criteria is sometimes difficult to define in signs and symptoms. The mixture of the actual clinical findings and data from history and laboratory make the application of Hanifin and Rajka's criteria in the daily practice difficult.

Table 2.6 Diagnostic criteria for atopic dermatitis according to Hanifin and Rajka (1980)

A minimum of three major criteria	+3 or more "minor" criteria
Itch	Dry skin
Typical morphology and distribution: Big flexures and linearity in adults Facial and extensor sites in infants and children Chronically relapsing dermatitis	Ichthyosis (palmar-/hyperlinearity, keratosis pilaris) Skin test reactivity of the immediate type (type I) Increased serum IgE Onset in early life Tendency to skin infections (especially *S. aureus* and herpes simplex/decreased cell-mediated immunity) Itch when sweating Incompatibility of wool and solvents
Personal or family history of atopy (asthma, allergic rhinitis, atopic dermatitis)	Perifollicular accentuation Food hypersensitivity Influenced by environment or emotional factors White dermographism/delayed blanch

2.8.1.2 Criteria of the UK Working Party

With regard to epidemiological trials, an English working group around H. Williams came up with the UK Working Party's diagnostic criteria in 1994 which were based on clinical examination and validation of dermatological criteria, whereby sensitivity and specificity were around 90 % (Williams et al. 1994a, b, 1996; Möhrenschlager et al. 1998; Williams 2005) (Table 2.7).

According to this definition, the diagnosis "atopic dermatitis" can be made when there is an itchy skin rash together with three or more criteria from Table 2.7.

2.8.1.3 Criteria According to Ring

In 1982, Ring published a list of diagnostic criteria for atopic eczema (Ring 1982a) (Table 2.8) which in the daily practice allow the diagnosis in a simpler way, namely, when four of the six criteria are fulfilled.

2.8.1.4 Other Criteria

These diagnostic criteria have been studied in a recent systematic review (Brenninkmeijer et al. 2008).

Table 2.7 Diagnostic criteria for atopic dermatitis according to the UK Working Party (Williams et al. 1994a, b)

The diagnosis of atopic dermatitis can be made when there is an itchy skin rash together with three or more of the following criteria:
History of flexural involvement (elbow, anterior foot, neck, in childhood also cheeks)
History of asthma or hay fever in patients with one atopic disease in a near relative first grade (mother, father, brother, sister) in children under 4 years
History of general skin dryness in the last year
Actually existing flexural eczema (or eczema of cheeks, forehead, or extensor sides of extremities in children under 4 years)
Onset during the first years of life (not relevant for children under 4 years)

Table 2.8 Diagnostic criteria for atopic eczema according to Ring (1982a, b)

The diagnosis of atopic dermatitis can be made when at least four of the following six criteria are fulfilled:
Age-specific morphology
Itch
Age-specific distribution of skin lesions
Stigmata of atopic eczema (typus neurodermitis or atopic diathesis)
Personal or family history of atopy
Detection of IgE-mediated sensitization (in vitro or in skin test)

It has to be mentioned that apart from these three mentioned criteria, several other authors with excellent clinical and scientific merits have come up with good criteria (Bos et al. 1998; Wüthrich 1999a).

2.8.2 Evaluation of Severity of Eczema

When the diagnostic criteria had been established, the problem of variable severity of the disease in different patients became apparent. It is obvious that there are mild and very severe courses which are not exactly defined beforehand. Several attempts were made to quantify the severity (Charman and Williams 2000; Emerson et al. 2000; Queille-Roussel et al. 1985; Ring 1982a). Therefore a task force of the European Society for Pediatric Dermatology (European Task Force on Atopic Dermatitis ETFAD) developed a scoring system for atopic dermatitis (SCORAD) at the beginning of the 1990s (Stalder for European Task Force on Atopic Dermatitis 1993; Kunz et al. 1997).

2.8.3 Objective and Subjective Signs and Symptoms (SCORAD)

The SCORAD consists of an objective score which quantifies both the extent of the body surface involved and the intensity of the relatively different skin lesions together with a subjective evaluation of the intensity of suffering. The latter is measured as intensity of itch and sleep loss in a visual analog scale. The various qualitatively different skin lesions registered in the SCORAD are:

- Erythema
- Edema/papules
- Oozing/crusting
- Excoriation
- Lichenification
- Skin dryness

These different skin lesions are semiquantitatively evaluated from 0 (absent) to 3 (maximal). The subjective complaints are registered on a visual analog scale (VAS) from 0 to 10 by the patient (or the parents, respectively). In order to measure the SCORAD, there are standard figures and forms (Figs. 2.42 and 2.43). Special training sessions are offered.

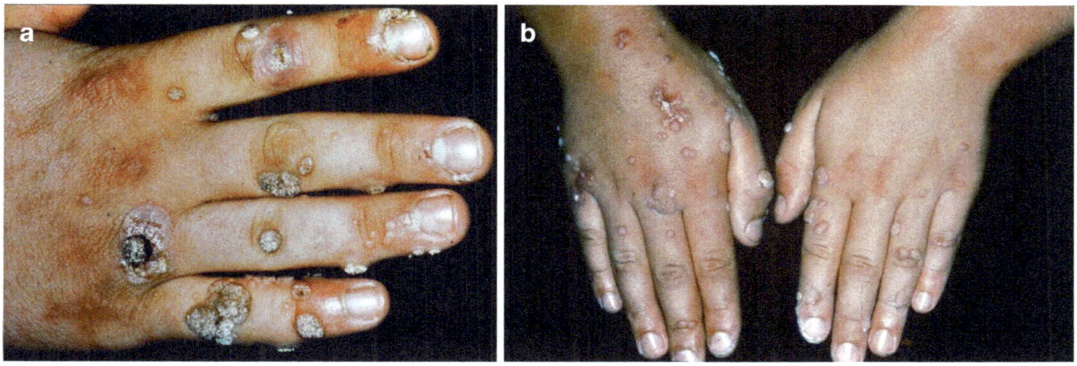

Fig. 2.42 Eczema verrucatum. (**a**) Intensive warts on the hands, especially periungual, in atopic dermatitis. (**b**) Massive appearance of warts on both hands

SCORAD European task force for atopic dermatitis (EFTAD)

Patient: Name/First name | Birth Date | Date of Investigation

Topical steroid used

Active Substance (brand name, concentration) | (g) Amount/Month | Number of flares per month

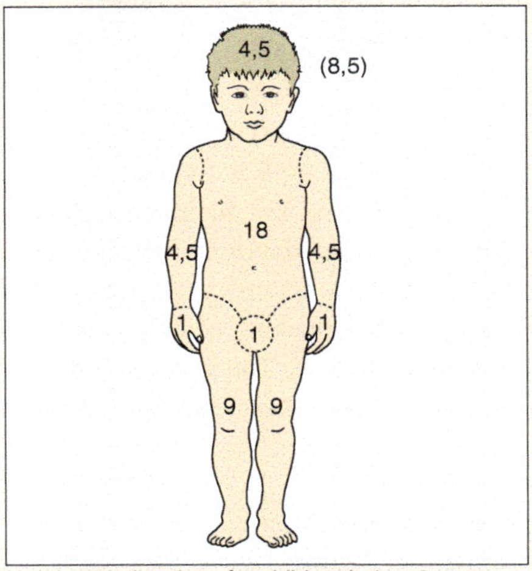

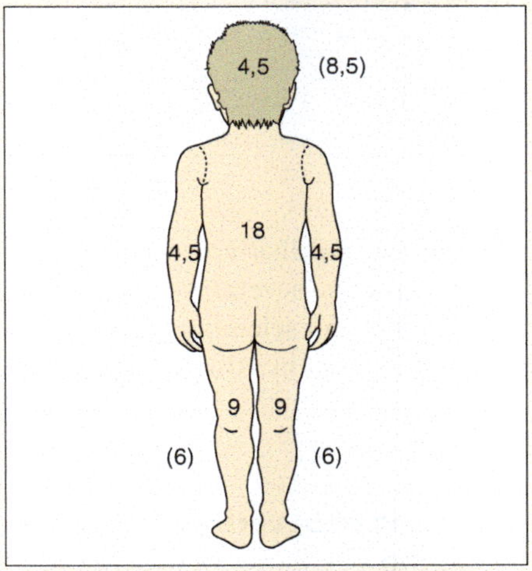

Numbers in brackets for children below 2 years

A: Extent
Please add the sum of affected skin areas

B: Intensity
Values for intensity
(on maximal affected skin location)

0 = non 1 = mild 2 = moderate 3 = severe

Criteria	Intensity	Criteria	Intensity
Erythema		Excoriation	
Edema/Papules		Lichenification	
Oozing/Crusting		Dryness (evaluated at non-lesional skins)	

C: Subjective symptoms

Itch and loss of sleep | SCORAD A/5 + 7B/2 + C

Visual analogue scale (average the last 3 days or nights)

Pruritus (0–10) 0 1 2 3 4 5 6 7 8 9 10

Loss of sleep (0–10) 0 1 2 3 4 5 6 7 8 9 10

Treatment | Remarks

Fig. 2.43 Scoring system for atopic dermatitis (SCORAD) with objective and subjective scales

Recently in a clinical trial, the validation of a patient-oriented (PO) SCORAD has been shown valuable so that patients themselves or parents can measure the severity of atopic eczema over time (Stalder et al. 2013; Vourch-Jourdain et al. 2009).

2.8.4 Evaluation of the Clinical Course

Using the SCORAD it is possible to follow the actual severity of the disease objectively and reproducibly over long time periods. Especially for clinical trials with regard to the effect of therapeutic strategies, the SCORAD has been proven valuable.

It should be mentioned that various groups (partly authors of the original ETFAD group) started to develop more simple versions of SCORAD for faster analyses. However, for the experienced the examination of the SCORAD means 10 min of time. In specialized hospitals the SCORAD belongs to the routine diagnostic procedure in every eczema patient.

The SCORAD offers the advantage that it can also be used for single parts; thus, it is possible to measure the clinical course of certain symptoms independent of the total score over time. So the effect of therapeutic treatment can be studied with regard to effect upon different morphologic skin lesions.

The SCORAD was developed by the ETFAD and studied in several hundred patients in 11 European countries over several years before it was finally established and refined. In these studies the statistical analysis came to a maximum of 103 points for the most severe patient. Many have not understood why one could not more simply come to 100 points as a maximum. This is due to the fact that the SCORAD was not developed only arbitrarily, but really studied in hundreds of patients and measured and evaluated in a statistical analysis.

2.8.5 Eczema Area and Severity Index (EASI)

In some countries the Eczema Area and Severity Index (EASI) is more popular than SCORAD. The EASI was developed in analogy to the Psoriasis Area and Severity Index (PASI); however, it is not measuring the major symptom of atopic dermatitis which is the itch sensation. Currently there is a debate going on as to which outcome measure should be used in clinical trials, the SCORAD or the EASI (Williams, personal communication).

2.8.6 Summary

The diagnosis of atopic dermatitis can be made on the basis of various diagnostic criteria. The most commonly used ones are those of Hanifin and Rajka (1980). For daily practice in epidemiological trials, the UK Working Party's criteria (Williams et al. 1994a) and those of Ring (1982a, b) have proven valuable.

In a task force of the European Society for Pediatric Dermatology (European Task Force on Atopic Dermatitis ETFAD), a scoring system to measure the severity of atopic dermatitis (SCORAD) has been developed which not only registers the extent of skin lesions over the body surface, but also the intensity of six different morphologically apparent skin lesions together with the subjective impairment due to itch or sleep loss. The SCORAD can also be used with regard to single parameters for scientific studies or therapeutic trials.

3 Pathophysiology of Atopic Dermatitis/Eczema

3.1 Genetics

3.1.1 Classical Genetics of Atopic Dermatitis

Since the introduction of the term "atopy" by Coca and Cooke in 1923 and the inclusion of the correspondent skin disease atopic dermatitis or atopic eczema by Wise and Sulzberger in 1933, the familiar occurrence of these diseases is common knowledge in textbooks (Schnyder 1960). Classical genetics examine the occurrence of diseases or symptoms of certain phenotypes within family trees. Twin studies allow the clear-cut estimation of genetic factors versus environmental influences when monozygous and dizygous twin populations are compared (Schultz-Larsen 1985) (Fig. 3.1). Since Gregor Mendel, various hereditary models can be determined.

When the determination of the phenotype is not exactly precise, difficulties may arise, e.g., history with the definition of family with regard to positive family history or with regard to the degree of relationship, the attribution of paternal versus maternal hereditary factors ("mater semper, pater numquam constat"), the overexaggeration of ascendant (retrospective) versus descendant (looking into the future) family history, as well as unprecise definitions of atopy versus atopic disease (Moffatt and Cookson 1998; Uehara and Kimura 1993).

The first detailed investigations with regard to family history and genetic risks of atopic diseases were done by Urs Schnyder in Zurich, where he found that the risk of a child to develop atopic eczema is around 15 % when both parents are healthy while it is 25–30 % when one parent is atopic and 66 % when both parents are atopic (Schnyder and Klunker 1957; Schnyder 1960). Twin studies showed a concordance rate of 80 % in monozygous twins compared to 25–30 % in heterozygous ones (Blumenthal and Jaffe 1933; Schultz Larsen and Holm 1985; Wüthrich 1975).

Unfortunately there are only few similar studies with regard to the phenotype "atopic dermatitis" alone. Family studies with long-term observation from Linköping (Kjellmann 1977) have shown that the atopy risk for children of atopic parents is then highest when both parents suffer from the same atopic manifestation (e.g., both parents suffer from atopic eczema) (Table 3.1). Apart from the "tendency to IgE formation," also the organ manifestation is somehow inherited.

Atopic eczema as a complex disease does not follow the simple Mendel heredity, but shows a polygenic inheritance under multifactorial influence and partly genomic imprinting (maternal influences stronger than paternal ones). This maternal dominance can be explained by epigenetic effects. There are critical opinions with regard to the methods and data analysis of family history. When parents are asked for early childhood diseases (e.g., cradle cap or infantile eczema) in their own personal life, it may be that

J. Ring, *Atopic Dermatitis: Eczema*, DOI 10.1007/978-3-319-22243-1_3

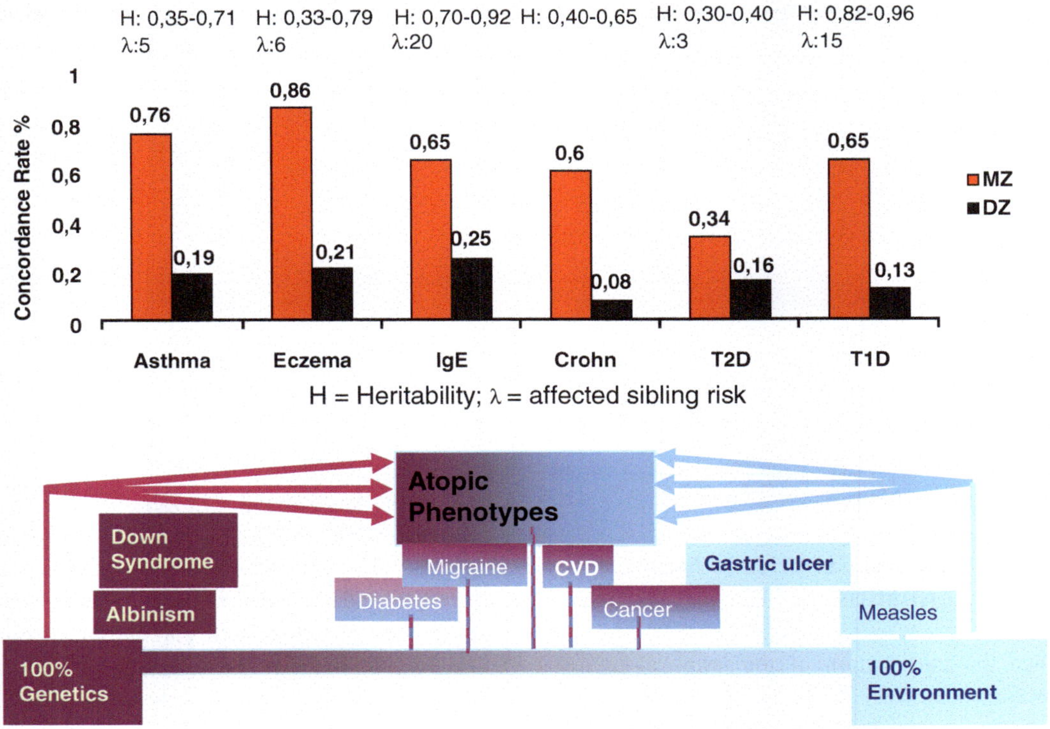

Fig. 3.1 Atopic eczema as genetically determined disease. *MZ* monozygous, *DZ* dizygous

Table 3.1 Atopy prevalence in children and parental atopy (Kjellmann 1977) (percent in the 12th year of life)

Parents	Atopy prevalence (%)
No atopy	10–15
One parent is atopic	20–30
Two parents are atopic (different manifestation)	30–40
Two parents are atopic (same manifestation)	60–80

Table 3.2 Incidence of atopic eczema in children from families with atopic eczema in one or both parents (Uehara and Kimura 1993)

Partners of patients with atopic eczema	*N* (families)	*N* (children)	Children with atopic eczema
Parents of partners non-atopic	164	321	180 (56 %)
Atopic eczema	26	59	48 (81 %)
Respiratory atopy	80	149	88 (59 %)
Total	270	529	316 (60 %)

women have a better memory since they may be more somatically oriented than boys already in youth and spend more time to external appearance while boys and men probably remember sports or traffic accidents better. Therefore studies using descendant family history are interesting as they have been performed by Uehara in Japan who compared parents with atopic eczema and asked them about the diseases of their children (Uehara and Kimura 1993). In 270 parents with a total of 529 children, the rate of atopic eczema was 60 % with absolute equality regarding gender (59 % boys, 60 % girls). In subclassification of adults with regard to the atopic diathesis in the spouse, the highest eczema rates were found in children from parents in whom both father and mother were suffering from atopic eczema (Table 3.2). There was no difference in eczema prevalence between parents in whom one partner was non-atopic or suffered from respiratory atopy. In another study, Uehara compared the paternal and maternal effects and found that for 285 adults with atopic eczema who were married to a non-atopic partner and had at least one child, there was no difference in the prevalence of atopic eczema in their children between families in which the father was suffering from eczema compared to families in which the mother was affected. Totally 57 % of children suffered from atopic eczema (Uehara et al. 1999).

Another problem of classical genetics can be seen in the decreasing number of children in many countries of the world; it is obvious that the frequency of a positive family history is higher in larger families than in one-child families.

In so-called "pure" eczema patients who are not affected by respiratory atopy neither in the personal nor in the family history, lower IgE levels and a higher percentage of "intrinsic" eczema can be found. It might be interesting to study specially this patient group with regard to molecular genetics. Schultz-Larsen found in a Danish twin study similarly high concordance rates for intrinsic atopic dermatitis as for IgE-associated cases (77 % monozygous versus 15 % dizygous) (Schultz Larsen and Holm 1985).

3.1.1.1 Summary

Atopic diseases are strongly genetically influenced. This is evident from twin studies where monozygous twins show a concordance of 80 % of atopic eczema while dizygous twins only show ca. 20 %. The risk to develop atopic eczema is 40 % for children with one atopic parent. When both parents are affected by the same manifestation of atopy (e.g., father and mother with atopic eczema), the risk is between 70 and 80 %. Similar high concordance rates can be found for extrinsic (IgE-associated) and intrinsic (non-IgE-associated) atopic dermatitis.

3.1.2 Molecular Genetics

Since it became clear that atopic dermatitis as a complex disease cannot show monogenous hereditary traits following Mendel's laws, there was the hope to define an atopy gene (Cookson and Moffatt 2002; Cookson et al. 1992; Marsh et al. 1981). In the meantime we know that a multitude of gene loci on various chromosomes are involved in the manifestation of the many phenotypes of atopic diseases. The modern methods of molecular genetics use naturally occurring DNA sequences which are distributed as polymorphous markers (microsatellites) over the whole genome and allow the determination of gene loci. In various studies, coupling analyses were performed when genetic markers and defined clinical signs and symptoms cosegregate within families (e.g. affected peer), while association studies use larger populations of affected persons and compare them with non-affected individuals with regard to allele distribution patterns of polymorphous gene markers. Principally there are two strategies for investigations:

- Candidate gene analyses
- Genome-wide association studies (GWAS)

In candidate gene analyses, genes are selected on the basis of their known function in encoding pathophysiologically relevant products for the disease investigated. It is thought that changes in the function of certain substances determine the susceptibility of an organism to the occurrence of a certain disease.

The best suitable model here is the Family Trio study using the transmission disequilibrium test (TDT). Here the transfer of a sign from heterozygous parents to an affected child is investigated; a disease-relevant allele should be more common in the affected child than a non-relevant gene.

3.1.2.1 Genome-Wide Association Studies

Using the microsatellite markers, the whole genome of many affected individuals can be screened and compared to non-affected controls. Associations are determined with certain disease-specific phenotypes. With this approach, totally new until now unknown genes with unknown functions can be detected which then can be further investigated.

Table 3.3 shows a review over the known gene loci with association to markers of atopy or atopic eczema. The progress in this area is so rapid that almost monthly new results are published (Kabesch et al. 2003, 2006; Moffatt et al. 1994, 2007; Vercelli 2008; Bussmann et al. 2011).

Table 3.3 Atopy and atopic eczema: associated *Candida* genes

Region	Candidate gene	Associated phenotypes
1q31-32	?	Psoriasis
1q21	EDC: filaggrin	Ichthyosis vulgaris, atopic eczema, asthma?
3p24	Chemokine RANTES	–
3q21	COL 29A1	Atopic eczema
4q35.1	IRF-2	–
5q31	SPINK5	Netherton syndrome
Common loci with IBD	IL-4 cluster	Asthma, rhinitis, SPT, total IgE
Common loci with IBD	IL-13	Asthma, BHR, SPT, total IgE
Common loci with IBD	CD14	Asthma, rhinitis, SPT, total IgE, specific IgE
11q13	FCER1B, FCER1A	Atopy, asthma, total and specific IgE, atopic eczema
13q12-14?	–	–
14q11.2	Mast cell chymase	–
16p11.2-12.1	IL-4-receptor A	Asthma, BHR, rhinitis, total IgE
17qcen-q11	NOD 2a	Asthma, SPT
17q11-q12	RANTES	Asthma, eosinophils
–	MCP1	Asthma, eosinophils
17q21	Eotaxin	Asthma, BHR
19b13.3	TX2	Total IgE
19q13.1	TGFB1	Asthma, SPT, total and specific IgE

EDC epidermal differentiation complex, *BHR* bronchial hyperreactivity, *SPT* positive skin prick test, *IBD* inflammatory bowel disease

The critical parameter for successful molecular genetic analysis is the exact characterization of the phenotype investigated; here the experienced clinician and exact observation and determination of morphology are crucial.

In the following, some gene loci will be shortly discussed. In the GWAS it became apparent that overlaps of relevant gene loci between atopic eczema and asthma but also between atopic eczema and psoriasis have been observed (Lee et al. 2000) and also to Morbus Crohn. This lets us speculate that there are common risk factors for inflammatory diseases of barrier organs like skin and gut. The most exciting results can be seen in the discovery of polymorphisms and deficiency mutations of the filaggrin gene as causal factor for ichthyosis vulgaris by the group of McLean and Irvine which also showed highly significant associations with atopic eczema (Palmer et al. 2006; Smith et al. 2006; Weidinger et al. 2007, 2008a) (see Sect. 3.2).

Another important factor in the evaluation of genetic effects is interactions between environmental influences and genetic factors: So certain genetic alterations only become clinically relevant after exposure to certain environmental factors such as allergens or pollutants (tobacco smoke) acting together.

3.1.3 Genes of Skin Barrier Function

Among the many genes associated with markers of atopy or atopic dermatitis, specially interesting associations were found with genes on chromosome 1 in the area of the so-called epidermal differentiation complex (EDC) (Fig. 3.2).

3.1.4 Filaggrin

Apart from many proteins of the so-called S100 group, filaggrin is crucial in the development of a normal skin barrier. This protein is formed from profilaggrin within the keratohyalin granules by proteolysis and plays a role in the aggregation of keratin filaments in the upper epidermis, keeping lipids and proteins together in between the dead keratinocytes of the stratum corneum (Fig. 3.3).

When a filaggrin loss of function mutation had been shown to be causal for the autosomal dominant variant of ichthyosis vulgaris, the most common genetic keratinization disorder, it was logical to study this mutation also in patients with atopic eczema. Indeed, and numerous studies have shown this, it was found that also over ethnic groups, Caucasians and Asians, highly significant associations have been found between filaggrin loss of function mutation and atopic dermatitis with high significance rates (Baurecht et al. 2007; Rodriguez et al. 2009).

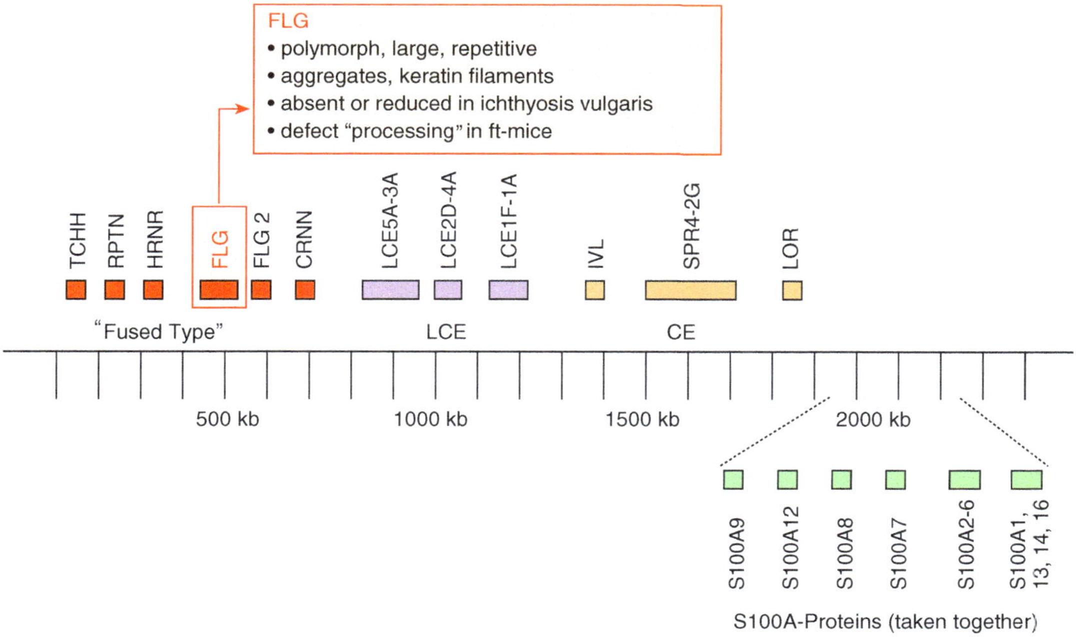

Fig. 3.2 Epidermal differentiation complex (EDC) on chromosome 1, part 1p.21, with various gene loci relevant for epidermal barrier function (Modified after Weidinger (2009))

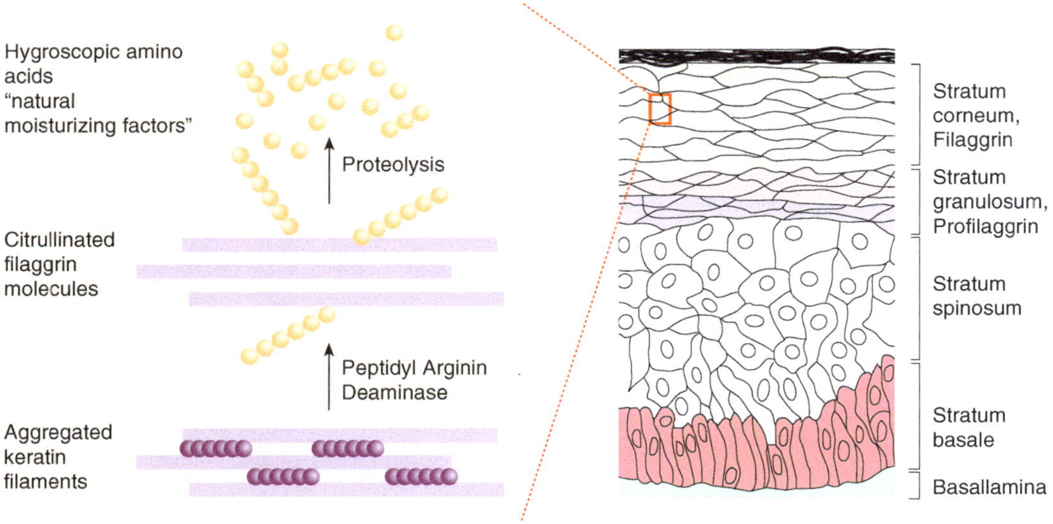

Fig. 3.3 Filaggrin processing (From Rodriguez et al. (2009))

In Caucasians, two most common filaggrin variations (R501X, 2282de14) as well as 18 less common variants have been described in European patients and controls. In addition, there are many mutations most commonly seen in Asian patients, but all these variations lead to loss of function mutations in the filaggrin molecule with consecutive disturbance of skin barrier function.

While filaggrin mutations have been found in almost all ethnic populations studied worldwide, there was a lack of information with regard to Africa (George 1989). Recently a study was performed in Ethiopia in 103 patients with clear-cut AD and seven patients with ichthyosis vulgaris compared to controls. No carriers of filaggrin mutations of the four most common FLG mutations were found; only in one patient with eczema, a new heterozygous mutation was detected. The authors concluded that filaggrin loss of function variants are less common in the Ethiopian population and maybe other factors are more important in this group of patients (Winge et al. 2011).

In a meta-analysis of 24 studies in a total of 6448 patients with atopic eczema and 26,787 controls in 1993 as well as 17 studies with 3138 cases of asthma, there was a high evidence for the role of filaggrin in the development of atopic eczema (Baurecht et al. 2007).

It is of interest that filaggrin mutations also are associated with the marker "increased IgE" as well as with "eczema plus asthma." There is no association for asthma alone.

The prevalence of filaggrin mutations in Europe in heterozygous carriers is 15 %; homozygous carriers of the filaggrin mutations develop ichthyosis vulgaris; heterozygous carriers have a three- to fourfold increased risk for atopic eczema.

It remains to be stated that there are patients with atopic eczema without filaggrin loss of function mutation; therefore, filaggrin cannot be regarded as a definite and single causal factor. Furthermore, there are many (around 7 %) filaggrin mutation carriers without any skin problems.

While at the beginning of the filaggrin mutation discovery one had hoped to find a positive marker for the diagnosis of intrinsic (non-IgE-associated) atopic eczema, this was not the case; especially the extrinsic variant is associated with filaggrin mutations (Weidinger et al. 2008a). Exposure to cat allergen in early life increases the risk of atopic eczema in children, especially in a subgroup carrying the filaggrin mutation (Bisgaard et al. 2008). Therefore, it has been speculated that the filaggrin mutation leading to a disturbed skin barrier facilitates the penetrance of exogenous noxious substances or allergens, then inducing IgE responses.

Filaggrin concentrations are decreased in patients with atopic eczema. There are clear-cut relations between the severity of eczema and filaggrin mutations (Nemoto-Hasebe et al. 2009) which are controversially discussed (Hubiche et al. 2007).

Filaggrin is further degraded in the epidermis into amino acids and thus represents a large part of so-called natural moisturizing factors contributing to skin barrier and smoothness.

Right next to the filaggrin locus within the EDC, the S100 calcium-binding protein S100A7 (= psoriasin) is encoded which is highly significantly associated with psoriasis (Gläser et al. 2009a).

Filaggrin seems to be expressed particularly in the epidermis. With regard to mucosal surfaces, it can be found in the oral mucosa, but neither in the airway nor in the esophagus (De Benedetto et al. 2008).

Filaggrin mutations not only confer the most significant risk for atopic eczema, but also associations with allergic rhinitis and asthma have been found in several studies. However, in large-scale studies it has been found that asthma per se and allergic rhinitis per se are not connected with FLG mutations, yet such loss of function mutations increase the risk to develop asthma plus eczema (Weidinger et al. 2008a, b).

In animal experiments with knockout mice for filaggrin, these showed very dry and scaly skin, but normal stratum corneum hydration and transepidermal water loss. Antigen penetration was found to be increased, so it might be that the increased TEWL only occurs secondary to skin inflammation (Kabashima et al. 2013). Similarly, in the spontaneous mouse mutant model of the flaky tail mice (ft), it could be shown that topical penetration of allergens is significantly increased, resulting in cutaneous inflammation (Vallon et al. 2009).

The loss of function of filaggrin not only leads to dry skin and increased sensitization, but also seems to be involved in the development of photosensitivity. This was studied in a three-dimensional skin model in vitro by the group of

Tschachler using small interfering RNA (siRNA) to specifically suppress filaggrin formation at different levels.

Indeed, there were keratohyalin granules reduced in number and size and disturbed lamellar body formation. However, the absence of filaggrin did not affect the susceptibility to urea extraction; however, a reduced concentration of urocanic acid in the epidermis was observed, rendering the skin more susceptible to UVB-induced apoptosis (Mildner et al. 2010).

In a large epidemiological trial, it was interesting to find significantly elevated vitamin D concentrations in serum to be associated with filaggrin mutation status, possibly due to increased UV effects (Thyssen et al. 2010).

With regard to food allergy, filaggrin loss of function mutation did not predict clinical food allergies; however, it was associated with an increased risk of food sensitization in the first year of life, making it likely that food sensitization may occur through impaired skin barrier function (Tan et al. 2012).

Filaggrin loss of function mutations are associated not only with an increased risk of eczema, but also of fissured skin on the hands, as has been shown in a large cross-sectional population study in Denmark (Thyssen et al. 2012) as well as the severity of occupational irritant contact dermatitis of the hands. These authors found that in the presence of atopy, filaggrin mutations may be a marker for more severe manifestation of the clinical course of irritant dermatitis.

Also allergic contact sensitization to nickel has been found to be associated with filaggrin mutations (Novak 2009; Thyssen et al. 2010). However, compared to other causal factors, the filaggrin mutation was a weaker contributing factor than the well-known effect of early ear piercing. Also chronic hand eczema was studied in a German cohort and found to be significantly associated with heterozygosity for filaggrin mutations (Molin et al. 2009).

The connection between ichthyosis vulgaris, filaggrin and allergic sensitization was studied in a group of 26 patients with ichthyosis vulgaris, where a high presence of CD1a-positive cells in the epidermis was found in a subgroup of IV plus atopic sensitization or atopic eczema and found to be significantly increased compared to ichthyosis vulgaris patients without atopy (Oji et al. 2010).

Filaggrin mutations are the strongest genetic determinants of atopic dermatitis and may help to define risk profiles of children as an early prognostic marker. Unsurprisingly, there was no association with filaggrin mutations when patients with ophthalmic complications such as keratoconus were investigated which was even below the expected frequency (Droitcourt et al. 2011).

Equally, filaggrin loss of function mutations have been found not to be protective against acne vulgaris as might have been speculated with regard to the dichotomy of dry versus greasy skin.

3.1.5 Protease Inhibitors

On the basis of the protease inhibitor defect in Netherton syndrome (SPINK5), which encodes an important serine protease inhibitor LEKTI, corresponding investigations have been performed in atopic dermatitis (Hubiche et al. 2007). There were decreased levels of kallikrein (KLK)-dependent peptidases. In a transgenic mouse model with overexpression of KLK7 with chymotryptase activity, skin changes similar to atopic dermatitis developed (Cork et al. 2009). In a candidate gene analysis, however, no significant association of KLK7 mutations to atopic eczema was found in humans (Weidinger et al. 2008a, b).

On the other hand, associations of polymorphisms of mast cell chymase have been shown with infantile atopic eczema (Mao et al. 1996).

Epidermal serine proteases act via signal transduction of protease-activated receptor (PAR)2 G-protein-coupled receptor which plays a role in innate immunity, but also in mediation of itch sensation (Steinhoff et al. 2003). Activation of PAR2 leads to inhibition of "lamellar" bodies and stratum corneum formation. The change in potassium gradients with concomitant activation of PAR2 receptors leads to a rapid transformation of the external keratinocytes in the stratum granulosum to terminally differentiated corneocytes (Hachem et al. 2003).

The thickness of epidermis, the thickness of stratum corneum, and the size of the corneocytes also influence barrier function. Hölzle and Plewig found smaller corneocytes in atopic dermatitis compared to healthy controls (1977). The smallest corneocytes were found in the retroauricular area and on the forehead, sites commonly affected by atopic eczema.

Other studies found an association of SPINK5 gene mutations to atopic eczema (Cork et al. 2009; Weidinger et al. 2008a, b).

In addition to the SPINK5 locus, a mutation in cysteine protease inhibitor cystatin A (CSTA and chromosome 3q21) was described which shows association to atopic dermatitis (Lee et al. 2000).

3.1.6 Genes of Innate Immunity

The innate immune system is the oldest active defense system in the evolution and protects the organism against a variety of exogenous intruders with a rather rapid reaction which somehow is able to recognize and differentiate pathogenic structures on microbes or other "danger" signals (Matzinger 1994; Janeway and Medzhitov 2002). Apart from the physicochemical barrier at the surface, various cellular and secretory elements are involved which are activated after stimulation of so-called pathogen-related receptors (PRR) (Akira 2006); all of them may be altered in a sense of being "defective" or "less efficient" in atopic dermatitis such as the response of the following PRRs:

- Toll-like receptors (TLRs)
- Nucleotide-binding oligomerization domain (NOD)
- Leucine-rich repeat-containing proteins (NLR) as well the endotoxin receptor CD14
- Some soluble PRRs (De Benedetto et al. 2009)

Thus major cells of the innate immune response like polymorphonuclear leukocytes, natural killer cells, and dendritic cells, especially pDC, have been found to show reduced functions (De Benedetto et al. 2009). Also the production of antimicrobial peptides (AMPs) from keratinocytes is reduced as well as the secretion of CCL20/MIP-3-α or CXCL8/interleukin-8.

Functioning innate immune responses are the basis of the establishment of a specific adaptive immune response. When the innate immunity is weaker, dysregulation of T-cell reaction patterns may occur. Toll-like receptor activation after epicutaneous allergen sensitization plays an important protective role in allergy development (Haapakoski et al. 2013). Impaired innate immune reactions can give rise to Th2-dominated reaction patterns (Mrabet-Dahbi and Maurer 2010).

These findings may lead to a new understanding of the mechanisms of the so-called "hygiene" hypothesis with regard to allergy and eczema development (Frei et al. 2012; Kemeny and Szabo 2013).

An association of polymorphisms of TLR2 gene with severe atopic eczema and common bacterial infections has been found (Ahmad-Nejad et al. 2004). There was no association between TLR4 and TLR6 (Weidinger et al. 2008a, b); however, there was significant association to a polymorphism in TLR9 (Novak et al. 2007) similar to the NOD1 gene, a molecule of signal transduction in innate immunity against bacteria (Weidinger et al. 2005).

3.1.6.1 Antimicrobial Peptides

An important part of innate immunity in the skin is antimicrobial peptides in the epidermis, such as defensin or cathelicidin. A study from Korea found significant polymorphisms for Defensin Beta1 (DFB1) in atopic eczema (rs5743399 and C haplotype) which are especially common in the extrinsic variant of atopic eczema (Kim et al. 2009).

3.1.7 Genes of Adaptive Immunity

In the beginning of the era of molecular genetics, associations between atopic disease and genes on chromosome 5 were already discovered, where the so-called cytokine cluster is located between 5q31 and 5q33 and encoding for a variety of candidate genes such as interleukin-4, interleukin-13, interleukin-9, and interleukin-5, but also for CD14 (receptor for endotoxin) (Marsh et al. 1994; Rosenwasser et al. 1995). Many gene associations in this cluster were found for atopy in general, IgE, but also respiratory atopic diseases; for atopic dermatitis, they have to be specially considered and only associations for certain subtypes were found (Novak 2009).

Similar findings have been observed for the STAT6 signal transduction marker (signal transport and activation in T cells) (Weidinger et al. 2004a).

The genes encoding for the chemokine RANTES or the transcription factor GATA equally were found to be associated with atopic eczema (Lee et al. 2000).

Another interesting association between polymorphisms of the high-affinity IgE receptor FcεR1 (Cookson and Moffatt 2002; Weidinger et al. 2008b) has been found. Obviously mutations in the alpha chain of the high-affinity IgE receptor have a special importance with regard to IgE production (Weidinger et al. 2008b, 2010).

3.1.8 Gene Loci with Yet Unknown Function

In one of the first GWAS, Lee et al. observed a highly significant association between atopic eczema and a region on chromosome 3q21 where the proteins CD80 and CD86 as costimulation molecules in T-cell activation are encoded (Lee et al. 2000).

On chromosome 11, recently a gene variant was identified as significantly associated with a risk for atopic eczema. Here a protein named EMSY is encoded which is present in various tissues, however, especially in the skin and in immune cells. There was a highly significant association also to inflammatory bowel disease (Esparza-Gordillo et al. 2009).

A meta-analysis of meanwhile numerous GWAS with a total of approx. 40,000 individuals, among them close to 10,000 patients with atopic eczema and 30,000 controls, first studied the ten most significant associations and then in a second set tried to reproduce these in other cohorts. Apart from filaggrin, which was significant in all studies, three loci were found to be consistently and reproducibly associated with increased risk of eczema, namely, OVOL1, KIF1A, and ACTL9 (Paternoster et al. 2012).

In a genome-wide association study (GWAS) combining Caucasian and Asian patients in a total of over 20,000 patients, altogether 11 susceptibility loci for atopic dermatitis have been described, many of them without known function at present (Ellinghaus et al. 2013 *neu*). In a GWAS in China, also previously undescribed loci with high association to atopic dermatitis have been identified (Sun et al. 2011 *neu*).

It has become clear that the future of molecular genetic research will be in close conjunction with precise clinical phenotyping and functional analysis of gene environment interactions. Now we know that in the manifestation of symptoms, a multitude of genes is involved.

Animal models with knockout mice or transgenic mice with overexpressed genes may help to elucidate the pathophysiological processes (e.g., flaky tale mouse with a combined defect in filaggrin and hornerin and eczema-like symptoms).

Figure 3.4 shows results of linkage studies with associations of gene loci on various chromosomes (Cookson et al. 2001).

3.1.9 Summary

With the new methods of molecular genetics, it was possible to identify certain loci on various chromosomes associated with specific phenotypic markers of atopic eczema. Some of these genes already have been positionally cloned. Genes of the epidermal differentiation complex (EDC) on chromosome 1 seem to have special importance (such as filaggrin and possibly hornerin) which are highly significantly associated with increased risk for atopic eczema. Homozygous carriers of filaggrin mutations develop ichthyosis vulgaris; heterozygotes have a three- to fourfold increased risk for atopic eczema. Also genes of epidermal proteases or protease inhibitors seem to play a role, like SPINK5 in the Netherton syndrome, a monogenic disease. Also genes of innate and adaptive immunity are involved in the

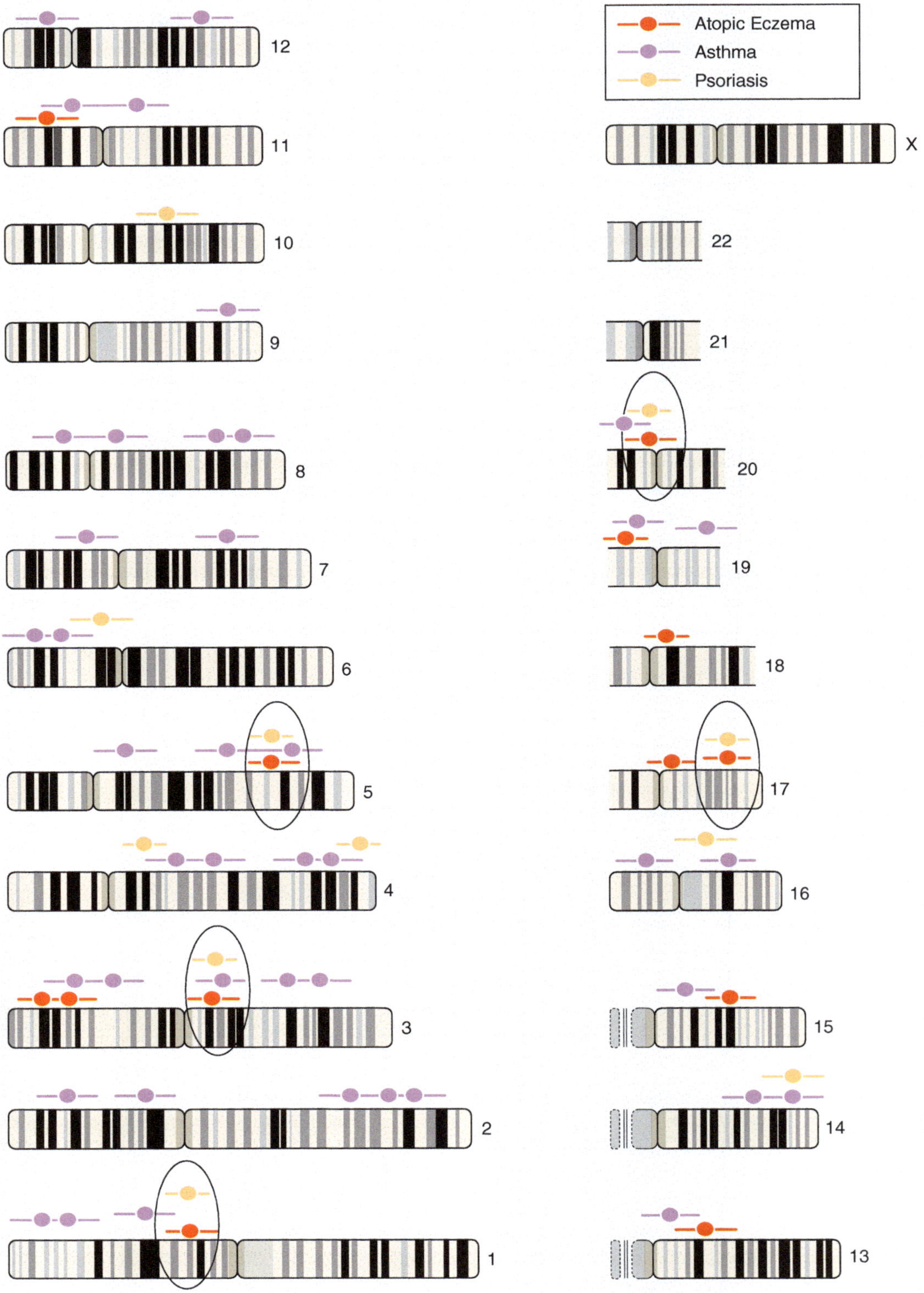

Fig. 3.4 Results of linkage studies showing associations of gene loci on various chromosomes with atopic diseases (After Cookson and Moffatt (2002))

pathophysiology of atopic dermatitis. Genome-wide association studies (GWAS) help to discover new gene associations whose function is not yet clear, such as on chromosome 11q, but also mutations in the area of the alpha chain of the high-affinity IgE receptor. It is clear by now that there is not only one atopy gene, but that in the development of the phenotype of an atopic disease, a multitude of genes on several chromosomes have to act together with environmental influences.

3.2 Disturbance of Skin Functions: "Sensitive" Skin, "Dry" Skin, and Disturbed Barrier Function

3.2.1 Structure and Function of the Skin

In order to better understand the processes in the pathophysiology of atopic dermatitis, it is important to understand the structure and function of normal skin. The skin with a size of 1.5–2 m^2 is the largest organ of the body. Many are astonished that the skin is called an "organ"; they feel it is more of a "cover" for the other "true" organs.

3.2.2 The Skin in Evolution

When the species *Homo sapiens* is regarded with respect to particularly advantageous development of certain organs over the millions of years of evolution, normally the research focuses on the nervous system and the development of the brain. Few studies take the development of the human skin with regard to evolution into account. Therefore, a short reflection of this aspect will be given. The earliest correlate of a "skin" can be found in the Metazoa (e.g., Porifera [sponges]) which have not yet really separated their internal body from the external aqueous environment densely. A structure called pinacoderm represents a very thin one-cell layer which is often disrupted to allow water flow. The Coelenterata (e.g., hydra) already show real epithelium closing the internal part of the body with a one-layered ectodermis overlaying an endodermis.

Further specialization with the development of a mesoderm or entomesoderm between the two other layers can be found in helminths. Arthropods have an important feature, namely, an exoskeleton consisting of chitin and proteins as cuticula connected to the underlying epidermis via hemidesmosomes. This cuticula becomes even more pronounced in Echinodermata (e.g., sea urchin).

Fish also produce an exoskeleton with a multilayered epithelium and the development of scales in the upper dermis (placoid scales). The major change occurred in Amphibia when they as the first animals conquered the land and had to cope with a dry environment. Here cornification of the most upper layers of the epidermis occurs; the secretory glands migrate down to the dermis. Cornification is more pronounced in Reptilia with a dry epidermis which periodically is shaded off sometimes within minutes as in the gecko species.

In birds, the skin developed feathers important for the temperature equilibrium and for movement in the air. The avian epidermis only consists of two layers: the stratum germinativum and the stratum corneum. There are no sweat or sebaceous glands. Feathers develop from a protrusion of epidermis with a central dermal pulpa. Finally they consist completely of keratin, only showing connective tissue rests in the papilla.

Mammalians finally have a wide variability from reptile-like corneal scales via dense furs until the relatively thin and reduced skin of humans. *Homo sapiens*, among all members, has the most reduced type of skin with regard to thickness, scales, or adnexal tissues, except for innervation which is rather well represented with many sensory cells and free nerve endings over the whole skin surface.

This part has been taken from the excellent reviews of Jablonski (2004) and Schempp et al. (2009).

3.2.3 Functions

However, the skin is much more than a bag which keeps the human being together so that he does not break apart similar to a sausage—as primitively

Table 3.4 Functions of the skin

Frontier
Barrier (physical, chemical, biological)
Metabolic organ
Immune organ
Organ to express psychologic changes
Aesthetic function

suspected. The skin is a highly complex system with a multitude of functions (Table 3.4).

The skin protects us from wind, cold and sun, noxious substances, and parasites. It ensures that the temperature in the body is kept in a way that the necessary metabolic processes can take place.

Only via the skin we can get into direct contact with our environment. Sometimes this contact is painful. The skin is a sensory organ and is the organ where psychologic processes are expressed as is seen, e.g., in erythema e pudore (to become red for emotional reasons which can be embarrassing). Poets have named the skin "mirror of the soul." There are many proverbial sentences of everyday use involving the skin like "to save one's skin," "this gets under my skin," "to jump out of one's skin," etc.

The skin is also an immune organ; all cells and cytokines necessary for the establishment of an immune response are contained in the skin. Similarly to the gut (gut-associated lymphoid tissue (GALT)), one can speak of a skin-associated lymphoid tissue (SALT) (Bergstresser and Takashima 2001; Granstein and Askari 1986).

3.2.4 Structure

Anatomically one can classify the skin from outside to inside into epidermis, dermis or corium, and subcutis (Fig. 3.5).

The epidermis is not of the same thickness on all sites of the body. Dependent upon the localization, the thickness of the epidermis varies between 0.014 and 1.5 mm. The epidermis is formed from inside to outside in four layers:

- Stratum basale or stratum germinativum (basal layer)
- Stratum spinosum (spinal layer)

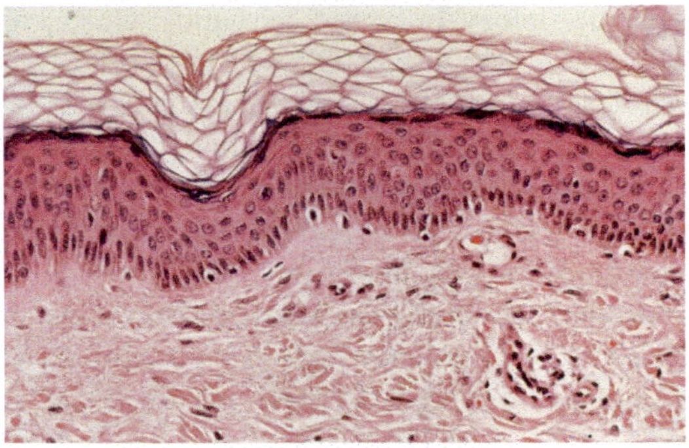

Fig. 3.5 Histological structure of normal skin with dermis and epidermis (hematoxylin-eosin staining) (With friendly permission from Volker Steinkraus)

- Stratum granulosum (granular layer)
- Stratum corneum (corneal layer)

Within the epidermis, fine dendritic cells can be found (Langerhans cells) which represent the most external sentinels of the immune system. They act as antigen-presenting cells together with dendritic cells in the dermis which take up foreign substances and present them after migrating to lymphocytes in lymph nodes.

The multitude of cells in the epidermis are formed in the basal layer as keratinocytes producing the most important protein of the epidermis, keratin, but also other proteins (see below). Also keratinocytes are immunologically active and able to produce important cytokines such as interleukin-1 and -6 as well as defensins and other antimicrobial peptides.

The corium, or dermis, consists of connective tissue with collagen and an extracellular matrix produced by fibroblasts. Here also lymphocytes, nerves, and blood vessels are embedded. In the corium reaching into the subcutis are the adnexal structures of sweat glands and sebaceous glands plus hair follicles.

The adipose tissue forms the mass of the subcutis above the fascia of the muscle.

3.2.5 Barrier Function and Stratum Corneum

The barrier function of the skin is important to form a frontier between the organism and the environment. Physiologically it protects the body from pathogenic noxes and is anatomically realized mostly in the stratum corneum. This barrier is not totally impermeable but has permeability to a degree to allow transport between the internal milieu of the organism and the outside. The corneal layer is not "dead skin" but is the end product of a highly differentiated epidermal process where skin cells transform into corneocytes from inside to outside with increasing numbers of keratin filaments which, together with lipids, form the stratum corneum according to the model of "bricks and mortar" (Elias and Menon 1991; Piérard 1989; Seyfarth et al. 2011).

The structural integrity of the stratum corneum is guaranteed by so-called modified desmosomes (corneodesmosomes) which bind corneocytes together and thus build a defense against tangential forces and mechanical trauma. In the model of Peter Elias, corneocytes can be compared to bricks, while the lipid lamellar layers can be compared to mortar. Corneal desmosomes could be regarded as iron rods (Cork 1997; Cork et al. 2005) which supply resistance against mechanical stress (Proksch et al. 2003).

3.2.6 Corneocytes

Corneocytes are flat cells in the terminal differentiation of epidermal keratinocytes which takes place in the stratum granulosum. Here the cells lose their nuclei as well as intracytoplasmic organelles and are connected densely with keratin fibrils. The human stratum corneum consists of approximately 20 layers of corneocytes, each 30 μm in diameter. The keratinocytes of the stratum granulosum release the contents of the keratohyalin granules which then together with keratin filaments form the lipid lamellar matrix of the mortar. The lipid layer consists of cholesterol, ceramides, fatty acids, and cholesterol esters which represent as a coherent lamellar layer in the stratum corneum (Fartasch et al. 1989). In the terminal differentiation of keratinocytes, the cell membrane changes into an insoluble protein matrix, called cornified envelope, to which the lipid layer binds. The cornified envelope consists mainly of structural proteins such as loricrin, involucrin, filaggrin, and smaller proline-rich proteins which are bound together by transglutaminases.

3.2.7 Filaggrin

Filaggrin, which is formed from profillagrin, plays a special role in the aggregation of keratin filaments in the cellular cytoskeleton. Finally filaggrin is further degraded to small peptides and free amino acids which form part of the well-known natural moisturizing factors (NMF) together with lactic acid, sodium pyrrolidone, urocanic acid, urea, and others. The natural moisturizing factors play the decisive role in the binding of moisture in the stratum corneum by binding water to corneocytes. Sodium pyrrolidone and lactic acid are specially hygroscopic and absorb water and thus prevent the formation of fissures between corneocytes (Cork 1997).

Probably the most important causal factor in explaining disturbed skin barrier function in atopic dermatitis may be seen in loss of function mutations in the structural protein filaggrin, which leads to also diminished hydration of the stratum corneum and adhesion of corneocytes. This allows an increased penetration of noxious substances, be it microbial, chemical, or allergenic in nature (Fig. 3.6) (see also Sect. 3.1.4).

Besides filaggrin, other proteins may be involved, such as desmoglein, desmoplakin, but also proteins of the "tight junctions" like claudin-1 and claudin-23 as part of the corneodesmosomes (Fujita et al. 2011).

Furthermore, disturbances of protease and protease inhibitor metabolism have been described in atopic eczema especially based on the gene defect in SPINK5 with diminished LEKTI known from Netherton syndrome.

3.2.8 Corneodesmosomes

The corneodesmosomes are part of corneocyte envelopes and consist mainly of proteins of the cadherin family, a group of extracellular transmembrane glycoproteins. Corneodesmosin is a 52kD protein specially expressed in cornifying epithelia, which, after its secretion in the extra-

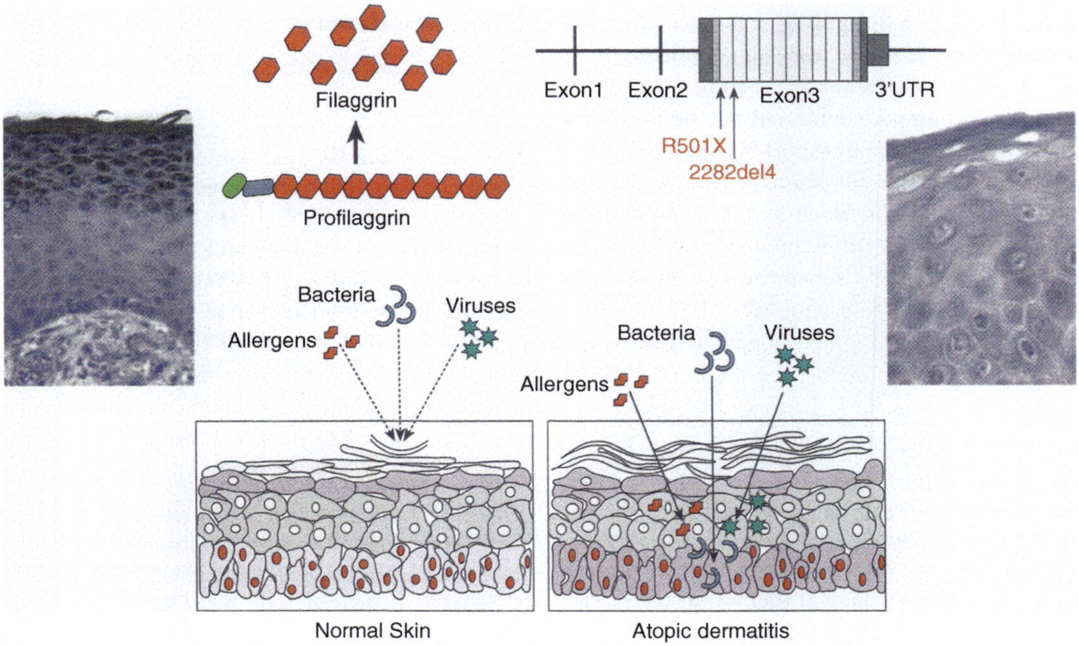

Fig. 3.6 "Loss of function" mutations in the filaggrin gene predispose to atopic dermatitis. With inefficient function of filaggrin, noxious substances make penetration more easily through the disturbed barrier of the epidermis (With friendly permission from S. Weidinger)

cellular space between stratum granulosum and stratum corneum, is integrated into the desmosomes in a way that corneodesmosomes develop.

A very rare disturbance of cornification and skin barrier function has been described as "peeling skin disease" which shares some features with Netherton syndrome, but without "bamboo hair" and SPINK5 mutation. In a family with this rare autosomal recessive ichthyosiform erythroderma, a defect in corneodesmosin has been found to be relevant and another very important factor for epidermal barrier integrity (Oji et al. 2010).

3.2.9 Desquamation

A natural decay of superficial corneocytes leads to a continuous process of desquamation in an equilibrium between keratinocyte proliferation in the stratum basale and desquamation on the surface. The process of desquamation depends upon a net of active proteases and protease inhibitors which degrade extracellular corneodesmosomal structures and thus allow the desquamation of superficial corneocytes. In this process, kallikrein-associated peptidases such as stratum corneum chymotryptic enzyme (SCCE) KLK7 as well as stratum corneum tryptic enzyme (SCTE) KLK5 are involved (Egelrud 1993). Apart from serine proteases, also cysteine proteases like cathepsin L2 (SC thiol protease) and aspartate protease cathepsin D with a pH optimum in the acid range are active. KLK-related serine proteases have their activity optimum in the mild alkaline pH.

All the activities of these proteases are regulated by a mixture of protease inhibitors such as serine leukoprotease inhibitors, but also cystatin protease inhibitors. Cystatin A is formed in sweat and forms a protective film against exogenic proteases from microbes or parasites (*S. aureus* or house dust mite) on the skin surface. The lymphoepithelial Kazal-type 5 protease inhibitor (LEKTI), which is encoded via the serine protease inhibitor Kazal-type 5 gene (SPINK5), is a special pH-dependent regulator of desquamation. LEKTI is formed in the stratum granulosum and secreted into the intracellular space between stratum granulosum and stratum corneum (lamellar bodies) where it is found colocalized with the above-mentioned kallikrein peptidases in the neutral pH. The more acid the pH to the outside, the weaker the inhibitory potential of LEKTI, thus allowing a normal desquamation in the most superficial layers.

3.2.10 Acid Mantle

Since the germinal work of Marchionini in the 1930s, the concept of the acid mantle of the skin explains a major part of skin barrier function (Marchionini and Hausknecht 1938). The mildly acidic skin surface pH develops together with stratum corneum in the neonatal period with acidification of the stratum corneum that goes along with normal functioning lipid-processing enzymes which are acidic pH-dependent such as the beta-glucocerebrosidase (Behne et al. 2003).

It is a well-known fact that seasonal changes in atmospheric conditions can affect the epidermis and trigger some skin diseases. In hairless mice, various environmental humidity conditions were studied with regard to skin surface hydration and amino acid generation which was drastically decreased in environmental dry air (Katagiri et al. 2008). While the formation of the acid mantle in earlier work was mainly regarded to be due to exogenous substances from colonizing bacteria on the skin surface or free fatty acids from sebaceous glands and eccrine glands, it is known today that also by-products of keratinization together with free fatty acids and phospholipids through phospholipase A2 additionally contribute to the acid mantle.

The acidic pH of the skin surface exerts strong antimicrobial effects (Leyden et al. 1975;) and improves the adhesion of nonpathogenic bacteria. Furthermore, it plays a role in influencing the above-mentioned proteases and protease inhibitors in the process of desquamation (Schmid-Wendtner and Korting 2007).

3.2.11 Alteration in Epidermal Lipids

Alteration in epidermal lipids has long been regarded as a crucial characteristic of skin barrier dysfunction in dry skin or skin of patients with atopic dermatitis. Apart from lipids from sebaceous glands which have been studied intensively (Gloor et al. 1991) and were also found to be decreased in some patients, it is the intraepidermal ceramides which constitute the majority of epidermal lipids and are important in providing the skin barrier in the stratum corneum (Imokawa 2009). They represent 50 % of stratum corneum lipids. Alterations in ceramide concentrations and patterns have been described (Imokawa et al. 1991).

In this context, possible defects of sphingolipid-metabolizing (SM) enzymes like SM deacylase can contribute to ceramide deficiency in eczema, preferably SM glucosylceramide deacylase, which is an enzyme that cleaves the N-acyl linkage of sphingomyelin and glucosylceramide (Imokawa 2009).

Other lipids include cholesterol; a factor of possible importance for lipid homeostasis could be apolipoprotein C1 (APOC1). In a mouse model transgenic for human APOC1, development of dermatitis, disturbed skin barrier function, and pruritus was observed (Nagelkerken et al. 2007; Proksch et al. 2006).

Long-chain fatty acids contribute to the skin barrier, and fatty acid-binding proteins seem to play a role. In specifically deficient mice, the basal transepidermal water loss was increased with overexpression of fatty acid-binding proteins, and there was a decreased transepidermal water loss and a better repair after acetone treatment (Owada et al. 2002).

3.2.12 Disturbance of Skin Barrier Function in Atopic Eczema

The complexity in the formation of a normal skin barrier function makes it understandable that disturbances at various levels may lead to clinical consequences. Therefore, it is not surprising that many authors studying skin barrier functions observed quite different findings in atopic eczema such as disturbance of the acid mantle with increased pH on the skin surface (Eberlein-König et al. 2000; Seidenari et al. 1996), but also disturbances of lipids and lipid-synthesizing enzymes (Hara et al. 2000; Imokawa et al. 1991; Jungersted et al. 2010; Mustakallio et al. 1967) as well as alterations in protease or protease inhibitors, and structural proteins.

The variations and distribution of several subgroups among ceramides were studied in healthy volunteers and correlated to skin barrier function as measured by transepidermal water loss and a subjective questionnaire. There was no difference between young and old skin with regard to ceramide subgroups or ceramide/cholesterol ratios, although there was a higher ceramide/cholesterol ratio in males compared to females.

3.2.13 How to Measure Skin Function

In studies of skin physiology, a variety of methods are used in order to study the most important functions of the skin. Unfortunately, many of these techniques are only good for scientific investigations under very controlled conditions and not useful for daily clinical practice. Thus the clinically obvious parameter of "sensitive skin" cannot be measured in routine in the same way as bronchial hyperreactivity in respiratory airway disease.

The following methodologies are used to measure skin function:

- With the profilometry, the roughness of the skin can be measured. It is increased in atopic dermatitis (Eberlein-König et al. 1996).
- The water content of the stratum corneum can be measured with the corneometer and has been shown to only show small or little changes in atopic dermatitis (Eberlein-König et al. 2000)
- Secretion of sebaceous glands can be measured with lipid analyses of the skin surface with the sebumeter; some authors found decreased sebaceous secretion (Gloor 1991) which, however, is not consistently measurable.
- The best method to measure a functioning skin barrier is the estimation of the transepidermal water loss which determines the liquid water leaving the stratum corneum by passive diffusion as well as gaseous water vapor as a result of sweating. Normally measurements are done below the sweat thresholds so that there should be no eccrine sweat. With disturbed skin barrier, the TEWL increases, which can be measured by different devices, mostly open-chamber systems (e.g., Tewameter, VapoMeter, Germany, VapoMeter, Finland). Recently a new methodology has been described using a condenser chamber where a closed chamber is cooled below the freezing point just as a sink for water vapor; no recovery time is necessary (Farahmand et al. 2009). In patients with atopic dermatitis, also in uninvolved skin, but more marked in eczematous skin lesions, dramatic increases of TEWL can be measured (Gfesser et al. 1997).

Of special interest are studies who measure the repair activity of regenerative capacity of the epidermis after certain stimuli, such as tape stripping of stratum corneum or application of irritants, like sodium lauryl sulfate or dimethyl sulfoxide (DMSO). In many studies, abnormal reaction patterns have been found in patients with atopic dermatitis, sometimes also in patients with respiratory atopy, although the latter is discussed controversially (Cork et al. 2005).

3.2.14 Exposure Studies

In exposure studies measuring effects of indoor air chemicals or pollutants (e.g., formaldehyde or volatile organic compounds (VOCs)), we have found significant impairment of epidermal barrier function in patients with atopic eczema (Eberlein-König et al. 1998; Huss-Marp et al. 2007). Patients were exposed under conditions of normal indoor air with concentrations of the above-mentioned substances below toxic levels in a climate chamber.

Concomitantly epicutaneous application of house dust mite allergen was performed in the atopy patch test (APT): There was a significant increase in intensity of APT reactions after exposure to VOCs, without any clinical dysesthesias from the patients' side; the patients did not feel any discomfort (Huss-Marp et al. 2007). Tobacco smoke has been identified as the most common indoor air pollutant and can increase the risk of atopic eczema in genetically predisposed individuals, as has been shown in a study in preschool children with actual determination of cotinine in the urine (Krämer et al. 2004).

3.2.15 Clinical Relevance

It can be concluded that the obvious disturbance of skin barrier function already in subclinical levels is of pathophysiological relevance and may give rise to an enhanced penetrance of noxious substances in these patients. Patients with very sensitive skin often in their history tell the following symptoms:

Itch when sweating
Wool incompatibility
Incompatibility with solvents
Incompatibility with UV light

3.2.16 Skin Hygiene and Cleaning Habits

It is an open question whether the increasing hygiene procedures in the Western world have led to an increase in prevalence of atopic dermatitis. Cork et al. have found a significant increase of soap use from 67 million pounds in 1981 to 453 million pounds in 2001 in the UK (Cork et al. 2005). In the same time, also the personal use of water has increased from 11 L per person and day in 1961 to 51 L per person and day in 2001. Furthermore, the degree of hardness of water may influence directly, by irritation and increased soap use, the clinical course of atopic eczema (McNally et al. 1998; Miyake et al. 2004).

3.2.17 Summary

In order to guarantee adequate barrier function of the skin, a physiological exchange between organism and environment has to be possible. This is guaranteed by a complex interplay of proteins and lipids in the stratum corneum. In atopic dermatitis, several abnormalities have been observed; the most important one probably is a loss of function mutation in the structural protein filaggrin, which gives rise to a three- to fourfold increased risk for atopic eczema in affected individuals (see also Sect. 3.1.2). Disturbances in protease and protease inhibitor metabolism also may play a role.

The clinically measurable phenotype of "dry skin" or "sensitive skin" can best be explained as roughness of the skin or as increased transepidermal water loss (TEWL). The increased susceptibility to irritants has practical relevance. Environmental pollutants such as formaldehyde or volatile organic compounds in patients with atopic dermatitis can lead to increased eczematous reactions as has been shown in the atopy patch test with house dust mites. They also can lead to an increased transepidermal water loss.

However, until today there is no simple routinely available test to measure skin barrier function in the daily office such as that for measuring bronchial hyperreactivity in patients with asthma.

3.3 Immunodeviation in the Pathophysiology of Atopic Eczema

In order to better understand the complex mechanisms in the pathophysiology of atopic dermatitis, it makes sense to briefly recall the physiology of normal immune reactivity with the small round lymphocytes in the center; it is only 50 years that their fundamental importance as carrier of specific immunity has been discovered (see Bergmann and Ring 2014).

3.3.1 B and T Cells

In the process of maturation of lymphocytes from stem cells in the bone marrow, the first step of differentiation is the development of the large group of B and T cells. Both arise from undifferentiated stem cells (Fig. 3.7). T cells, which mature within the thymus, are the carriers of cellular immunity (e.g., cytotoxic cells) and immune regulation, while B cells differentiate into antibody-secreting plasma cells.

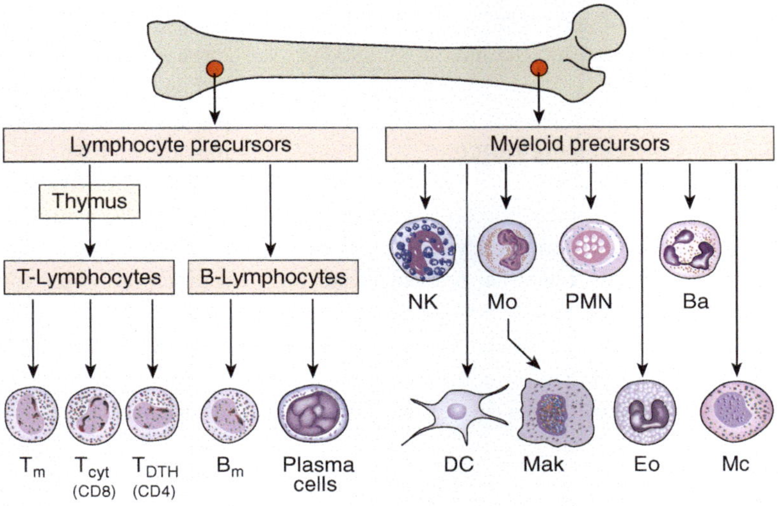

Fig. 3.7 Development of various lines of immune cells from the bone marrow. T_m T-memory cells, T_{cyt} cytotoxic T cells, T_{DTH} T cells involved in delayed-type hypersensitivity reactions, B_m B-memory cells, *NK* natural killer cells, *Mo* monocytes, *PMN* polymorphonuclear neutrophils, *Ba* basophils, *DC* dendritic cells, *Mak* macrophages, *Eo* eosinophils, *Mc* mast cells

T cells mature in the thymus, hence the name. The thymic epithelium provides the immunological identity of cells which helps to establish tolerance against autologous antigens. The precursors of B cells mature in the bone marrow, in birds in a special organ, Bursa fabricii, hence the name.

Mature T and B cells come into the blood and reach so-called secondary lymphatic organs (e.g., lymph nodes) where they come into contact with antigens via antigen-presenting cells, thus starting further steps of differentiation.

Both T and B cells, when specifically simulated, can finally transform into long-living memory cells which only become reactivated after renewed antigen simulation.

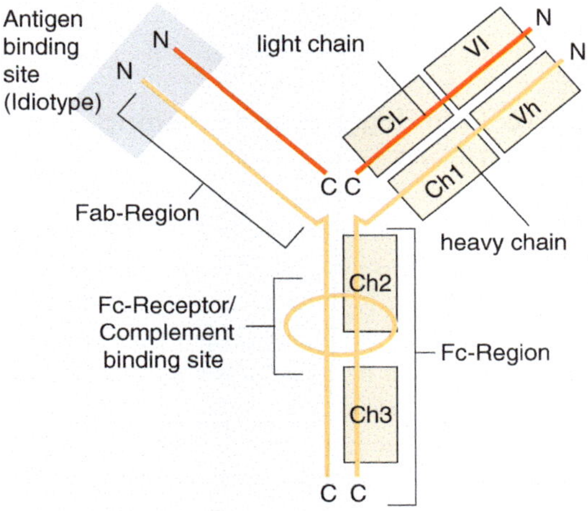

Fig. 3.8 Schematic structure of an immunoglobulin molecule with constant (*Fc*) and antigen-binding regions (*Fab*)

3.3.2 Antibodies

Antibodies are proteins—also called immunoglobulins—which are secreted by specially differentiated plasma cells from B-cell precursors. According to their primary structure, five different immunoglobulin classes (isotypes) are distinguished which can be defined according to the characteristics of their heavy chains as G, M, A, D, and E (Fig. 3.8).

IgE antibodies differ from IgG by a fifth domain; they are larger (190,000 kD compared to 150,000 for IgG) and can bind to specific receptors on the surface of mast cells and basophil leukocytes via high-affinity specific receptors (FcεR1) (Fig. 3.9).

3.3.3 IgE and Atopic Dermatitis

While the pathophysiological processes in other allergic diseases like hay fever or bronchial asthma are quite well understood, the etiopathophysiological concepts in atopic dermatitis still differ with regard to various dysregulations at several levels leading to a complex interplay between genetic predisposition and

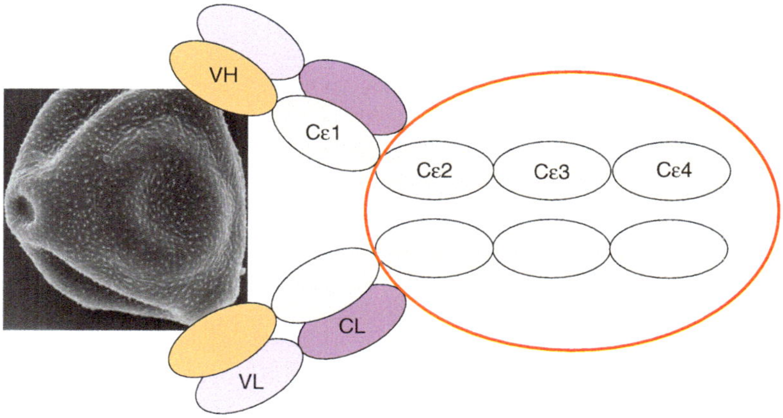

Fig. 3.9 Schematic structure of immunoglobulin E. *VH* variable heavy chain, *VL* variable light chain, *CL* constant light chain

Table 3.5 Atopic dermatitis: etiopathophysiological concepts

Genetic predisposition
Dry skin—disturbed skin barrier function
Microbial colonization
Vitamin D deficiency?
Dysregulation in autonomic nervous system
Psychosocial factors (stress)
Inflammation:
Non-immune (irritative-toxic)
Allergic DTH[a] (Th1)
Allergic atopic (Th2, IgE)
Autoimmune

[a]*DTH* delayed-type hypersensitivity

environmental influences in the development of the eczematous skin lesions.

As illustrated by the multitude of names for this disease (see Sect. 1.2.2), different hypothetical concepts are supported by different research groups—probably also by their subjective special focus (Table 3.5).

One of the most characteristic features of atopic diseases and especially of atopic dermatitis is the increased tendency towards IgE production. While in the normal organism only little amounts of IgE antibodies are formed (in the range of few ng/mL serum), atopic diseases are characterized by much higher serum concentrations of this immunoglobulin.

In the development of this "immune deviation," a complex interplay of several cells and cytokines is involved; the major players in this concert will briefly be introduced. It should be stressed that never one cell or subpopulation or mediator alone is sufficient, but it is the total interaction with target and receptors (Metzger et al. 1984) which practically determines the outcome of the immune response in the organism.

3.3.4 Dendritic Cells

Dendritic cells (DC) in the tissue are, next to monocytes in the blood, the major antigen-presenting cells in lymphoid and peripheral tissue; these are the cells which allow the first contact with a foreign substance (antigen) and, by processing, uptake, and presentation of specific structures to lymphocytes, initiate a specific immune response (Lanzavecchia and Sallusto 2001). Without adequate stimulation by dendritic cells, no specific effector T cells can develop.

There are various dendritic cells (Schaekel et al. 2002) which can be classified according to the topography in the skin where we can distinguish between epidermal and dermal DCs.

According to their function, dendritic cells can be classified into the following:

- Plasmacytoid dendritic cells (pDC)
- Myeloid dendritic cells (mDC)

which in the epidermis can be further classified into the following:

- Langerhans cells
- Inflammatory dendritic epidermal cells (IDEC)

Dendritic cells can be regarded as sentinels of the immune system and form part of the so-called innate immune response; they express specific receptors for danger-associated molecular patterns (pathogen-associated molecular patterns (PAMP)) as, e.g., the strongly conserved Toll-like receptors (TLR) in the evolution (Terhoorst et al. 2010). Stimulated by danger signals—as mechanic trauma, scratching, heat, etc.—dendritic cells may be activated (Matzinger 1994). Via the production of various cytokines, they influence the differentiation and polarization of T cells in the direction of specifically functional subpopulations.

3.3.5 Langerhans Cells

Langerhans cells have been described as the first group of dendritic cells in the normal human epidermis, originally by the medical student Paul Langerhans (1847–1888) in his doctoral thesis with Rudolf Virchow; because of their dendritic appearance, he believed them to be nerve cells (Langerhans 1868). Only in 1961 was the specific characteristic of Langerhans cells discovered in electron microscopy, the so-called Birbeck granule, which allows the morphological identification of Langerhans cells and can be immunologically detected by the expression of langerin (Silberberg et al. 1974).

Langerhans cells express on their surface markers of major histocompatibility complex (MHC) class II as well as CD1a. They originate from stem cells in the bone marrow via precursors (CD34-positive cells) and differentiate under the influence of certain growth factors such as granulocyte-monocyte colony-stimulating factor (GM-CSF) or TGF-beta (transforming growth factor beta). Langerhans cells can stay over longer time periods (weeks to months) in the epidermis before they migrate to lymph nodes where they present antigens to lymphocytes.

Langerhans cells often are regarded as the outermost sentinels of the immune system in the organism with the function of antigen recognition, uptake, and presentation (Enk and Katz 1992; Jakob et al. 2001; Stingl et al. 1977, 1978). Recently through modern techniques, it has become clear that for the initiation of an immune response, dermal dendritic cells play the crucial role while epidermal Langerhans cells have a more important role in regulatory aspects and tolerance induction (Von Buboff et al. 2004).

3.3.6 Inflammatory Dendritic Epidermal Cells (IDEC)

The second population of dendritic cells in the epidermis is the so-called inflammatory dendritic epidermal cells (IDEC) which do not contain Birbeck granules, but express CD1a and MHCII molecules on the surface and can be detected especially in inflamed skin as, e.g., in atopic dermatitis, psoriasis, and allergic contact dermatitis, but also in mycosis fungoides and other inflammatory skin diseases (Wollenberg et al. 1996).

In the kinetics of the development of an atopic inflammation—using the model of the atopy patch test (see below)—we could show that IDEC can be detected very early in the development of an eczematous skin lesion in the epidermis, both in extrinsic (IgE-associated) and intrinsic (non-IgE-associated) atopic dermatitis (Kerschenlohr et al. 2003a).

3.3.7 Role of Epidermal Dendritic Cells for Atopic Dermatitis

The first note that Langerhans cells may play a role in the pathophysiology of atopic dermatitis came through the detection of IgE molecules on the surface of LC by Bruijnzeel-Koomen (1989) and the detection of the high-affinity IgE receptor (FcεR1) on the surface by the groups of T. Bieber and G. Stingl (Bieber et al. 1992, 1995; Maurer et al. 1994; Wang et al. 1992) (Fig. 3.10). At this time the high-affinity IgE receptor was only recognized to be present on the surface of mast cells and basophil granulocytes, while lymphoid or dendritic cells only could express the low-affinity IgE receptor CD23.

Further investigations showed that there are differences in the expression of this receptor: Langerhans cells express the FcεR1 mostly intracellularly, while IDEC show the complete

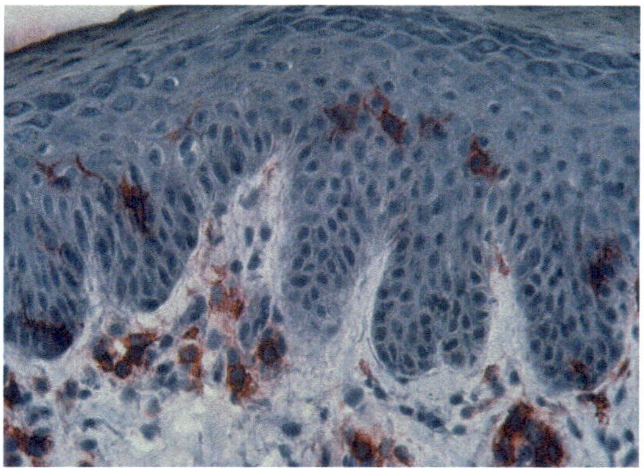

Fig. 3.10 Immunohistochemistry of immunoglobulin on epidermal Langerhans cells (With friendly permission from Thomas Bieber)

membrane expression of the high-affinity receptor. It is speculated that the membrane-bound IgE also plays a role in the antigen recognition.

A Japanese group showed in immunohistochemical analysis the concomitant presence of IgE antibodies and house dust mite allergen on the surface of epidermal Langerhans cells (Tanaka et al. 1990).

3.3.8 Plasmacytoid Dendritic Cells

The role of plasmacytoid dendritic cells is less well established; after activation, they mediate antiviral responses via production of pDC interferon and are present in peripheral blood of patients with atopic dermatitis. They also carry the three chains of the Fcγ receptor on their surface. They usually are not in the epidermis and seem to be rarer in the dermis of patients with atopic dermatitis, which might play a role in the decreased immune reactivity against viral infections such as eczema herpeticum (Wollenberg et al. 2003a, b).

3.3.9 T Cells and T-Cell Subpopulations

In the immunohistochemical analysis of eczematoid skin lesions, an inflammatory infiltrate can be found, consisting predominantly of T lymphocytes (Werfel 2000) and especially T helper cells (CD4 positive). The role of CD8-positive cells in atopic dermatitis is controversial; however, they can be detected and may play a role in the development of spongiosis (Trautmann et al. 2000). A delayed maturation of T cells in atopy has been discussed as a possible feature (Holt et al. 1992; Prescott et al. 1999, 2003).

Table 3.6 T helper cell subpopulations

Type	Cytokines secreted	Function
Th1	Interferon-γ Interleukin-2 TNF-α	Delayed-type hypersensitivity (DTH) Allergic contact dermatitis Tuberculin reaction Chronic atopic eczema
Th2	Interleukin-4 Interleukin-13 Interleukin-5	IgE formation Parasite defense Atopic eczema initiation
Treg	Interleukin-10 TGF-β	Tolerance, inhibition of Th1 and Th2 responses
Th17	Interleukin-17	Neutrophil activation Pustular dermatosis Defense of infection
Th22	Interleukin-22	Tissue signaling Wound healing

The thymic function was studied in atopic dermatitis and psoriasis, using the detection of T-cell receptor excision circles (TREC) which are produced during the rearrangement of the T-cell receptor and represent a possible marker for recent thymic immigrants (RTI), cells freshly migrating from the thymus. In psoriasis, TREC levels were significantly reduced in atopic dermatitis and showed significantly greater variation compared to healthy controls, especially within the CD8 T subpopulation. This suggests that eczema patients have a higher capacity to develop compensatory mechanisms, especially involving CD8 cells, compared to psoriasis patients (Just et al. 2008).

3.3.10 CD4-Positive Cells

Major progress in the understanding of the atopic immune response came through the recognition of highly differentiated subpopulations of T cells, especially T helper cells, starting with the concept of Th1 and Th2 cells (Mossmann and Saat 1996; Coffmann and von der Weid 1997). Table 3.6 lists some of the most important T helper cell populations.

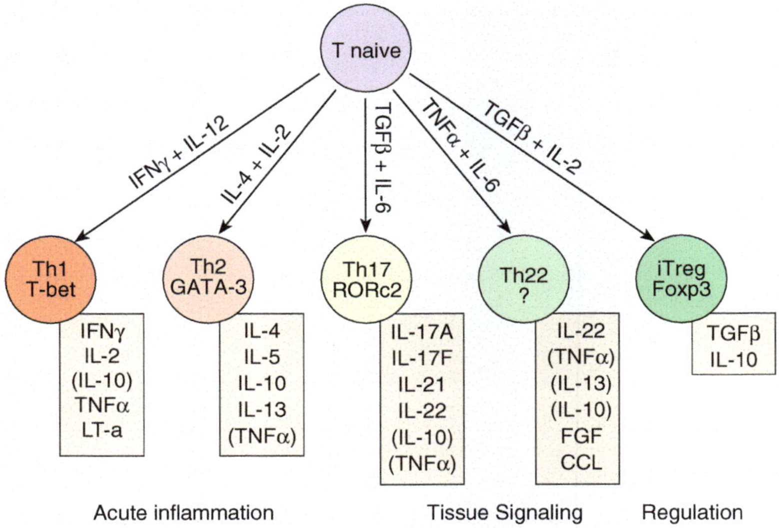

Fig. 3.11 New concept of T helper cell interaction of various T-cell subpopulations (With friendly permission from K. Eyerich)

Th1 cells are the classic carriers of delayed-type hypersensitivity (DTH) and allergic contact dermatitis (type IV allergy according to Coombs and Gell). They produce interferon-γ and tumor necrosis factor alpha (TNF-α).

Th2 cells are characterized by the secretion of interleukin-4, interleukin-5, and interleukin-13 and are the responsible cells for the development of IgE production. IL-4 induces the differentiation from B cells into IgE-secreting plasma cells by activating a recombinase which in the nucleus brings the γ domain of the heavy chain in contact with the junction and light-chain domain and thus allows the production of antibodies of the IgE class ("isotype switch").

For a long time, the paradigm of Th1/Th2 balance dominated the concepts of pathophysiology of immune deviation in atopic diseases with increased Th2 and decreased Th1 response (Romagnani *neu*). The decreased Th1 responses were interpreted as explanatory of the tendency towards more common skin infections in the sense of a "minimal immunodeficiency" (Neumann 1991; Ring 1979; Busse and Lantis 1979). From there also the concept of a lower prevalence of contact allergy in atopic dermatitis was developed (see Sect. 2.7.7).

Indeed, in the early phase of an atopic inflammation, one sees predominantly Th2 cells in the inflammatory infiltrate (Hamid et al. 1994). Great progress was possible through the model of the atopy patch test (see Sect. 4.1) where it became possible in an experimental situation to elicit atopic eczema locally on the back of an affected individual by application of a specific allergen, e.g., house dust mite (Ring et al. 1989; Darsow et al. 1996). Using this model, one can see that in the early phase an influx of Th2 cells and eosinophils occurs, while in the more chronic phase of the skin lesion, Th1 cells with secretion of interferon-γ and TNF become more prominent.

The role of T cells in the eczematous inflammation was especially studied by C. and M. Akdis in Davos: They found lymphocyte-dependent apoptosis of epidermal keratinocytes as important parameter in the development of the dermal-epidermal inflammation (Akdis et al. 1999; Trautmann et al. 2000). Similar results were found by Girolomoni and others (Cavani et al. 2001; Girolomoni et al. 2001).

The concept of T-cell subpopulations and their functions is illustrated in Fig. 3.11.

Recent research has shown that the simple Th1/Th2 paradigm for the description of the pathophysiology of atopy might be too simple. Through the discovery of new subpopulations, especially the influence and role of regulatory T cells have been supported (Sakaguchi et al. 2000). In a "balancing square model" of at least four different T-cell subpopulations keeping the balance, this complex interaction has been made more understandable (Orihara et al. 2008).

Table 3.7 Chemokines and receptors with possible relevance for atopic dermatitis (Homey et al. 2006)

Chemokine	Earlier name	Receptor	Source
CCL2	MCP-1	CCL2	Keratinocyte
CCL3	MIP-1α	CCL1, CCL5	?
CCL4	MIP-1β	CCL5	
CCL5	RANTES	CCL1, CCL3, CCL5	Keratinocyte
CCL11	Eotaxin	CCL3	Fibroblast, T cell, eosinophil
CCL13	MCP-4	CCL2, CCL3	Keratinocyte
CCL17	TARC	CCL4	Endothelium, Keratinocyte
CCL20	MIP-3 α	CCL6	Keratinocyte
CCL22	MDC	CCL4	Macrophage Dendritic cell
CCL26	Eotaxin-3	CCL3	Keratinocyte
CCL27	CTACK	CCR10	Keratinocyte
CXCL1	Fractalkine	CXCR1	Endothelium

Also a specific subpopulation of dendritic cells and even B cells has been described to play a crucial role in this complex disease (Eyerich and Novak 2013). As Thomas Bieber stated, the old wisdom "Many ways lead to Rome" also holds true for the immunopathophysiology of atopic eczema (Bieber 2013; Pilette et al. 2013; Fujita et al. 2011).

The better understanding of pathophysiology at the gene and molecular level may allow a better diagnosis and phenotyping from the gene via pathophysiology to an endo-phenotype resulting in a clinical phenotype and finally offering possibilities of personalized management (Bieber 2013).

3.3.11 Recruitment of T Cells in the Skin

T cells are recruited from the blood into the skin via certain "homing" factors, the most important of which is the cutaneous lymphocyte antigen (CLA) (Santamaria Babi et al. 1995). This is a neuraminic acid-containing carbohydrate structure corresponding to the P-selectin glycoprotein ligand-1 (PSGL-1). CLA binds on the vessel wall to E-selectin (CD62) which under inflammatory conditions then is expressed in postcapillary venules and endothelia.

By further stimulation, e.g., with superantigen-producing staphylococci (Boehncke and Zollner 1999), the expression of CLA, but also of E-selectin on the endothelia, can be increased via the cytokines interleukin-1 and interleukin-12. Thus an increased recirculation of lymphocytes into the inflamed tissue is the consequence. In atopic dermatitis, CLA-positive T cells with special secretion of Th2 cytokines have been detected immunohistochemically, together with factors preventing eosinophil apoptosis (Simon et al. 2003).

Among the chemotactic factors recruiting T cells, there are predominantly chemokines and cytokines which can be detected in atopic dermatitis (Table 3.7), namely, CCL2 (earlier MCP-1), CCL5 (earlier RANTES), CCL17 (earlier TARC), and CCL27 (earlier CTACK) (Homey and Zlotnik 1999). Sometimes serum levels of these cytokines or chemokines—especially CCL17—seem to correlate with the intensity of the actual skin inflammation. Cytokines of the Th2 class (interleukin-4 and interleukin-13) also influence keratinocytes and make them attract CCL4-positive Th2 cells via CCL22 (Purwar et al. 2007).

Interesting findings show an interaction between filaggrin expression and cytokine secretion: keratinocytes under the influence of IL-4 and IL-13 show a significantly reduced filaggrin gene expression in the medium (Howell et al. 2007) (see Sect. 3.2).

3.3.12 Cytokines and Itch

In the development of itch sensation, a cytokine, namely, interleukin-31, which is Th2 associated and can be found especially in the acute phase

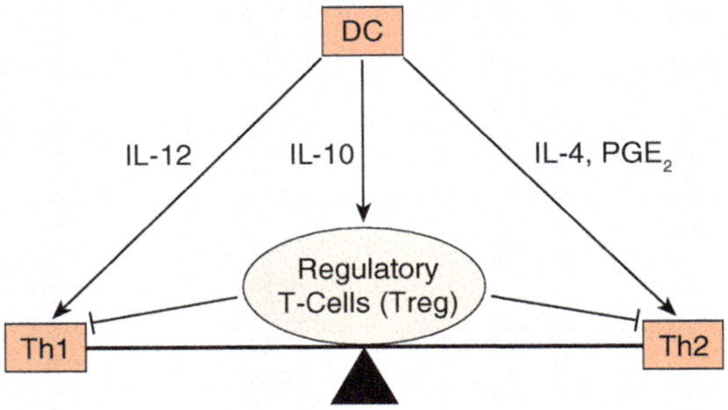

Fig. 3.12 Balance of immunological reactivity with regulatory T cells. *DC* Dendritic cells (Eyerich et al. 2009a)

of eczematous inflammation both of atopic and contact-allergic origin, seems to play a critical role (Neis et al. 2006). In the mouse model, interleukin-31 is associated with itch development (Sonkoly et al. 2006). In extremely itching skin areas, there was an increased IL-31 expression (Raap et al. 2006). Furthermore, some autacoids but also superantigens from microbial colonization can lead to an increased interleukin-31 expression (Gutzmer et al. 2009).

3.3.13 CD8-Positive Cells

While in the 1980s CD8 cells were called suppressor cells and were regarded as mediators of immunological tolerance or suppression of immunity (Tada 1975; Tada et al. 1997), they suddenly disappeared in immunological congresses over many years, and they came "out of fashion." Only through the work of Sakaguchi (Sakaguchi et al. 2000; see Blaser 2008) were T cells, which not only stimulate activation but which also can show inhibitory effects, rediscovered as "regulatory T cells" (Treg) (Fig. 3.12).

Blaser and Akdis' group was able to show that this population is critical in the regulation of the immune response and characterized by the secretion of cytokine IL-10 and transforming growth factor β (TGF-β). Regulatory T cells need for their maturation the signal transduction marker Foxp3 while Th1 cells use T-bet and Th2 cells GATA (Akdis et al. 2000; Blaser 2008). There is a rare autoimmune disease with polyendocrinopathy and gastrointestinal disturbance and extremely elevated IgE levels based on an X chromosome-associated mutation of Foxp3. In atopic dermatitis, decreased numbers of regulatory T cells have been found in the skin (Verhagen et al. 2006).

3.3.14 Other Subpopulations of T Helper Cells

A new subpopulation of lymphocytes has been described as CD4+ IL-17-producing Th17 cells (Ochs et al. 2009) which can be clearly distinguished from other subpopulations and are predominantly found in Th1-mediated reactions (Table 3.6). They are involved in the defense of microbial infection, especially *Candida* (Eyerich et al. 2008, 2009b). In inflamed skin of patients with atopic dermatitis, Th17 cells are present in the atopy patch test after house dust mite application; however, their activity in atopic eczema seems to be diminished.

The role of the recently described Th22 cells, which besides Th17 cells can be regarded as tissue-signalling cells and possibly have relevance for overcoming the sequels of immune reactions, is a matter of future research (Eyerich et al. 2009a).

In patients with the rare disease of chronic mucocutaneous candidiasis (CMC), for a long time the immune defect was unknown. They have normal T-cell functions as measured in mitogen or antigen stimulation. The only defect which could be clearly identified was the absolute lack of interleukin-17 secretion after *Candida* stimulation (Eyerich et al. 2008). Recently it has been shown that the underlying defect may be a gain of function mutation of the STAT1 gene.

3.3.15 B Cells

The decision to produce IgE instead of IgG occurs early in naive B cells and even resides in a subpopulation of "memory" IgE-positive B cells later developing into IgE-secreting plasma cells (Akdis and Akdis 2012).

In humans, the switch from intrinsic to extrinsic atopic eczema seems to occur very early in life (Dondi et al. 2013).

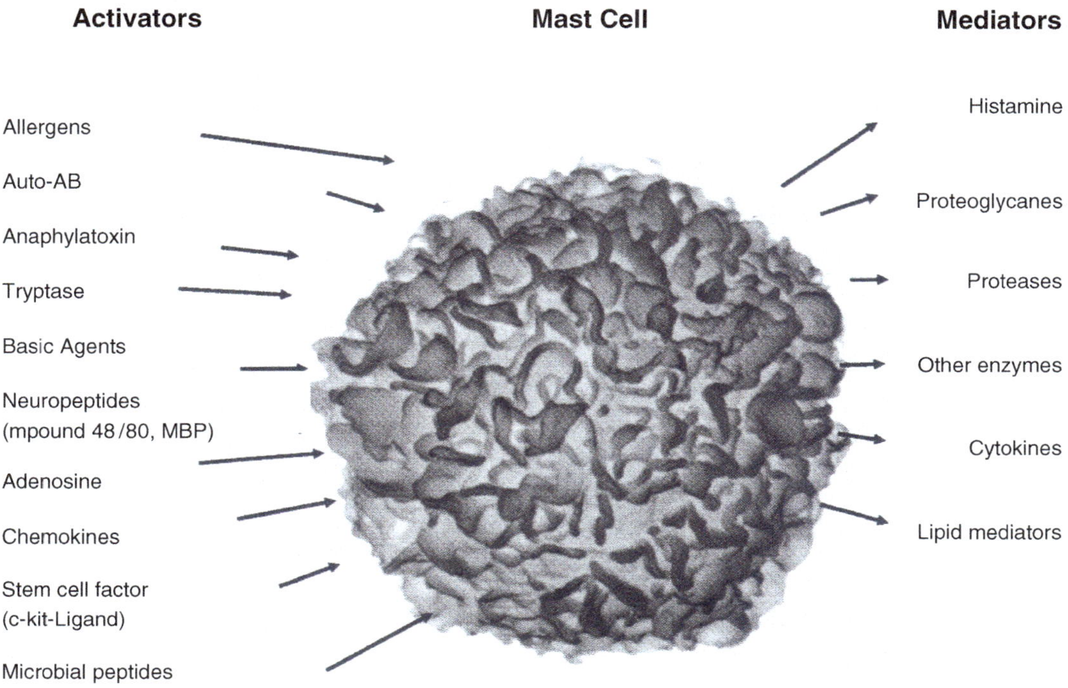

Fig. 3.13 Scanning electron microscopic image of mast cells (With friendly permission from H. Behrendt). Stimulating activating factors of mast cells and mediators released or secreted by mast cells

3.3.16 Mast Cells

Mast cells are commonly associated with the pathophysiology of urticaria, angioedema, and anaphylaxis. They represent a heterogeneous group of tissue cells localized predominantly around vessel or adnexal structures and have been first described by Paul Ehrlich in 1877 and named because of their well-fed impression stuffed with granules (Ehrlich 1877).

Mast cells develop from CD34-positive precursor cells in bone marrow and carry a receptor for stem cell factor (SCF) which together with interleukin-6 plays a role for the differentiation and growth (Galli et al. 2004, 2005).

Mast cells can be differentiated phenotypically into bone marrow mast cells and connective tissue mast cells. Dependent on the type of neutral proteases secreted, one distinguishes tryptase-positive mast cells from mast cells secreting tryptase and chymase (MC_{TC}).

All these phenotypes express the high-affinity IgE receptor on the surface and play a role in the acute allergic reaction, releasing mediators after antigen contact with the surface-bound IgE. Recently it is speculated that tryptase-secreting mast cells play a more prominent role in allergy development while chymase- and tryptase-secreting mast cells are involved in chronic inflammation and fibrosis. Increased mast cell numbers have been found in atopic dermatitis (Mihm et al. 1976) in the tissue.

Numerous stimuli are able to activate mast cells; mast cells also secrete numerous mediators, not only histamine, but also a variety of other mediators, cytokines, heparin, and proteases and proteoglycans and platelet-activating factor (PAF) (Benveniste and Arnoux 1981). Furthermore, mast cells secrete carboxypeptidase and cathepsin G (Fig. 3.13). Among the cytokines secreted by mast cells, interleukin-3, interleukin-4, interleukin-5, interleukin-10, and TNF-α should be named (Galli 2004).

After contact with allergen, bridging of at least two IgE molecules on the surface of mast cells or basophil leukocytes gives rise to activation of a signal cascade with consequent degranulation and mediator release (de Weck 2008).

Table 3.8 Receptors and mediators of eosinophil granulocytes

Receptors
High-affinity IgE receptor?
IgG receptors
Mediators (content of granules)
Cationic proteins (eosinophil cationic protein (ECP))
Eosinophil-derived neurotoxin (EDN)
Eosinophil peroxidase (EPO)
Major basic protein (MBP)

As to what extent the IgE receptor on Langerhans cells or other cells like eosinophil granulocytes or platelets plays a role in atopic inflammation is a matter of speculation. Various authors favor the concept of an increased releasability of mast cells in atopic dermatitis (Conroy et al. 1977; Lichtenstein 1975; Ring and Thomas 1989; Ring 1979). According to these concepts, increased plasma histamine concentrations have been found in severe atopic eczema (Amon et al. 1994; Ring and Thomas 1989).

There is no doubt that histamine is not the critical proinflammatory mediator of atopic dermatitis since antihistamines used in the therapy of atopic eczema only have a limited effect (see Sect. 5.4). Nevertheless, by initiating acute allergic reactions—e.g., against foods—mast cells also can play a role in atopic dermatitis by initiating an allergic immediate inflammation with consequent facilitation or triggering an eczematous flare.

3.3.17 Eosinophil Granulocytes

Increased numbers of eosinophil granulocytes in the peripheral blood are a hallmark of atopic diseases. For a long time, the role of eosinophils has been discussed controversially between "good" and "bad" from "early dawn of overcoming inflammation" in pathology textbooks to tissue-destructive toxic dangerous cells.

By secreting enzymes degrading or inactivating proinflammatory mediators such as leukotrienes or platelet-activating factor (PAF), eosinophils might have a protective role (eosinophils as "police").

There is no doubt that eosinophils can act as proinflammatory cells by the release of highly active basic and cationic proteins which have a tissue-destructive effect (Elsner and Kapp 1999; Simon et al. 2003) (Table 3.8).

Gleich and Leiferman first detected eosinophil products in eczematous skin (Gleich 1982). Eosinophil cationic protein (ECP) is a marker of eosinophil inflammation and can be used as parameter of severity in the clinical course during exacerbations (Jakob et al. 1991, Kapp 2002).

In the blood of patients with atopic dermatitis, elevated interleukin-5 levels and decreased or delayed eosinophil apoptosis have been found. The fact that in routine histology of atopic dermatitis rarely eosinophils can be seen may be explained by the fact that eosinophil recruitment occurs in the very early phase of atopic inflammation, as can be studied in the atopy patch test (Bruijnzeel et al. 1993; Bruijnzeel-Koomen 1989); secretory products such as eosinophil cationic protein can still be detected, while whole eosinophils are no longer found (Wedi et al. 1997). The marker "thymus and activation-regulated chemokine (TARC)" also seems to be suitable as a parameter of severity of atopic dermatitis.

3.3.18 Keratinocytes

Ninety-five percent of epidermal cells consist of keratinocytes which produce the characteristic protein of the epidermis, the keratin. For a long time, keratinocytes were regarded as immunologically uninteresting structure material like a scaffold, but not playing any role in allergic or inflammatory phenomena. In the last decades it became clearer and clearer that keratinocytes are fundamentally involved in immune reactions; they produce a whole variety of chemokines (CCL2, CCL5, CCL18, CCL22, CCL27) and cytokines (interleukin-1, interleukin-8, interleukin-18, interleukin-23, interleukin-27). Keratinocytes play a fundamental role in innate immunity; they express TLR and secrete antimicrobial peptides (defensin, cathelicidin) as well as thymic stromal lymphopoietin (TSLP). The latter seems to be especially important in atopic dermatitis (Soumelis and Liu 2004) and is involved in the Th2 dominance of the micromilieu. Keratinocytes from lesional skin of atopic dermatitis produce increased amounts of certain cytokines such as GM-CSF. Via interaction with lymphocytes and a secretion of proinflammatory cytokines, they are actively involved in the maintenance of eczematous inflammation. Furthermore, the epithelial barrier is intrinsically connected with skin immune reaction patterns, e.g., Th1 immune reactions seem to strengthen the barrier by enhancing ceramide production in the epidermis, while Th2 cytokines have a deteriorating effect (Sawada et al. 2012).

Th2-dominated immune responses after protein antigen application induce thymic stromal lymphopoietin (TSLP) receptor on epidermal Langerhans cells, leading to production of interleukin-31 known to evoke itch and at the same time decrease filaggrin expression in the upper epidermal layer (Kabashima 2013).

On the other hand, mutations in the interleukin-6 receptor (IL6R) may predispose to more severe phenotypes of atopic eczema (Esparza-Gordillo et al. 2009).

Tumor necrosis factor can also lead to epithelial barrier disruption in the bronchial system and seems to be regulated by a special group of kinases, namely, the Src family (Hardyman et al. 2013).

The apoptosis factor B-cell leukemia 3 (Bcl-3) is an important modulator of secretion of antimicrobial peptides from keratinocytes (Massoumi 2009) and can be induced by Th2 cytokines such as interleukin-4 and interleukin-13, finally leading to downregulation of antimicrobial peptides (Büchau et al. 2009).

3.3.19 Animal Models

While some years ago there was a general complaint that for atopic dermatitis there was a lack of animal models, this can no longer be stated. Mice, and here the Nc/Nga mice with spontaneously occurring atopic dermatitis lesions, but also models induced by epicutaneous allergen application or transgenic mice with overexpression of certain factors, have provided excellent tools to study specific mechanisms of atopic inflammation (Yin et al. 2009).

Also canine models may be very useful. Atopic dermatitis is extremely common in dogs, with a prevalence of 10–15 %; it is a common phenomenon in veterinary practice. This disease is very similar to human atopic dermatitis with regard to the clinical appearance. Especially in air-exposed areas in the face and in the skin folds, it goes along with severe itch and IgE responses. The major difference is that in dogs there is no atopic march and airway allergy is rare (Marsella and Girolomoni 2009).

3.3.20 Autoimmune Phenomena (IgE Autoantibodies) in Atopic Dermatitis

Many, especially chronic cases of atopic eczema, are very difficult to treat; in spite of changes in environment with avoidance of relevant allergens, they do not respond to treatment.

Already in the early twentieth century, observations of "allergy" against human dandruff have been reported and gave rise to the exploration of other possible autoimmune phenomena (Simon 1947; Uehara and Ofuji 1976). The author remembers very well from early allergen skin test kits that there were special allergen extracts besides pollen, house dust mites, and animal dander with the label "human dander"; they only disappeared with the emergence of HIV and AIDS. However, when these reactions were positive, nobody really knew how to interpret.

It was Rudi Valenta's group who investigated this phenomenon scientifically and found IgE antibodies against human epidermal proteins in sera of patients with variably severe conditions of atopic dermatitis. The authors found that especially in severe atopic eczema (SCORAD over 40) there was a high percentage of patients with antibodies of the class IgE against human epidermal proteins (Natter et al. 1998) (Table 3.9). The hypothesis is attractive that by the destruction of keratinocytes, be it through inflammation or by scratching, autoantigens may be released which can stimulate autoreactive lymphocytes and contribute to the allergic reaction in the sense of a perpetuation (Valenta et al. 2000). Recently these epidermal autoantigens have been more closely characterized as calcium-binding proteins and so-called Hom s 1 to Hom s 5.

That IgE autoantibodies found in severe atopic eczema also may play a pathogenic role was

Table 3.9 Possible autoantigens with relevance for atopic eczema (Valenta et al. 2000)

Allergen	Molecular weight (kD)	Source	Function
Hom s 1 (SART-1)	73.4	Skin, lung, liver	Recognized by cytotoxic cells from cancer patients
Hom s 2 (α-NAC)	23.2	Skeleton, muscle, liver	Sorting and translocation of intracellular proteins
Hom s 3 (BCL7B)	?	Bile, skeletal muscle, liver, placenta, liver, ciliary body	Putative oncogene
Hom s 4 (CALC)	54	Skin, brain, lung, breast, liver, heart, calcium-binding protein	
Hom s 5 (KER)	42.6	Epithelial tissue	Production of intermediary filaments

shown in vitro when the recombinant IgE-reactive autoantigen Hom s 2 was able to stimulate interferon-gamma production in peripheral blood mononuclear cells and induced an effect in culture supernatants that caused disintegration of respiratory epithelial cell layers and apoptosis in skin keratinocytes (Mittermann et al. 2008).

Apart from these epidermal autoallergens, also cross-reactivities between well-known allergens from the environment and human proteins have to be considered. This has been described for profilin, a well-known allergen from plants (Bet v 2) which is produced by all eukaryotic cells, but also cross-reactivities between mammalian allergens (dog, cat) and fungal allergens (manganese superoxide dismutase (MnSOD)) from *Aspergillus fumigatus* have been described (Crameri et al. 1996).

3.3.21 Summary

The skin is not only a bag keeping the body together but exerts a variety of important functions, among others also the function of an immune organ. Besides the physical-chemical barrier of the stratum corneum, there is an immunological barrier of the skin as an important part of defense against microbial invaders. First the innate immune systems play the primary role via formation of antimicrobial peptides (human beta-defensin (hBD)), and then dendritic cells come into the play. T cells via Th17 will be attracted by keratinocytes. These primary immune reactions seem to be weakened in atopic dermatitis. On the other hand, there is a dominance towards a Th2 response which after antigen recognition via dendritic cells lead to the formation of IgE antibodies from plasma cells and via Th2-dependent cytokines (interleukin-4, interleukin-13, interleukin-5) to further attraction of inflammatory cells. IL-5 recruits and activates eosinophil leukocytes. Interleukin-31 seems to play a role in the induction of itch. Regulatory T cells seem to be weaker in atopic dermatitis. The thymus and activation-regulated chemokine (TARC, today CCL17) may be a marker showing a correlation to the severity of the eczematous inflammation. Patients with severe atopic eczema form autoantibodies of the IgE class against epidermal proteins which possibly play a role in the chronification and perpetuation of the inflammatory reaction.

3.4 Role of Infection and Microbial Factors

An increased susceptibility to infections is a well-known clinical feature of atopic diseases. While in rhinoconjunctivitis and asthma mostly the upper respiratory tract is affected, atopic dermatitis is characterized by an increased incidence of skin infections. The first published observations date back to Kaposi when he described the varicelliform eruption (today eczema herpeticum) (Kaposi 1891). Already the allergist Urbach concluded that infection may be a predisposing initiator for allergy (Urbach 1939). Special microbes are particularly associated with atopic dermatitis such as among bacteria *Staphylococcus aureus*, among viruses herpes simplex virus, and among fungi *Candida albicans* in the intertriginous areas and *Malassezia furfur* in the head/neck region. The clinical characteristics have been discussed in detail in Chap. 2.

3.4.1 *Staphylococcus aureus* and Atopic Dermatitis

While the normal skin surface due to the well-known physiological conditions with a mildly acidic pH is covered mostly with *Staphylococcus epidermidis* and rarely *S. aureus*, the skin of patients with atopic dermatitis is colonized in over 90 % (also in non-lesional skin) with *S. aureus* (Bode et al. 1982; Hauser and Saurat 1985, Leyden et al. 1975; Mempel et al. 1998; Stalder and Sourisse 1989). On lesional skin, the density of *S. aureus* has been measured as 105 CFU/cm^2 (CFU = colony-forming unit) up to 10^7 (Leung 2003). Causal to this phenomenon is a complex interplay between virulence factors, bacteria, and adherence mechanisms in the upper epidermis in atopic dermatitis.

S. aureus produces a variety of adhesion factors, among them protein A, coagulase, but also certain proteins binding to other proteins such as fibronectin-binding protein. With increasing pH between 7 and 8, this adhesion is facilitated. The fibronectin expression, among others, is enhanced by interleukin-4 which is prominent in atopic dermatitis. Also fibrinogen is binding to clumping factors from staphylococci. This may play a role in inflamed skin with regard to plasma exudation.

Furthermore, *S. aureus* strains produce several toxins which may damage or activate keratinocytes (e.g., exfoliative toxin); also constituents of the cell wall like peptidoglycans or lipoteichoic acid play a role. Among the virulence factors, especially superantigens like staphylococcal enterotoxins have to be mentioned; they act as danger signals and activate not only the innate immune response, but also directly the T-cell receptor; besides, they can act as antigen and induce specific IgE antibodies (Boehncke and Zollner 1999, Bunikowski et al. 1999; Neuber et al. 1995; Novak 2009).

There seem to be no specific staphylococcal strains with particular affinity to atopic dermatitis in general; however, we have found specific strains in individual patients which could be detected over a long period of time (Schnopp et al. 2008). Also the formation of staphylococcal toxins in 70 % was corresponding for at least one superantigen in the PCR analysis for several seg-seo genes in the enterotoxin gene cluster. There was no direct relation to the clinical severity as measured in the SCORAD.

Staphylococci stimulate the innate immune system via Toll-like receptors on keratinocytes which then activate various defense mechanisms such as production of interleukin-8 and inducible NO synthase (iNOS) and formation of antimicrobial peptides (human beta-defensins 2 and 3) as well as antimicrobial peptide LL-37 (Mempel et al. 1998). All these defense mechanisms seem to be weaker in atopic dermatitis compared to healthy controls or in psoriasis (Leung 2003).

Even if the mechanisms are not fully established, it is a fact that the common colonization of the skin with *S. aureus* and especially the mucosal parts of the nasal entrance plays a role in patients with atopic eczema and should give rise to the recommendation of an antimicrobial treatment as part of therapeutic strategy (see Sect. 5.3).

3.4.2 Viral Infection and Atopic Dermatitis

3.4.2.1 Smallpox (Variola Vera) and Vaccination

From the era of smallpox infection and vaccination, it is known that patients with atopic dermatitis have an elevated risk to suffer from a rapidly spreading infection with a vaccinia virus ("eczema vaccinatum"), which may end lethally (Plaut and Tinkle 2003). Thus, the diagnosis atopic eczema was a contraindication for smallpox vaccination in many countries. Therefore, the development of an attenuated virus as "modified vaccinia virus Ankara MVA" was a great progress.

It could be shown that the risk of side effects was markedly diminished by prior application of the MVA vaccine. Unfortunately this MVA vaccine was no longer produced or studied, although over 100,000 patients had been successfully treated when the WHO announced in the 1980s that smallpox had been eradicated in the world. There are only two laboratories—one in Russia and one in the USA—where Variola vera strains are still kept for research purposes. The concern regarding bioterrorism rejuvenated the thinking about smallpox vaccination. In a study with the new MVA vaccine, we were able to show that patients with atopic dermatitis, also with actual skin lesions, can, in comparable doses, tolerate this vaccine (Darsow et al. in prep., von Sonnenburg et al. in prep.). Measured in vitro in antibody titers and cellular reactions, this vaccine seems to be effective.

Even if hopefully these thoughts are no more than a nightmare, it is good to know that, in an eventual case for people at risk—soldiers, dermatologists, nurses, and infect tiologists—there would be an effective and safe prevention.

3.4.2.2 Herpes Simplex Virus

The major problem regarding viral infection in atopic dermatitis is eczema herpeticum. Already in the nineteenth century, Kaposi described this eruptive event as varicelliform eruption (Kaposi 1891).

After an incubation period of 5–12 days, multiple, extremely itching, vesiculopustular skin lesions occur which are easily scratched and turn hemorrhagic or appear as point-like erosion. Rapidly these areas are also superinfected with bacterial germs such as *S. aureus*, but also streptococci. When eczema herpeticum spreads, there is usually a severe exacerbation of eczema in general. Most commonly eczema herpeticum is transferred by kissing from persons with labial herpes (see Chap. 2).

Pathophysiologically, possibly plasmacytoid dendritic cells (pDC) which are less active in atopic dermatitis may be involved (Wollenberg et al. 2003a, b).

3.4.2.3 Other Viral Infections

Also other viral infections may be more prevalent in patients with atopic dermatitis or show a more intense clinical course such as verrucae vulgares, mollusca contagiosa, but also chickenpox (varicella) (see Chap. 2). One also could speak about "eczema verrucatum," "eczema molluscatum," and more.

3.4.3 Fungal Infection and Atopic Dermatitis

There may be an increased susceptibility to *Candida* infection, especially in the intertriginous area, in children with atopic dermatitis.

More common is the presence of *Malassezia furfur* (earlier *Pityrosporum orbiculare*), a saprophytic yeast, in the head and neck region which in normal individuals may give rise to pityriasis versicolor during summertime or when sweating (Nenoff et al. 2001). The Danish dermatologist N. Hjorth observed that the skin of patients with atopic eczema, especially with involvement of head and neck region, often was colonized with *M. furfur* (head and neck dermatitis, Hjorth et al. 1983). It was interesting that skin test reactions of the immediate type, but also specific IgE antibodies, against *Malassezia furfur* can be detected in patients with atopic dermatitis (Devos and van der Valk 2000; Rokugo et al. 1990, Tengvall Linder et al. 2000). Positive atopy patch test reactions with *M. furfur* have been described (Johansson et al. 2003; Schmid-Grendelmeier et al. 2002).

Also immediate-type reactions against dermatophytes, e.g., *Trichophyton*, have been reported (Jones et al. 1973a, b; Woodfolk et al. 1998).

It has been speculated that IgE reactivity against microbial organisms such as *S. aureus* or *M. furfur* might explain the so-called "intrinsic" variant of atopic eczema (Leung et al. 1993); however, this has not been found (Novak et al. 2003). IgE antibodies against *M. furfur* are especially detected in patients with elevated total IgE and IgE antibodies against common allergens (Schnopp et al. 2008).

When there is predominantly head and neck involvement, patch test with the yeast *Malassezia sympodialis* may be helpful as has been found for predominant involvement of the axillary line, but sparing the axillary vault and the areas under snug garments—the so-called textile pattern (Ramirez de Knott et al. 2006).

3.4.4 Summary

Infectious diseases of the skin are common in patients with severe atopic dermatitis as infections with herpes simplex virus in the form of eczema herpeticum. From the era of smallpox vaccination, the possible fatal complication of eczema vaccinatum is known. Bacterial colonization and infection with *S. aureus* are common in patients with atopic dermatitis, even on uninvolved skin. Via the secretion of superantigens, but also the induction of specific IgE antibodies, staphylococci may contribute to the maintenance of atopic inflammation. The yeast *Malassezia furfur* can play a role in patients with special head and neck involvement.

3.5 Psychological Influence in Atopic Dermatitis

Already in 1891, the French dermatologists knew about the close connection between nerves and eczema when they coined the term "neurodermite," which nowadays is used commonly in Germany (see Sect. 1.2.2). It is a well-known clinical experience that nerval or psychological factors can play a role in triggering or maintaining atopic eczema. The German term "Neurodermitis" illustrates the involvement of nerval reaction patterns in the pathophysiology of this disease (Bosse and Gieler 1987). The sentence "without nerval interaction there is no eczema" contains a lot of truth (Mitschenko et al. 2008).

I myself have fought against this term since I did not like my patients to become stigmatized as having a "neurologic" or "psychiatric" disease when they were suffering from a clear-cut skin disease (Ring 1982a, b). However, I admit that, looking at recent research in the field of psycho-neuro-allergology (Ader et al. 1991; Bienenstock 2013; Iamandescu 2007; Raap et al. 2003, 2006; Sugiura et al. 1992), it is a fact that psychological influences play a role in the actual clinical course of the disease; whoever denies this will not be a good doctor for these patients. However, it is crucial not to give the patient the feeling to be "put into the psychological corner." It is annoying how often the term "psychosomatic" is used to only describe psychological effects on certain diseases; it is essential to know the influence of a somatic disease—especially with such tormenting itch—upon the psychological condition of the patient. We always should keep in mind that psychosomatic is also somatopsychic in a complex interplay (Chida et al. 2008)!

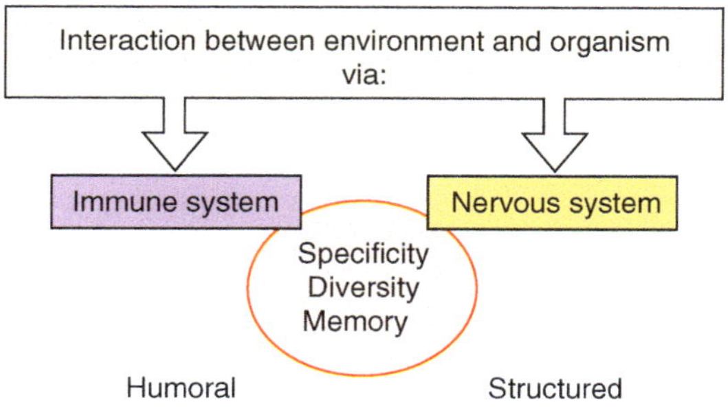

Fig. 3.14 Analogy of nervous system and immune system in the reactivity of the organism with its environment

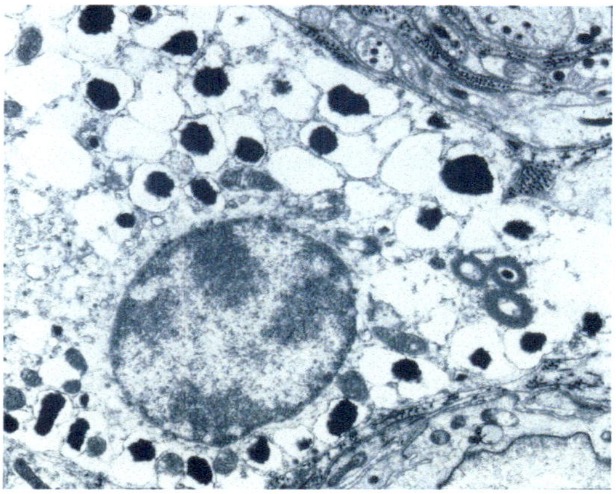

Fig. 3.15 Electromicroscopical picture of a mast cell in close contact with a sensory nerve (With friendly permission from H. Behrendt)

The immune system and nervous system are two systems that interact with the environment (Fig. 3.14). They cooperate in manifold ways, as, e.g., mast cells and nerves (Fig. 3.15). The group of J. Bienenstock has done seminal work studying this interaction and has shown that there are direct contacts—almost synaptic—between nerves and mast cells or basophil leukocytes in tissue culture; furthermore, they showed that it is possible, in a Pavlovian setting, to induce anaphylactic shock in ovalbumin-sensitized rats by just applying the conditioning audiovisual stimulus (Rolling Stones music and flashlight) (Bienenstock 2013).

The analogy of nervous and immune system describes not only the high degree of specificity, but also the large amount of diversity of specific reactions together with a long-lasting memory. The difference can be seen in the nervous system as sensory, and we can feel most of its actions, and it does its function via clear cellular and tissue structures; the immune system in contrary cannot be felt when it is active; it works in the blood and in the organs with only few specific structures (thymus, lymph nodes).

One of many lifestyle factors also includes the psychosocial interaction which may influence the development of allergy and atopic eczema. In an ongoing birth cohort study, also parameters of "life events" were investigated such as severe disease or death of a family member, unemployment, marital problems, or divorce of parents. There was a reduced risk for atopic eczema in families with other severely sick family members. At the same time, there was a significantly increased risk for developing atopic dermatitis when parents were separated or divorced (OR 3.59, CI 1.6–7.6) (Bockelbrink et al. 2006).

Another study showed a clear-cut association of stress with symptoms of atopic dermatitis by increased expression of nerve growth factor-reactive cells in epidermis and dermis and intensity of neuropeptide Y-positive cells as a parameter of anxiety and stress inducing pruritus (Oh et al. 2010).

3.5.1 Pruritus

Itch as a major symptom of atopic dermatitis actually occurs in the brain—it initiates in the skin! There is no itch under anesthesia; the new methods of imaging like positron emission tomography (PET) or functional magnetic resonance imaging (fMRI) allow objective examination of the itch sensation in the brain; itch can be visualized (Darsow et al. 2000; Pfab et al. 2010a).

3.5.2 Autonomic Nervous System Dysregulation

Due to the rapid progress in immunology, some aspects of atopy and atopic dermatitis have been forgotten which are a well-known clinical fact and had been studied in the early 1950s, namely, that these patients show an altered reactivity in several autonomic nervous system functions. These aspects have been studied intensively by G. W. Korting in his thesis "Endogenous Eczema" (Korting 1954). Much of this work has been forgotten. In asthma, Szentivanyi developed the theory of beta-adrenergic blockade in the pathophysiology.

In summary, atopic patients and also eczema patients exhibit weaker beta-adrenergic reactions while alpha-adrenergic and cholinergic responses seem to be increased (Szentivanyi 1968; Ring 1979).

Patients with atopic dermatitis show altered responses to certain pharmacological stimuli which can be shown in vivo (Zirbs et al. in press) and in vitro: These phenomena can go along with an altered activity of phosphodiesterase (PDE) and alterations of the cyclic nucleotide metabolism (Butler et al. 1985; Chan et al. 1993). In vitro stimulation with cholinergic stimuli can enhance histamine release (Ring 1981).

Altered reactivity patterns in the autonomic nervous system not only affect immune reactions, but quite normal physiological phenomena such as pupillary reaction in the eye, orthostatic cardiovascular reaction (Schellong-Grote test), and sweating (Korting 1954; Warndorff 1970). In a Japanese study, atopic eczema patients suffered less frequently from hypertonic blood pressure than controls (Uehara M, personal communication 1998).

In a Swedish study, heart rate variability, deep breathing, and orthostatic tests were performed in patients with severe atopic dermatitis, who showed an autonomic dysbalance with higher values for parasympathetic modulation than controls (Boettger et al. 2009).

Elevated intracellular phosphodiesterase levels have led to development of specific PDE inhibitors in the treatment (see Sect. 5.9.19). For a long time, theophylline was also used in eczema treatment; papaverine was used with a clear-cut activity against itch. All these agents are no longer used because of limited specificity and small therapeutic index (see Chap. 5).

The well-known white dermographism and the abnormal delayed blanch reaction to acetylcholine may also be regarded as signs of altered autonomic nervous system reactivity.

Weakened beta-adrenergic reactions can lead to an enhancement of allergic phenomena (Hemels 1970). It is a well-known fact that beta blockers increase asthmatic bronchoconstriction and anaphylactic reactions.

Patients with atopic dermatitis may release vasoactive mediators to minimal stimuli leading to elevated plasma histamine levels, but also to increased secretion of other mediators like leukotrienes (Ruzicka and Ring 1987). These mediators not only have effects as proinflammatory agents, but also act via histamine receptors on lymphocytes, especially regulatory T cells (Jutel et al. 2001) in a way that increased IgE, increased mediator releasability, and decreased regulatory T-cell function can form a vicious cycle (Ring 1981).

On the basis of this autonomic nervous system dysregulation, one may also understand some of the above-mentioned psychological influences, both positive and negative, for the clinical course of eczema since stress and anxiety are able to release the same mediators (histamine) which also are involved in itch and inflammation (Szentivanyi et al. 1980; Giannetti et al. 1992; Grewe et al. 2000; Renz et al. 2006).

3.5.3 The Problem of an "Atopic" Personality (or "Atopic Eczema Personality")

Many doctors—probably on the basis of some remarkable experiences with certain patients—have the prejudice of a typical "atopic eczema personality" (Borelli 1950; Bosse 1990; Hölscher 1998), especially prominent also for mothers of an atopic eczema child; however, this prejudice is not really evidence based. Each of us can tell a story about a very unpleasant meeting with a mother of an eczema child—e.g., a mother who is a teacher and member of the Green Party who knows everything better than the doctor and nurse, demanding a lot of patience—all in all a very subjective and wrong prejudice! There is abundant literature regarding characteristic personality profiles in allergic individuals (Borelli 1950); when studied closely, however, it is surprising how controversial the descriptions are with attributes such as "lack of ability to surrender," "shy," "passive," "introverted" and at the same time with "hyperactive," "need for recognition," "pedantic," "hypercorrect," and "outgoing" (quoted at Whitlock 1976).

Recent literature, however, does not support the existence of a typical atopic or atopic eczema personality profile. Longitudinal examinations found normalization of previously abnormal personality profiles going along with improvement of clinical symptoms (Rechardt 1970).

More psychoanalytically oriented literature supports—sometimes in the early childhood—sexual conflicts as causal for the development of allergy; they see an autoerotic component in the orgiastic scratching against itch (Marty 1958).

Whether psychological factors are actually causal, i.e., relevant in the development of the disease, is still a matter of scientific debate. However, there is no doubt that psychological influences like stress or emotional excitation can trigger and exacerbate eczema flares.

Half of the patients are reporting this experience without doubts.

There are new studies showing that parental partner problems may be a risk factor for the development of atopic dermatitis (see Chap. 1, Sect. 1.5.3).

3.5.4 Parent-Child Relation in Atopic Dermatitis

Family dynamics are of special importance when dealing with children with atopic eczema (Hölscher 1998).

Several studies have shown that atopic dermatitis in childhood goes along with a very negative impact on the family life by inducing physical and mental health problems in mothers especially of severely affected children (Hohao et al. 2010).

In psychodiagnostic tests, we investigated personality profiles of children with atopic eczema and found no statistically significant differences between children with atopic dermatitis and children with other skin diseases with regard to the parameters "neuroticism" and "extraversion" (Ring et al. 1986). In the tests according to the Freiburg Personality Inventory (FPI), mothers of children with atopic eczema were found to be a little "less spontaneous," "more controlled," and "less emotional" than normal. Fathers of atopic children, however, showed no significant differences. There was a trend to increased "irritability."

Since the chronic disease and especially the itch/scratch cycle sometimes are used by the child as "weapon" in order to get his or her will against parental education, it is of interest to study the parental educational style in this disease. Using the educational tables according to Stang, we found that, in the educational style perceived from the eyes of the children, the parameter "strictness" of the mother was stronger noted than in controls, while the educational style of the fathers was equal. Looking in detail, it was interesting that, from the eyes of the eczema children, mothers of eczema children more often would reward "adult behavior" while the parameter "affective warmth" or "shared joy" was less strongly expressed (Ring et al. 1986).

When we made the children draw the family—either as persons or as animals—eczema children in their drawings showed a less friendly atmosphere than was normally seen in control children (note: they suffered from other skin diseases leading to hospitalization!) (Fig. 3.16). Of special interest was that the body size of the mother usually was drawn larger than that of the father in atopic eczema children: The father to mother ratio was 0.7–1, while control children showed 1.1–1, which probably corresponded to the physical reality (Ring et al. 1986) (Fig. 3.17). In an audio play written together with Prof. Schröpl (Ring and Schröpl 1989), typical scenes in the doctor's office were performed by actors: A family enters the office with the affected 10-year-old girl, and the doctor asks history questions which are only answered by the mother like "we have this since birth," "we suffer from terrible itch," "we cannot sleep at night," etc. The father stays in the background, asks whether there is extra payment necessary, and then retreats in the corner. After a while, the doctor asks the mother, looking intensively at her: "My lady, don't you notice that I am not talking to you?" With that, the girl smiles for the first time and the mother blushes. By such a "blow," one can achieve that the child takes over some responsibility for herself or himself. Of course, I never want to insult a mother, and I immediately apologize after the visit. But sometimes many weeks or months later a mother comes to me telling "this was really tough, doctor, at the first visit in your office—but you were so right; it's not *my* skin. I should be more relaxed!"

In a study investigating the psychosocial adaptation in Korean schoolchildren, it was found that allergic children had more problems when they had acute symptoms of atopic dermatitis; these children exhibited more "internalizing problems"; this was increasingly observed with an increasing number of IgE-mediated sensitizations. Boys seemed to be more prone to show these alterations than girls (Park et al. 2011).

It is clear that most likely the maternal behavior is not the cause, but the result or the consequence of the eczema of the child, the mothers usually bearing much more work in taking care of the children and of the disease than the fathers. So as a very practical advice, I sometimes say "Daddy, take over and let's send Mommy to the Caribbean for a holiday!" Unfortunately the insurance does not pay this.

One could go on for hours with these stories; my recommendations regarding various attitudes of parent-child affection in atopic dermatitis are briefly summarized in Table 3.10.

3.5.5 Stress and Atopic Dermatitis

Gieler and coworkers found that patients with atopic dermatitis and especially some subgroups show markedly elevated values for "anxiety," "depression," as well as "hostility" which, however, in general are suppressed by the patients (Gieler et al. 1992; Wright 2005).

Conflict situations (private problems, occupational stress) or special situations (examination, wedding) may trigger eczema flares. Itch as a

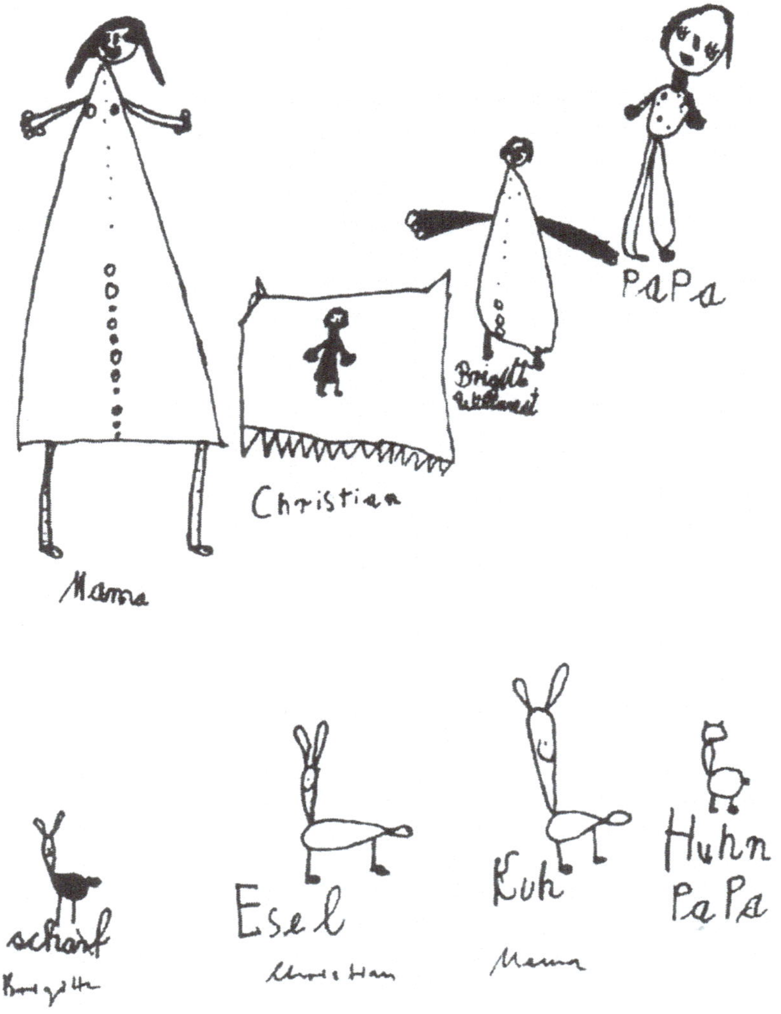

Fig. 3.16 Children's drawing of a girl with atopic eczema illustrating the family in a rather rigid mode with little contact (From Ring et al. (1986))

symptom can go along with aggressive behavior. Today the term "stress" is used to describe these psychosocial interferences. Doctor and patients use it without thinking; however, when asked for a definition, there is often silence or stuttering.

It is helpful to look at the history: The term "stress" was coined by Hans Selye in 1936 when he as a medical student was asked by the professor in the big lecture while presenting a case, "What do you notice about the patient?" and Selye answered, "He looks sick," generating laughter in the audience. However, Selye wanted to describe better this phenomenon so obvious as "looking sick." In trying to do this, he created a new term which meant an "unspecific response of the body to some challenge."

For many years the phenomenon was regarded to be purely biological; however, over the decades, it has also been used in the psychological area.

Based on various authors (von Eiff 1984; Young et al. 1986), we define

> Stress as a "primary unspecific psychobiologic reaction to a threat for the individual physico-chemical or psychological well-being." (Ring 2005)

It does not make sense to talk of "stress reaction" since the reaction is already contained in the

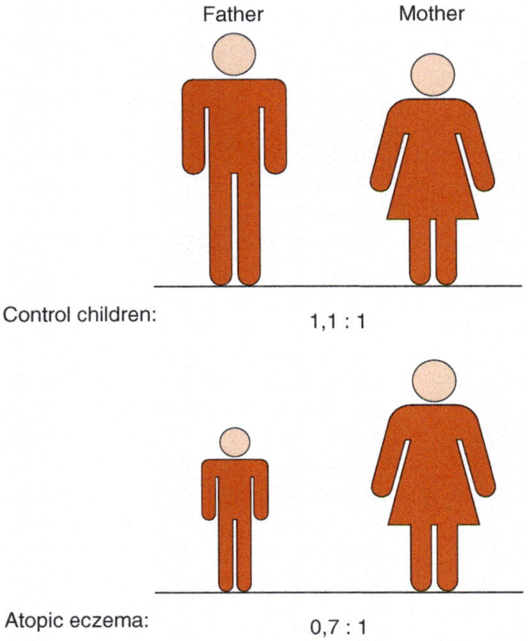

Fig. 3.17 Family dynamic in the psychosomatic interactions in atopic eczema. Comparison of size of father and mother of children with atopic eczema and control children with other skin diseases. In children with atopic eczema, the mother seems to be too tall compared to the father

Table 3.10 Ways of parental affection and educational style of particular relevance in atopic dermatitis

Bad	Good
Tenseness—no	Concern—yes
Rigorousness—no	Consequence—yes
Dominance—no	Strength—yes
Overpowering—no	Motivation—yes
Indifference—no	Relaxedness—yes
Ambition—no	Love—yes

term stress. Elicitors of stress are also called stressors and can be of various origins (Table 3.11).

Regarding the timely course, one can distinguish between acute and chronic stress. Especially the latter may induce psychosomatic complaints such as anxiety, loss of activity, impairment of self-confidence, and vasovagal reactions and hyperventilation (Sapolsky 1992).

Stress also can alter skin barrier function. Studies have shown that the local production of corticotrophin-releasing factor (CRF) may influence the integrity of stratum corneum (Kokao et al. 2003).

Table 3.11 Various kinds of stressors

Physical	Chemical	Biological	Psychosocial (life events)
Trauma	Environmental pollution	Nutrition	Grief
Pain		Infection	Anxiety
Exhaustion		Allergens	Depression
Heat			Emotional excitation
Cold			
Noise			

Stress may act via various mechanisms and induce physiologic or pathophysiologic changes which lead to symptoms in the nervous or endocrine system or in several organs.

Also modulation of the serotoninergic neurotransmitter system may play a role. In patients with severe atopic dermatitis, increased expression of several serotonin receptors has been found in the epidermis (Lonne-Rahm et al. 2008).

Also the expression of nerve growth factor (NGF) discovered 50 years ago (Levi-Montalcini 1987; Yamaguchi et al. 1991) has been found altered in inflammatory skin diseases such as psoriasis, but most expressed in atopic dermatitis, where it was found to correlate with the severity of itch and objective signs of eczematous inflammation (Yamaguchi et al. 1991).

There are different methodologies to measure and quantify stress (Ravens-Sieberer and Bullinger 1998) (Tables 3.12 and 3.13).

3.5.6 Psychosocial Stress

Stress is also dependent on sociocultural aspects since many stressors come from psychosocial environment. Aleksandr Solzhenitsyn criticized the culturally accepted drive for profit of the Western world which leads to exaggerated competition, personal isolation, and beyond to a more and more egoistic attitude with a vicious circle of stress (quoted in Young et al. 1986).

Observations from Japan after the big earthquake in Kobe (Hanshin) of 1995 have shown that 38 % of patients with atopic dermatitis showed marked deterioration of eczema compared to 7 %

Table 3.12 Possible mechanisms of stress influence upon allergic reactions

Tissue	Cells/mediators	Clinical consequences
Nervous system	Nociceptors Neurotransmitters Autonomic impulses (weak beta-adrenergic, increased cholinergic)	Effects upon immune and inflammatory cells as well as manifestation organ
Endocrine system	Hypothalamus (CRF) Adrenal glands (catecholamines)	Hormone effects
Immune system	Th1 NK cells Th1/Th2 deviation Inflammatory cells	Immunodeficiency Susceptibility to infection IgE formation (allergy) Mediator release
End organ (airway, skin)	Mucous secretion Bronchoconstriction Vasodilatation Itch	Rhinopathy Asthma Urticaria Eczema

Table 3.13 Techniques to measure and quantify stress

Chemical	Physiological	Psychological
Determination of hormones or autacoids	Pulse	Cognitive activity
Adrenaline	Blood pressure	Affect resonance
Noradrenaline	ECG	Psychodiagnostic tests (e.g., STAI)
Metabolites	Muscle tension (electromyogram)	
Adrenocorticotropic	Skin temperature	
Hormone ACTH	Skin perfusion	
Corticotropin-releasing factor (CRF)	Electrical resistance	
Neurotrophin	EEG changes	
Nerve growth factor (NGF)		
Aldosterone, renin		
Angiotensin		
Histamine		

in a control group without earthquake. Nine percent of the patients from the earthquake region experienced marked improvement of the eczema (Kodama et al. 1999).

In a multivariate regression analysis, the subjective stress was the best indicator to predict an eczema flare. Everyday stress situations can influence atopic dermatitis considerably. Many studies show that stress can trigger exacerbations of atopic eczema (Hünecke 1993, Kilpelainen et al. 2002; Münzel 1999).

Especially in adult atopic eczema, psychosomatic interaction and psychological problems are common. In a case control study, affective- and stress-related behavioral and psychiatric conditions were investigated; it was found that eczema was independently associated with several of these conditions (Schmitt et al. 2009a, b).

Münzel and Schandry (1990) have investigated several types of stress in patients with atopic dermatitis and healthy controls with regard to physiological effects on pulse rate, electrical skin resistance, and skin temperature. Thereby patients with atopic eczema reacted stronger to emotional stress (when they were asked to express an opinion in front of a group) than to mental stress (counting backwards).

There are several psychodiagnostic test procedures to evaluate various stress situations: there is the State-Trait Anxiety Inventory (STAI) as well as the "social readjustment rate scale." High values in these tests mean an increased risk for future disease.

When talking about psychological influence upon disease, one should never forget that the questions what is cause and what is sequel of a disease often remain open. It is a characteristic of skin diseases that they not only represent a disturbance of the function of one organ, but that they always also have a psychological component, since the skin is an expression organ of the psyche and has an eminent aesthetic function (Pallas et al. 2010).

3.5.7 Attention-Deficit/Hyperactivity Disorder (ADHD)

There is a long discussion and controversy as to whether atopic dermatitis children have an increased risk for ADHD or whether symptoms of ADHD are due to allergic reactions. In a birth cohort study followed over 10 years, it was found that indeed there was an association of ADHD and atopic dermatitis which, however, appeared to be partly explained by sleeping problems in early childhood, thus giving rise to ADHD (Romanos et al 2010; Schmitt et al. 2010).

3.6 Hormones

It is surprising that hormonal influences upon allergy development are only little investigated. It is common knowledge that some allergic diseases like asthma or atopic dermatitis in early childhood are more frequent in boys than in girls, while in adults the female sex is much more often affected. This gives rise to the speculation that sex hormones may play a role (Chen et al. 2008).

Indeed patients with severe atopic eczema may more frequently show signs of testosterone deficiency (Weidinger et al. 2004a, b). Substitution of testosterone in a patient with gonadal dysgenesis and concomitant severe nummular eczema leads to a marked improvement of the previously therapy-resistant eczema (Neuber et al. 1993).

Mast cells have shown to carry androgen receptors, and androgenic hormones may inhibit mediator release (Chen et al. 2008). Estrogens seem to have an enhancing effect upon B cells with regard to transformation in IgE-secreting plasma cells (Kamml et al. in prep).

3.6.1 Summary

There is no doubt that patients with atopic dermatitis show altered reactivity patterns in the autonomic nervous system in the sense of a weaker beta-adrenergic and increased alpha-adrenergic and cholinergic reactivity. This not only holds true for cellular functions of lymphocytes and mast cells but also for cardiovascular parameters.

There is no specific "atopic" or "atopic eczema" personality as is often quoted in a prejudice of many doctors. However, psychological influences play a distinct role in the elicitation and maintenance of allergic and eczematous skin reactions. Stress can influence allergic reactions and trigger or worsen atopic dermatitis. Psychological influences can also be observed within families with atopic eczema children. Family dynamics are therefore important to be studied and considered in the management, which is part of some educational programs in "eczema school."

Management of Patients with Atopic Eczema

4

Many patients with atopic dermatitis are desperate, change doctors, and visit "witchcraft" and "shaman" gurus because they have heard that atopic dermatitis is incurable. Many physicians use this sentence to finally be left in peace by demanding patients or parents. Of course they feel correct with this sentence stressing the genetic predisposition which is inborn and which cannot be altered at the moment. However, one has to clearly distinguish: The genetic disposition of atopy or atopic dermatitis cannot be changed today; however, molecular genetics may soon be valuable in predictive diagnostics.

These genetic markers, however, are not the disease; the disease "atopic dermatitis" can very well be treated and very often disappears over long periods or for lifetime. Therefore, I never use the term "incurable"; I prefer to tell the patients that they have a problem and a tendency to develop hypersensitivity reactions of the skin and maybe elsewhere but that these clinical conditions can very well be treated. I tell my patients that streptococcal tonsillitis cannot be called "incurable" just because there may be a relapse. The angina can very well be treated.

Based on the complex etiopathophysiological mechanisms involved, it becomes clear that therapeutic management in most patients requires a complex program of management including aspects of diagnostics, prevention, and actual treatment.

Therapeutic procedures focus on the one hand on the acute treatment of the inflammatory skin disease; on the other hand and at the same time, they have to include preventive aspects regarding the disturbed skin barrier function and individual provocation factors which can be avoided (Abeck and Ring 2002; Abels and Brocks 2006; Akdis et al. 2006; Braun-Falco and Ring 1984; Ellis et al. 2003; Harper et al. 2002; Leung and Barber 2003; Przybilla et al. 1994; Schnopp and Ring 2003; Ring et al. 2012; Darsow et al. 2013; Wollenberg et al. [in press]). The acute eczema flare can be treated very well; it is difficult to predict the intensity and frequency of new flares.

The tendency to develop hypersensitivity reactions of the skin requires special care and may be time-consuming.

Thus, management of atopic dermatitis is much more than writing a prescription for a tablet or an ointment. Rather, it requires intense diagnostics including allergy diagnosis for individual provocation factors and needs a confidential cooperation between physician and patient so that behavioral changes can be induced. The motivation of the patient or the parents to take responsibility for the disease has to be slowly developed (patient "empowerment") and often needs special educational programs. These aspects will be covered in Sect. 6.4 (Eczema School). I like to call the whole bunch of procedures to be done in order to improve the clinical condition "patient management" (Ring et al. 1996). These procedures comprise much more than diagnostics and treatment and include recommendations regarding nutrition, style of living, leisure activities, occupational counseling, etc.

J. Ring, *Atopic Dermatitis: Eczema*, DOI 10.1007/978-3-319-22243-1_4

4.1 Diagnostic Procedures

There are few diseases where diagnostics and therapy are so closely connected as in allergy and especially atopic dermatitis.

This chapter does not deal with the actual diagnosis "atopic dermatitis" and considerations for differential diagnosis, but it reflects the ongoing diagnostic procedures necessary in the individual patient after the diagnosis "atopic dermatitis" has been made (Prucha et al. 2013). Like in all other allergic diseases, the procedure can be classified into four steps (Darsow and Ring 2000; Høst et al. 2003) which are connected to each other (Ring 2005) (Fig. 4.1):

- History
- Skin test procedures
- In vitro allergy diagnostics
- Provocation tests

At the moment there is no standard routine procedure for provocation testing with aeroallergens in atopic eczema such as an exposure in a standardized chamber (pollen chamber) with varying concentrations of aeroallergens (Heratizadeh et al. 2015). Thus, provocation tests at the moment are restricted to food and food additives (see below).

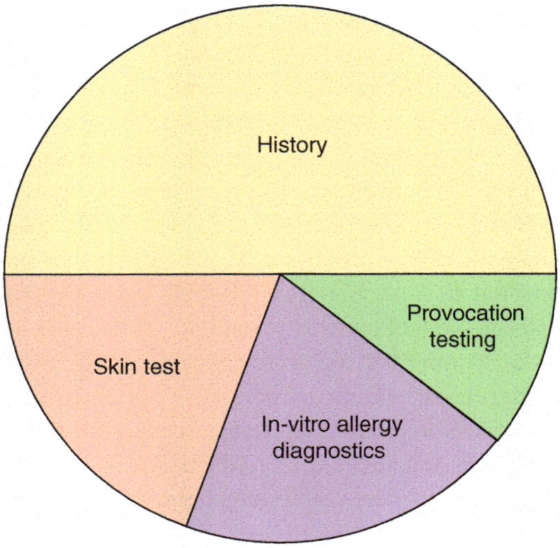

Fig. 4.1 The four major parts of allergy diagnosis

4.1.1 History

A very careful history not only considers the clinical course of the disease but also includes questions regarding the symptoms, the onset, the duration, the timely course, and the circumstances with regard to possible triggering factors like seasonal, local, and occupational conditions. Activities in holidays or leisure, application of drugs, hormonal situation, and stress all have to be included in a careful history in atopic dermatitis (Brockow et al. 1999a) (Table 4.1).

Table 4.1 Contents of a good history in atopic dermatitis

Symptoms
Onset (first onset, acute disease)
Duration
Timely course (circadian, around the year, seasonal)
Intensity (severity)
Frequency
Response to therapy
Exacerbation by therapy
Hospitalization
Concomitant diseases
Personal history (atopy)
Family history (atopy)
Other diseases (gastroesophageal reflux, skin or airway diseases)
Eliciting factors and environmental aspects
Season
Local environment (indoor, outdoor)
Occupation
Holiday
Hobby
Drugs
Foods
Exercise
Stress, emotional excitement
Common cold (viral infection)
UV light
Hormonal situation (menstruation, pregnancy)
Lifestyle
Living, apartment
Animal contact (also passive)
Tobacco smoke (active, passive)
House dust mite, molds
Chemicals
Plants
Cosmetics
Snarling, breathing through the mouth

4.1.2 Skin Test Procedures

Among various skin test procedures, primarily those which are done percutaneously (scratch test, skin prick test) as well as patch test procedures are discussed.

4.1.3 Prick and Intradermal Test

The most commonly used skin test is the skin prick test where a drop of an allergen extract is applied to the skin and pricked with a special lancet, preferably without bleeding. After 15 min, it is read. Positive prick test reactions are typical for atopic diseases; occasionally, they are exclusively used for the diagnosis of atopy. It is estimated that 90 % of atopics show positive skin prick test reactions against common aero- or food allergens (especially cat, house dust mite, and grass pollen) (Guillett and Guillett 1992; Schäfer et al. 1997a). In the intradermal test, 0.02–0.05 ml of an allergen dilution are injected strictly intradermally, using a small needle. Intradermal tests are necessary when prick tests remain negative in spite of a suggestive history.

The interpretation of the test results has to be done with regard to possible clinical relevance from detailed history or provocation test (see below).

4.1.4 Atopy Patch Test (APT)

Positive skin prick tests or specific IgE antibodies against aeroallergens or foods almost routinely can be found in atopic dermatitis. The relevance of these sensitizations was controversial over decades. In the philosophy of this disease in the last hundred years, the estimation of allergy playing a role went up and down like modes of fashion. Decades where merely the dry skin or the psychological influence was in the focus alternated with phases where the role of allergy was put forward strongly. Mainly due to lack of methods, this uncertainty continued. It is a clear clinical experience that many patients develop flares after contact with animal dander or in dusty environments while they experience improvement in allergen-free rooms or under high-altitude conditions (Borelli et al. 1967; Storm van Leeuwen et al. 1926).

At the end of the 1970s of the twentieth century, several working groups wanted to develop a test procedure as a correlate for these clinical observations, since the skin prick test alone was not suitable. It correlated much better with the allergic airway reactions of hay fever or asthma than with the atopic dermatitis symptoms.

We first tried the intradermal test with a late reading and believed to find a correlate in the so-called late-phase reaction (LPR) similar to severe cases of bronchial asthma (Dorsch et al. 1982). This late cutaneous reaction (LCR) was regarded as a model of atopic eczema; however, the absence of epidermal involvement, which is so characteristic of the eczematous inflammation, was an argument against this idea (see Chap. 1).

Therefore, we and other groups tried to induce eczema by epicutaneous application of aeroallergens; we used intradermal and prick test extracts and remained unsuccessful for many years. Others tried to come to positive test reactions by manipulation of the test areas through tape stripping or preceding scratching with irritation. The breakthrough was done by the group of Thomas Platts-Mills (Mitchell et al. 1982; Platts-Mills et al. 1983) who were able to induce eczematous skin reactions after application of house dust mite extract on rather large skin areas. Therefore, in the future we used larger Finn chambers than normally used for the classical patch test in contact allergy and were equally successful in the procedure which we called "atopy patch test" (APT) (Darsow et al. 1996, 1999; Ring et al. 1989, 1997, 2001b; Vieluf et al. 1993).

In the 1990s, we standardized the APT with regard to methodology, skin test site, influence of medication, extracts used, etc., especially also considering the vehicles (Darsow et al. 1996; Langeveld-Wildschut et al. 2000). Today, we can say that the atopy patch test represents a standard procedure in allergy diagnostics for patients with atopic dermatitis (Darsow et al. 1999) (Fig. 4.2). Contrary to our theoretical considerations, where we thought that a hydrophilic emulsion would be

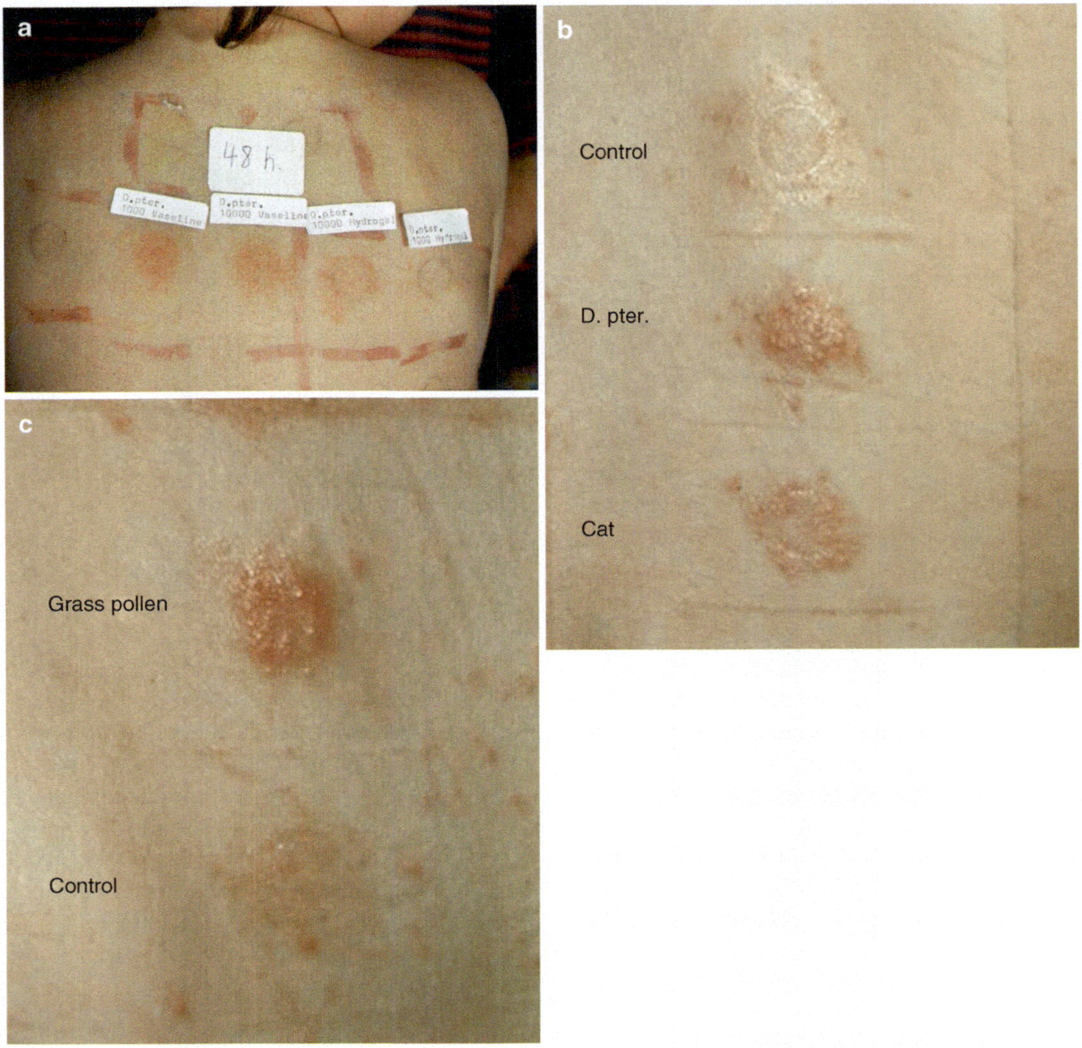

Fig. 4.2 Positive atopy patch test after 48 h. (**a**) Comparison of petrolatum and hydrogel as vehicle. (**b**) Allergen 200 IR/G (Index of Reactivity) in petrolatum. (**c**) Grass pollen and petrolatum control

better for the application of protein allergens, petrolatum proved to be the most reliable vehicle also for the atopy patch test (Fig. 4.2a) (Darsow et al. 1996).

4.1.5 Differences to Classical Patch Test

Apart from the methodology (use of larger diameter Finn chambers), there are differences between the atopy patch test and the classical patch test in contact allergy also in the reading of the test results (Table 4.2). In the atopy patch test, the substances used are protein allergens, while in the contact allergy patch test, small chemicals (haptens) are used. Furthermore, there are differences in morphology, dermatohistology, and time course. The classical patch test shows a typical crescendo pattern with a maximum of the reaction after 72 h; in atopy patch test, often a maximum is already reached after 48 h. The reproducibility of the atopy patch test is very good with 80–90 %. In the histopathology, an

Table 4.2 Difference between classical patch test in contact allergy and atopy patch test

Criteria	Patch test contact allergy	Atopy patch test
Nature of allergens	Low-molecular-weight chemicals	Proteins
Kinetic of the reaction	Maximum after 72 h (crescendo)	Often after 24 h
Morphology	Papulovesicular with spreading	Often follicular, rarely vesiculous
Dermatohistology	CD4 lymphocytes, Th1	CD4, Th2 Eosinophils
Indication	Allergic contact dermatitis	Atopic dermatitis

early influx of eosinophils and eosinophil products can be seen in the atopy patch test more commonly than in contact allergy. Clinically, often follicular patterns are observed; real vesicular or bullous reactions are extremely rare. The European Task Force on Atopic Dermatitis (ETFAD) has come up with a special reading guide for APT reactions (Darsow et al. 1999).

Unfortunately, test reagents are in many countries not routinely available; they have to be self-made by best using lyophilized allergens in petrolatum to be mixed by an experienced pharmacist (Darsow et al. 1996).

Pathophysiologically, the atopy patch test represents an artificially induced atopic inflammation after penetration of high-molecular weight allergens into the epidermis. These are recognized and taken up by dendritic cells (see Sect. 3.3). IgE and IgE-binding receptors have been recognized on the surface of epidermal dendritic cells partly in colocalization with house dust mite allergen (Maeda et al. 1992; Tanaka et al. 1990). From atopy patch test biopsies, specific T cell clones could be isolated which characteristically show a Th2 cytokine pattern. At a later point of time—after 48 h or in more chronic lesions—also in atopic inflammation Th1 patterns become visible (Bruijnzeel-Koomen et al. 1989; Kondo et al. 1998, van Reijsen et al. 1992; Wistokat-Wülfing et al. 1998).

In a common study of the European Task Force on Atopic Dermatitis (ETFAD), the atopy patch test was further standardized. Petrolatum was chosen as vehicle; the protein allergens from lyophilized extracts, together with minimal concentrations of an emulsifying agent, cetylpyridinium chloride, were mixed with petrolatum. In large Finn chambers (1 cm in diameter), they are applied to uninvolved and unaltered skin, preferably on the back. For the most common aeroallergens in central Europe, eliciting allergen doses between 5000 and 7000 protein nitrogen units (PNU) were used.

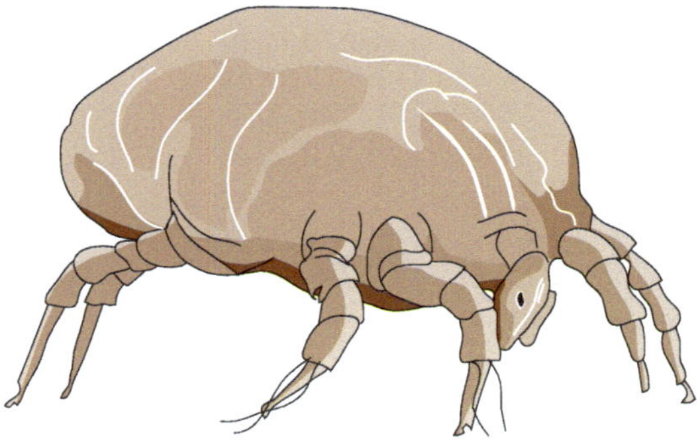

Fig. 4.3 The most common allergen positive in atopy patch is house dust mite *Dermatophagoides pteronyssinus*

4.1.6 Results

The most common positive APT reactions were found with aeroallergens like house dust mite (Deleuran et al. 1998; Gondo et al. 1986) (Fig. 4.3), but also cat epithelium and pollen allergens are often positive (Darsow et al. 1996). The APT is dose-dependent and especially positive in patients where the eczematous skin lesions occur in air-exposed areas as, e.g., face, hands, or forearms. In a comparison of various test procedures, the clear-cut history in disease exacerbation offers that allergen contact was taken as gold standard; the following sensitivities and specificities could be calculated (Table 4.3). In 75 % of patients who had an exacerbation during the last preceding pollen season, atopy patch test against grass pollen was positive compared to only 16 % in eczema patients without seasonal exacerbation.

Compared to skin prick test and radioallergosorbent test (specific IgE antibodies), APT showed a lower sensitivity (75 %) compared to almost 100 % for the skin prick test, which is natural when we regard the atopy definition (see above). However, the specificity was much higher (80–90 %) for the atopy patch test compared to 40–60 % for skin prick test or RAST. It is possible, using the APT, to evaluate the relevance of an IgE-mediated sensitization for the actual eczematous skin changes and not for general allergy (see Fig. 4.4).

Considerations regarding the concordance of the various test results are of special interest. There are patients with negative prick test and RAST and positive atopy patch test (Kerschenlohr et al. 2003b). In 53 of 314 patients (14 %), at least one allergen was positive in APT without corresponding sensitization in skin prick test or RAST (Table 4.4). This is interesting with regard to the question regarding intrinsic versus extrinsic atopic eczema (see Chap. 1). According to our understanding, positive atopy patch test reactions should be regarded as a sign of extrinsic atopic dermatitis, even if skin prick test and IgE are negative. Possibly the IgE reaction takes place without involvement of mast cells or circulating IgE antibodies but with involvement of IgE on the surface of dendritic cells.

The atopy patch test meanwhile has become a routine diagnostic procedure starting as a merely scientific instrument. We only recommend house

Table 4.3 Sensitivity and specificity of various test procedures in patients with atopic dermatitis using clear-cut personal history as gold standard (Darsow et al. 1999)

Test	Sensitivity (in %)	Specificity (in %)
Grass pollen (*n*=79) Skin prick test	100	33
Specific IgE	92	33
Atopy patch test	75	84
European Multicenter Study (*n*=314) Skin prick test	68–80	50–71
Specific IgE	72–84	2–69
Atopy patch test	15–45	64–91
German Multicenter Study (*n*=253) Skin prick test	69–81	44–53
Specific IgE	65–94	42–64
Atopy patch test	42–56	69–92

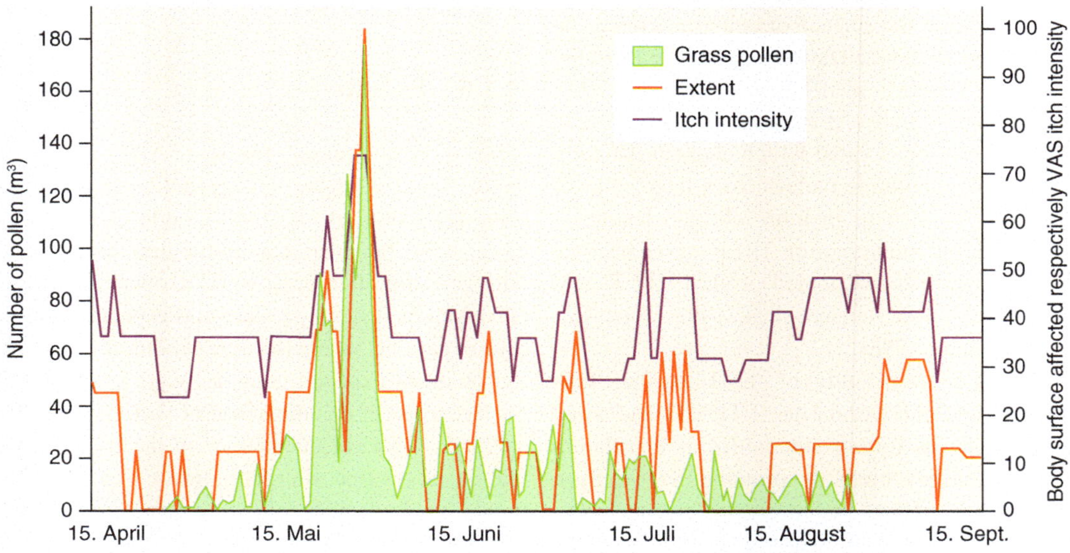

Fig. 4.4 Relevance of pollen exposure for exacerbation of atopic eczema in children (From MIRIAM-Panel-Study Augsburg, see Krämer et al. (2005))

Table 4.4 Positive atopy patch test in patients with negative prick test and negative RAST (43 out of 314 patients)

N	Allergens
31	*Dermatophagoides pteronyssinus*
7	Cat epithelium
8	Grass pollen
16	Birch pollen
11	Hen's egg
16	Celery
18	Wheat flour

dust mite avoidance with corresponding living and bedroom changes when the atopy patch test is positive.

4.1.7 Problem Food Allergens

The use of the atopy patch test with food allergens remains difficult (Werfel et al. 2007). While some years ago there was the big hope that, by using APT, one could replace time-consuming provocation tests in eczema (Niggemann et al. 2000; 2001), the nature and quality of food allergen extracts seem to be problematic. Direct application of native wheat flour, e.g., may be irritative. Atopy patch test with food is still a matter of scientific studies. However, in our and others' experience (A Taieb et al., personal communication 1998), there are clear-cut positive APT reactions with foods especially in children who are negative in skin prick test and RAST and where this reaction is of clinical relevance.

4.1.8 Classic Patch Test for Contact Allergy

While some years ago allergic contact dermatitis was not regarded to be a problem in atopic eczema or was expected to occur much less frequently, recent studies have shown that contact allergy also represents a problem in atopic dermatitis. A recent study shows that in 6 % of over 600 patch-tested children with atopic dermatitis, positive epicutaneous tests were found especially for topical preparations such as emollients and antiseptics, particularly in children with severe atopic eczema (Mailhol et al. 2009; Lipozenzic and Wolf 2007).

Many studies have shown that allergic contact dermatitis can occur in patients with atopic dermatitis, especially in chronic hand dermatitis (Lipozencic and Wolf 2007; Rysted 1985; Schnuch et al. 2006; Dinkloh et al. 2015) (see Sect. 2.7.7 Contact Allergy). There are numerous studies showing that patients with atopic eczema also suffer from contact allergy. In our own study, we found 41 % (Enders et al. 1988) positive patch test reactions in atopic eczema patients. This also holds true for children who have been rarely tested epicutaneously so far. In an epidemiologic study, we found in preschool children up to 15 % allergic contact individuals, especially prominent to nickel, whereby there was a clear-cut correlation to ear piercing and nickel allergy in small girls (Kunz et al. 1990). But also chronic foot eczema can be due to contact allergy against shoe materials.

4.1.9 Testing of Corticosteroids

It is recommended to test patients with atopic dermatitis also with classical patch tests in order to rule out contact allergies. Special consideration should be given to the testing of topicals used, especially corticosteroid topicals which in chronic eczema can also act as contact allergens. This is often not easy to diagnose, since the pharmacological effect of anti-inflammatory cortisone acts against the inflammation while at the same time the nature as contact allergen maintains the inflammation. Therefore, in therapy-resistant eczema, the testing of topical corticosteroids is recommended also in children (Mailhol et al. 2009; Rycroft et al. 1991; Rystedt 1985, 1986; Susitaival and Hannuksela 1995; Uehara and Sawai 1989).

4.1.10 In Vitro Allergy Diagnosis

In vitro allergy diagnosis plays an important role in the management, especially in cases of severe atopic eczema with generalized skin lesions or under systemic medications.

4.1.11 Specific IgE Antibodies

The determination of specific IgE antibodies in serum is in the focus and represents the major progress in allergy diagnostics in the last fifty years. Since the introduction of radioallergosorbent test (RAST), a variety of procedures has been developed to measure circulating specific IgE antibodies in the serum in a quantitative or semiquantitative way (RAST classes or units kU/L).

Total serum IgE also should be determined; however, it is of less relevance. In extremely high serum IgE levels (above 1000 kU/L), mostly very severe cases of atopic eczema, the interpretation of specific IgE has to be modified because of the high background noise. Probably the ratio of specific IgE to total IgE may have a better diagnostic relevance with regard to the specific sensitization (Huss-Marp et al. 2011). Total IgE elevations can be regarded as general marker of the atopic diathesis. Atopic eczema is one of those diseases with the highest serum IgE levels measured, higher than in respiratory atopy (Wüthrich 1975; Ring et al. 2006).

4.1.12 Cellular In Vitro Allergy Testing

In rare cases, when no specific IgE is detectable in serum, the determination of basophil activation after allergen stimulation can be helpful, either as activation of basophil leukocytes by expression of CD63 (Basotest) or CD203 (flow CAST) (Sanz et al. 2002). Also the measurement of histamine or sulfidoleukotriene secretion from basophil leukocytes after allergen stimulation can give information (CAST-ELISA). With regard to delayed reactions of eczema exacerbation, also lymphocyte transformation tests have been used. The group around Thomas Werfel found food-dependent allergen-specific T cell clones (Reekers et al. 1996; Werfel and Kapp 2002; Werfel et al. 1996). All these methods are scientific in nature and have not found entrance into daily clinical use.

4.1.13 Oral Provocation Test in Food Allergy

Many patients with atopic eczema suffer from food hypersensitivity with variable manifestation, either as urticaria, angioedema, anaphylaxis (Jäger and Wüthrich 2001; Ring 1978), or exacerbation of an existing atopic dermatitis. The frequency of food allergy in atopic eczema is estimated around 20–30 % in childhood and considerably lower among adults (Ring et al. 2012). The most frequent food allergens in childhood atopic eczema are ovalbumin, cow's milk, soy, wheat, but also peanut and tree nuts.

In diagnostics of food allergy, the real art is—as general in allergy diagnosis—to evaluate the relevance of a sensitization for the clinical disease. Many children have positive skin prick tests to various foods without ever noticing any deterioration of the symptoms after intake. Therefore, especially in this area, dietary recommendations should be very well considered (Kleine-Tebbe et al. 2009). We recommend the avoidance of a food only when the relevance of a sensitization for atopic eczema or for another allergic disease is certain.

4.1.14 Double-Blind Provocation Test

The determination of relevance can be done by clear-cut history (rather rare) or by oral provocation test best performed in double-blind procedure. The groups around Werfel and Niggemann found, in studies with double-blind, placebo-controlled oral provocation test, clear-cut positive reactions in over 50 % of the children (Niggemann et al. 2001; Werfel and Breuer 2004), similar to the results of Sampson (2001, 2003).

The timely appearance of skin lesions occurred in a majority of cases relatively rapidly (30 min to 2 h). Ca. 15 % react only after 12–48 h, which sometimes is difficult to recognize under daily life conditions. A rather large number of patients also experience immediate-type reactions together with delayed-type reactions to foods.

4.1.15 Practical Performance

The performance of a placebo-controlled oral provocation test needs a good blinding of foods which mostly are applied in porridge form (Bindslev-Jensen et al. 2004; Werfel et al. 2008a). The selection of the vehicle has to be done on the basis of previous allergy tests (skin prick test, RAST) since occasionally there are also allergens against unsuspicious foods like St. John's bread. The foods to be tested are mixed with the placebo ground substance together with unsuspicious colorings and flavors (e.g., black currant juice) for blinding.

In the oral provocation test, food additives should not be forgotten since they also can trigger exacerbations in atopic eczema, especially in adults (van Bever et al. 1989; Vieluf et al. 1999). According to the schedule of the oral provocation test for idiosyncrasy (OPTI), as it is performed in chronic urticaria (Ring 2005) also in patients with atopic dermatitis, the detection of a pseudo-allergic hypersensitivity against food additives can be achieved (Ring et al. 1987; Worm et al. 2000) especially against sulfites.

With a history of severe anaphylaxis and positive skin prick test or RAST results, one can refrain from oral provocation.

In order to estimate the relevance of a sensitization for atopic dermatitis, however, provocation is often mandatory. The double-blind, placebo-controlled oral provocation test until now remains the gold standard and is usually done in specialized centers (Bindslev-Jensen et al. 2004). It can be further improved by the measurement of mediators in plasma during the provocation procedures (Ohtsuka et al. 1993). For the daily practice, a nutrition diary is recommended where the patient or the parents record the symptoms, together with the food intake (see Chap. 6).

4.1.16 Skin Test Versus RAST

Unfortunately, the predictive value of skin prick test and RAST with regard to food allergy in atopic eczema is limited. The positive predictive value (PPV) of food allergen-specific IgE is only around 30 % for eczematous skin reactions, while it is 60 % for clear-cut immediate-type reactions (Werfel et al. 2008a). Also the nature of the eliciting food allergen plays a role: The relevance of sensitization against hen's egg or peanut is much higher than that of positive test against cow's milk or cereals.

The role of atopy patch test in the diagnostic procedure for food allergy is controversial (see Sect. 4.1.4).

4.1.17 Microbiological Diagnostics

Based on the considerations regarding pathophysiology (see Sect. 3.4), microbial factors with colonization or infection of the skin surface should also be considered in the diagnostic procedure.

Microbiological examination makes sense and should cover the following aspects:

- Bacteriological swabs of lesional and uninvolved skin as well as nasal mucosa (especially *S. aureus*)
- Mycological examination of squamous material especially in the head/neck region (Malassezia furfur)
- Virus detection of HSV when eczema herpeticum is suspected

In infants and small children with oozing skin lesions, superinfection is common not only by staphylococci but also by streptococci (impetiginized eczema). These considerations will also find entrance into the therapy (see Sect. 5.3).

4.1.18 Psychological Diagnostics

The clear-cut influence of psychological factors upon the clinical course of atopic dermatitis should be considered also in the diagnostic steps, and if there is an indication, psychosomatic counseling together with the use of validated questionnaires is recommended (Stauder and Kovacs 2003) (see Sect. 3.5).

In particular the following instruments have proven helpful:

- Marburg Skin Questionnaire (Marburger Hautfragebogen MHF)
- Cognitive Itch Questionnaire (Juckreiz-Kognitions-Fragebogen JKF) (Stangier et al. 1996)
- Dermatology Quality of Life Index DQLI (Finlay and Khan 1994) (Deutsches Instrument zur Erfassung der Lebensqualität bei Hautkrankheiten, DIELH) (Schäfer et al. 2001; Staudt et al. 2002) (German Instrument for Quality of Life in Skin Diseases)
- Eppendorf Itch Questionnaire (Darsow et al. 1997a, 2001)

In addition there are specific questionnaires for children (Ravens-Sieberer and Bullinger 1998).

Often the motivation to write a diary for self-observation is very helpful for the patient in order to recognize the influence of psychological factors.

The most common psychological provocation factors comprise stress of any kind, both mental and emotional in nature (Richter and Dahme 1987). Furthermore, memories to significant life events which have not adequately been coped with, also too intensive concern with regard to the own skin disease, may have an enhancing or prolonging character (Hölscher 1998). The naive and well-meant question "How does your skin feel?" can occasionally trigger an intense itch crisis. Parents and relatives should be careful!

4.1.19 Summary

There are only few diseases where diagnostics and therapy are so closely connected as in allergy and eczema. Careful allergy diagnostics is standard in the management of atopic dermatitis and comprises the four steps from history and skin test to in vitro allergy diagnostics and provocation testing. The atopy patch test (APT) deserves special consideration; with this procedure, it is possible to evaluate the relevance of an IgE-mediated sensitization in patients with atopic dermatitis for the actual skin disease. The most common positive atopy patch test reactions are found against house dust mite, animal epithelia, and pollen. Also classic allergic contact patch test reactions should not be overlooked; contact allergy patch testing belongs to the standard diagnostic repertoire also in atopic dermatitis, also in childhood. Food allergy can often only be evaluated by placebo-controlled oral provocation tests. This also holds true for food additives which equally can elicit exacerbations of atopic dermatitis. We do not recommend an allergen avoidance diet unless the relevance of this food for triggering an exacerbation of the disease has been clearly established.

4.2 Avoidance of Individual Provocation Factors

Often patients complain that there is no "causal" therapy of this disease. However, in the individual case, one has to think about "cause" and "trigger factor" in daily life. The latter can very well be diagnosed and often be avoided in the sense of a causal therapy. This procedure, often called allergen avoidance, relies upon the results of careful allergy diagnostics (see Sect. 4.1). The recommendations regarding avoidance of individual provocation factors comprise much more; unspecific and specific stimuli often go together in the maintenance of severe eczema (Fig. 4.5).

4.2.1 Avoidance of Unspecific Irritants

Various influences and noxious substances from the environment are able to irritate the sensitive skin of patients with atopic dermatitis compared to healthy persons and trigger eczema flares (Table 4.5).

There are leaflets explaining these phenomena which should be given to the patients although this information is often regarded as trivial. Very often we see that especially in this so simple field

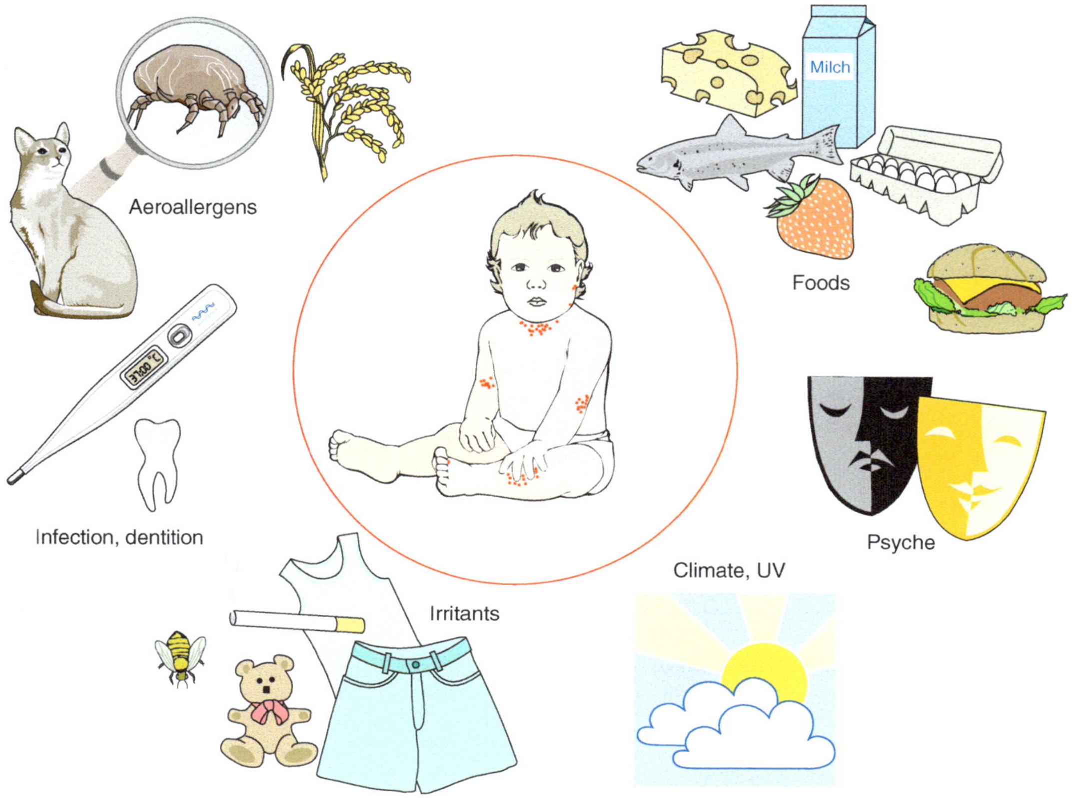

Fig. 4.5 Individual trigger factors of eczema flares (With friendly permission of C. Schnopp and C. Kugler, Arbeitsgemeinschaft Neurodermitisschulung)

Table 4.5 Atopic dermatitis: nonspecific irritants

Physical	For example, mechanical, exsiccation, UV light, temperature
Chemical	Detergents, solvents, acids, alkali
Pharmacologic	Vasoactive substances (alcohol, nicotine, amines)
Immunologic	Allergens, superantigens
Psychologic	Stress, emotional conflicts

of avoidance of irritants, heavy mistakes are made. People very early choose strong and possibly risky drugs before they even tried to start with simple avoidance of irritants and skin care. In our leaflet for patients (Table 4.6), we try to explain the importance of many so-called trivial things. A leaflet never replaces the dialogue which is very time-consuming and practically not achievable in the average office time of a practicing physician.

Therefore, this is a domain of eczema school and educational programs (see Chap. 6).

4.2.2 Nonspecific Procedures

Apart from adequate skin care (see Sect. 4.3), the consideration of certain principles regarding hygiene and clothing plays an important role (Ricci et al. 2004).

The so-called wool hypersensitivity of many patients is rarely based on a true allergy against sheep wool, but rather as typical marker of patients with atopic diseases shows the increased sensitivity of the skin to the mechanical stimulus of the small fibers.

Negative influences of environmental pollutants are also to be considered, like environmental tobacco smoke (also passive) as well as traffic

Table 4.6 Information leaflet for patients with atopic dermatitis

The disease is based on a genetic predisposition which can become manifest either as eczema, bronchial asthma, or allergic rhinoconjunctivitis, e.g., hay fever
The skin of patients with atopic dermatitis is dry, and the hair relatively brittle
There is an increased tendency to develop eczema, that is, red, squamous, itchy, sometimes oozing skin changes (the latter predominantly occur on the elbows, knee joints, hands, neck, and face)
The skin of children or adults with atopic dermatitis needs continuous care. The following aspects have to be considered:
Use mild detergents or soaps or syndets for cleaning
Avoid too often or too hot showering; no foam bath
Before showering or bathing, emollient additive (bath oil) should be given
After bathing or showering, the skin has to be creamed with emollients (lotion cream) prior to using the towel which should only be used as a mild touch, not as an intense rubbing!
Wool or irritant textiles never should get in direct contact with the skin (preferably use cotton or silk)
It is important that skin care is performed in the morning and in the evening in order to avoid itchy eczematous reactions
When there are red itchy or eczematous skin reactions, a doctor should be consulted, or anti-inflammatory therapy should be started
The treatment of itch is crucial. Itch and the automatically connected scratch reaction cannot be forbidden! The side effects of an anti-inflammatory treatment are definitely less damaging than the damage through injuring the skin by scratching. Especially children with strong itch should find sympathetic parents and teachers. Occasionally children who have problems in school need a special colloquium with the teachers in order to get the necessary understanding
Patients with atopic eczema principally can eat everything. In individual cases there is hypersensitivity against certain foods which have to be tested specifically. There is no general anti-eczema or anti-allergy diet. Obesity should be avoided. Newborns at risk should be breastfed if possible over 4 months. If this is not possible, hypoallergenic formula should be given
Pets (cats, dogs, birds, etc.) as well as house dust (old carpets, skirts, etc.) may lead to exacerbation of the disease. The living room should have normal humidity (less than 55 %)
Sea or high-altitude climate (above 1500 m) is well tolerated. Some rehabilitation programs in these climate zones can be helpful

exhaust. Also chemicals in indoor air, like volatile organic compounds or formaldehyde, can lead to deterioration of eczema (Huss-Marp et al. 2007; Eberlein-König et al. 1998).

Mechanic traumatization or exsiccation and contact to solvents are risky for atopic individuals. This also has a component with regard to occupational counseling and early diagnosis of occupational disease (see Chap. 6).

Vasoactive substances (e.g., alcohol) can trigger itch crises and thus contribute to eczema deterioration. In this context also psychological stress can be an unspecific irritant (see Sect. 3.5).

A special method for treatment of atopic dermatitis which considers both unspecific and specific stimuli is climate therapy which can be performed at sea level (e.g., North Sea) or at high altitude (above 1500 m, e.g., Davos, Switzerland) (Schuh and Nowak 2011; Borelli 1969, 1972, 1995).

4.2.3 Aeroallergens

The role of aeroallergens in eliciting eczema flares in atopic dermatitis has been covered in the Sect. 4.1.4. Thus, it makes sense that avoidance of these allergens should be recommended. The most common airborne allergens leading to eczema exacerbation derive from house dust mites of the species *Dermatophagoides pteronyssinus* and *Dermatophagoides farinae* (Tupker et al. 1996; Darsow and Ring 2000).

When talking about indoor air improvement, many measures are discussed leading to a decrease of allergen concentration in living rooms. Many of these procedures are scientifically not well investigated although they are based on rational considerations (van Leeuwen 1926; Diebschlag and Diebschlag 2000).

Thus, the avoidance of molds with its growth and spore formation belongs to general prevention measures not only for atopics. From epidemiologic studies, it is known that dampness and mold growth in living rooms go along with a higher prevalence of atopic dermatitis, which has also been considered in the most recent recommendations for primary prevention (Muche-Borowski et al. 2010).

4.2.4 House Dust and Storage Mites

House dust is a poorly defined mixture of sedimenting particles from the air whose consistency varies considerably depending upon the way it is collected. Only in 1964 the Dutch researchers Voorhorst and co-workers discovered small mites in the house dust and recognized them as elicitors of the allergic reactions (Voorhoorst et al. 1964). The most important mites in this context belong to the family of the Pyroglyphidae, like *Dermatophagoides pteronyssinus* and *Dermatophagoides farinae*, which occur all over the world except for the arctic and alpine altitudes. They are present in bed and upholstery, sometimes in concentrations of up to 4000 mites/g! Also old textiles, furs, and grain stores can contain considerable numbers of mites. In grain stores (flour, grains from different cereals, etc.), storage mites are common (*Lepidoglyphus destructor*, *Acarus siro*, etc.). The living conditions of house dust mites depend upon a complex ecosystem with factors like air humidity, concomitant mold growth, temperature, presence of human dander or organic fibers, etc. (Diebschlag and Diebschlag 2000). These mites are companions of humans and live from human dander.

In order to get rid of house dust mites, acaricides (benzyl benzoate, tannic acid, or hyperosmolar saline) are used, but these are of limited efficacy. The ecosystem has to be changed, e.g., by washable (60 °C) encasings of mattresses (Bauer 1985; Ehnert et al. 1992; Ricci et al. 2000; Schoenecker et al. 2001; Tan et al. 1996). Bedding and linen should be washed once a week at temperatures around 60 °C.

Stuffed animals, teddy bears, or textile toys can be kept over several hours in a deep freeze. Not only mattresses and beddings should be mite-proof, but there are also mite-proof pyjamas ("eczema overalls") which can be used overnight in severe atopic dermatitis (Schnopp et al. 2002). Also adequate basic therapy with emollient under closed conditions (wet wraps) and tube bandages has proven valuable.

The normal living room cleaning with vacuum cleaning or moist procedures (wiping) usually only minimally reduces the mite concentrations. While carpets were not recommended some years ago, today, with the development of new materials and adequate care, carpet floors are no longer definitely forbidden. However, there is consensus that in the bedroom floors which can be moistly cleaned are preferable when there are atopic diseases in the family.

There are several methods to detect house dust mite concentration or house dust mite allergen in a quantitative way which help in avoidance procedures (guanine coloring test "Acarex" or ELISA for house dust mite allergens (Ricci et al. 1999; Weber et al. 1997)).

Possibly other allergens are of relevance also for atopic dermatitis compared to airway atopy like allergens Der p 2 and Der f 2 (Lau et al. 1989; Nishioka et al. 1998; Tuft 1949).

4.2.5 Animal Epithelia

Many patients know from their own experience that contact with pets leads to an exacerbation of their skin symptoms. However, many patients do not know how to suppress this. When giving avoidance recommendations with regard to pets, it has to be distinguished strictly between primary prevention in order to avoid sensitization and development of atopic disease in risk families or individual prevention in an already sensitized or affected individual (for primary prevention, see Sect. 6.1). It is of interest that pets of allergic individuals may be allergic themselves (Schäfer et al. 2008). Affected individuals with animal dander allergy usually avoid animal contact; however, eczema does not improve after removal of the pet (e.g., cat). This may be due to the fact that cat allergen is kept over long periods in the indoor air since it is not connected to large particles which sediment faster, like house dust mite allergen. Therefore, it is typical that cat-allergic

Table 4.7 Recommendations to reduce airborne pollen exposure in patients with atopic dermatitis

Avoid staying in outdoor air at high pollen counts (see pollen information service broadcasting, newspaper, the Internet)
In cool weather or long-lasting rain, pollen counts are markedly lower
Daily exposure maxima (in rural environment) are early morning and evening. During this time, windows should be closed. The optimum time for ventilation of rooms is 0.00 h to 4.00 h in the night
With the use of pollen-protective foils, windows can be opened
On days with longer exposure in open air, persons should shower before going to bed (inclusively washing of hair). Then consequent skin care
Clothing should not be kept in the bedroom since many pollens get inside the room
Utmost care should be given to keep the bedroom cool and with low amount of dust
Regular vacuum cleaning with a fine particle filter and wet wiping and cleaning of surfaces in the living room during the pollen season are important; this work should not be done by the affected individual himself or herself
The use of skin care preparations prior to exposure in open air on air-exposed skin areas makes sense
Textiles should not be dried in the open air
Pets can carry considerable amounts of pollen into the living rooms
Use of cars: when cars are parked outside or under the trees, there may be a massive aggregation of pollen in the car ventilation which is then released when the motor is started. Pollen filters in cars are available and recommended
If possible, affected individuals should consider the pollen season when they make plans for vacation. Intelligent choice of time and location of holidays makes a partial or complete avoidance of allergen contact possible

individuals realize the presence of a cat in the indoor air much faster than other persons.

Allergies against dog seem to play a less important role, especially with regard to primary prevention. On the other hand, there are dog-allergic individuals with atopic dermatitis where the eczema exacerbates immediately after dog contact. These persons have to avoid dogs. By disciplined educational programs which are possible in dogs (control by education), it is often possible to reserve certain areas of a house to humans and keep them "dog-free." These strategies, however, need discipline from humans and animals!

Principally allergies can occur against all animals, however with variable frequency. Bird or amphibia in terraria are less often allergy inducers than furry pets. Fish in aquaria may be kept; however, there is allergy against fish food like red larvae of the species *Chironomus* (Baur et al. 1982). Rodents (like mice, rats, or hamsters) which are increasingly common in Western households (in Germany probably already in one million households) seem to be especially sensitizing. Against these animals, allergic reactions develop rapidly and abrase not only the skin, but also airways, and induce severe asthma attacks.

4.2.6 Pollen

It has been shown that pollen can trigger atopic eczema, as is reported by many patients during summer months and has been shown in a nested case-control epidemiological trial (Behrendt and Becker 2001; Krämer et al. 2005). It can be shown in a positive atopy patch test. Therefore, it makes sense to avoid pollen in patients with atopic dermatitis and grass pollen sensitization (Table 4.7) (Brockow et al. 1999a). It is important to know that closing the window does not guarantee the absence of pollen in the indoor air; to achieve this, air conditioning with adequate filters is mandatory. Pollen contain not only allergen but also proinflammatory lipids (Traidl-Hoffmann et al. 2005; 2009).

4.2.7 Foods

There is no general anti-allergic diet which could be recommended in atopic dermatitis (Behr-Voeltzer et al. 2008; Oranje and de Waard-van der Spek 2000; Przybilla and Ring 1990; Reese and Werfel 2006). Since the early experiments by Prausnitz and Küstner, it is known that food allergens can be absorbed after oral intake and elicit systemic reactions, e.g., flare-up at test sites (Prausnitz and Kästner 1921; Walzer 1927). Specific avoidance measures in the sense of a true allergy diet are recommended when they are specific and relevant. Temporarily general elimination diets can be recommended for diagnostic procedures (Atherton et al. 1978; Hide et al. 1994). However, they also go along with some risk (David et al. 1984; Roberts et al. 1979) when persons avoiding cow's milk inadvertently were exposed to cow's milk and developed anaphylactic shock.

Another situation is given in prevention: Breastfeeding and hypoallergenic formula are indicated (Bauer 2008; Exl et al. 2000; Falth-Magnusson and Kjellmann 1992; Halken et al. 2000; Hattevig et al. 1999). Normal nutrition avoiding vitamin or element deficiencies is crucial (Behr-Völtzer et al. 2008; David et al. 1990; Kreft et al. 2000; Schauber et al. 2007).

Knowledge about content of foods has been improved by better declaration rules which are very helpful for affected patients (Werfel and Reese 2009; Vieths et al. 2006).

4.2.8 Summary

The avoidance of individual provocation factors represents a basic feature of management of patients with atopic dermatitis. Apart from nonspecific irritants which have to be avoided generally like irritating textiles (wool), mechanical trauma, or pollutants, allergen-specific avoidance measures have been helpful in house dust mite but also in pollen allergy. Detailed counseling is mandatory and represents part of educational programs. In mite-free high-altitude climate, many patients experience improvement.

4.3 Basic Therapy of Disturbed Skin Barrier Function

All procedures to restore the disturbed skin barrier function which can be clinically regarded as "dry," "rough," or "sensitive" are often called "skin care," which has the consequence that they are not reimbursed by many insurances in many countries. Therefore, semantically it is better to talk about "basic therapy of disturbed skin barrier function" to help in understanding the basic defect. Unfortunately, for this type of treatment often the term "use of 'drug-free' vehicles" has become widely used in order to distinguish this type of treatment from specifically efficient pharmaceuticals like glucocorticosteroids or immunosuppressives. However, there is no doubt that these vehicle substances also have distinct effects upon the organ skin.

The major principle of this basic emollient therapy is the application of lipids in order to restore the skin barrier. The composition of these lipids is crucial for the effect.

4.3.1 General Considerations for Topical Dermatotherapy

4.3.1.1 How to Select Galenics

Galenics is the art to bring effective substances together with the desired vehicles into the correct mixture so that they reach the respective tissue. It is the most important aspect of topical dermatotherapy. It is the art of the experienced dermatologist, allergist, or pediatrician together with the pharmacist (Merk and Bickers 1992; Szczepanowska et al. 2008; Ring and Fröhlich 1985; Werfel et al. 2009).

In principle, there are different physicochemical characteristics of topical preparations which can be classified according to their nature with the so-called phase triangle according to Polano (Fig. 4.6) as:

Solid phase (e.g., powder)
Lipid phase (lipids of various origin)
Fluid phase (e.g., aqueous or alcoholic solutions)

By the mixture of these three different basic conditions, a variety of preparations with very different characteristics with regard to efficacy and acceptability can be derived (Merk and Bischof 1992, Ring and Fröhlich 1985; Thoma 1991; Gehring 2001).

Unfortunately, the common language does not patent exact scientific terms. The term "ointment" is used for any substance which can be

Fig. 4.6 Selection of vehicle according to disease acuity, localization, and individual skin type (From Ring and Fröhlich (1985))

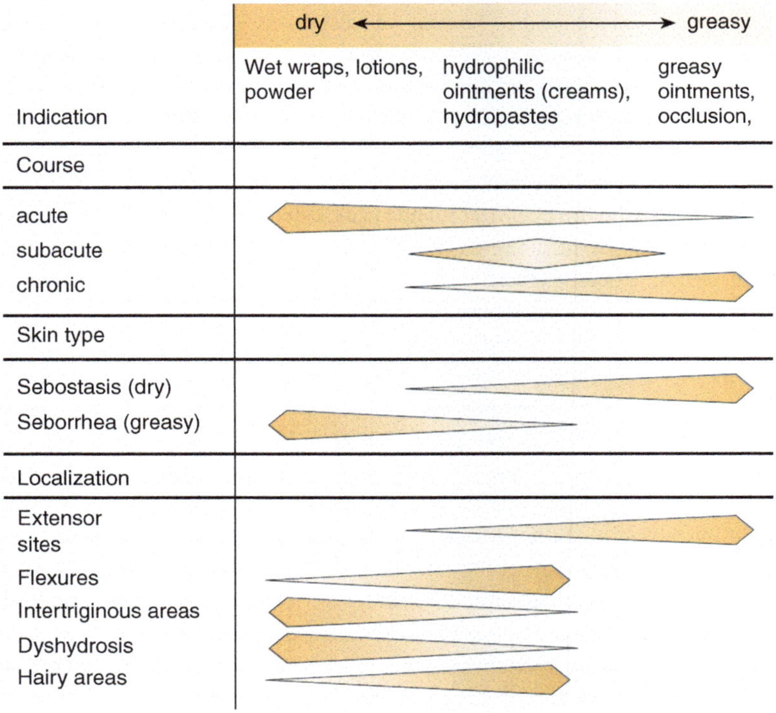

spread on the skin. In dermatological use, ointment describes a more greasy preparation, while cream has more hydrophilic constituents and lotion is even more aqueous in nature. Therefore, many preparations are advertised under dermatologically incorrect names.

The term "lotio" means a suspension of a solid, e.g., zinc oxide or titanium dioxide in a solution like water or alcohol, and lotio alba aquosa is an excellent topical preparation in acute skin inflammation or itchy conditions.

The contents of topical therapeutics can be of animal, plant, or mineral origin (Table 4.8) and show their effect already in the upper layers of the epidermis. It has to be considered that fatty materials form an occlusive film over the skin surface which prevents the loss of humidity but also the exchange of substances occurring normally through the skin barrier. This can be a disadvantage in very acute inflammatory conditions so that too greasy ointments should not be given in acute stages. The dermatological paradox describes that the opposite of moist is not "dry," but "fat"; a very moist preparation like an aqueous solution will—by increasing evaporation—lead to further dryness of the skin, while the application of a greasy ointment will contain humidity and moisture in the upper skin layers.

In this, the probably most famous physician in world history, Claudius Galenus (second century AD), who impressed medicine over a time of thousand years, is still considered modern today. In our more and more rapid and accelerating world, this art may be lost; however, it allows, with simple means and limited side effects and low costs, to achieve long-lasting improvement and avoidance of risky pharmaceutics. All you need is some patience and experience. I tell my patients: "The skin is not an organ which can be cured at the flick of a switch or at the push of a button."

The secret of every topical preparation is how to bring water and fat together to form a suitable emulsion. This amphiphilic system can be regarded on a spectrum between pure fatty constituents like petrolatum or paraffin and pure

Table 4.8 Vehicles for topical dermatotherapy

Fluid phase	Solid phase	Lipid phase
Water (aqua)	Mineral	Mineral
Alcohol	Zinc oxide	Paraffin, petrolatum (petrolatum album/flavum)
Ethanol	Titanium dioxide	Synthetic lipids
Isopropanol	Talcum	Polyethylene glycol
Ether	Plant	Propylene glycol
Acetone	Starch (amylum)	Plant
	Wheat starch (*Amylum tritici*)	Olive oil (*Oleum olivarum*)
	Cornstarch (*Amylum maysi*)	Peanut oil (*Oleum arachidis*)
		Animal
		Adeps suillus
		Beeswax (*Cera alba*)
		Cod liver oil (*Oleum iecoris*)
		Wool wax (*Adeps lanae*)

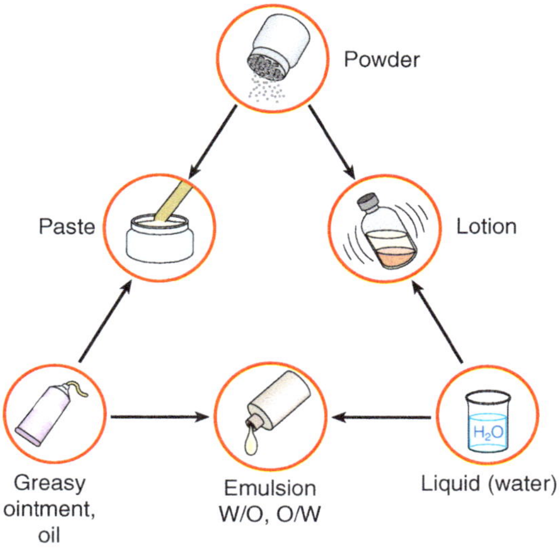

Fig. 4.7 Phase triangle according to Polano for selection of vehicle in topical dermatotherapy (Ring 2005)

solutions like water or alcohol and is characterized according to their nature constituent as either water-in-oil (W/O) or oil-in-water (O/W) emulsion. Creams are oil-in-water emulsions, while ointments in the dermatological terminology are water-in-oil emulsions. The larger the aqueous part of an emulsion, the more emulsifiers have to be used, which means that these are rather complex systems containing more substances than a rather fatty ointment with only petrolatum. Today, patients seem to prefer more hydrophilic preparations. When I compare old prescriptions of the ancestors in dermatology, I wonder how patients were able to tolerate these!

The best protection of the skin can be achieved by water-in-oil emulsions which form a fatty film on the skin surface and provide protection also in occupational context (itchy hand dermatitis). Maybe also the general shortage of time plays a role since creams or lotions can be applied faster than greasy ointments. I recommend my patients to take the time, every morning after the cleaning procedures (bathing or showering with adequate showering oils), for five minutes' skin care in the bathroom and let the ointments go in after application; one can read a newspaper during this time where the fatty fingerprints do not disturb. This finally saves a lot of costs, time, and adverse reactions and is a good prevention in atopic dermatitis.

In the selection of the right galenics, several aspects have to be considered, namely:

- The tissue inflammation which tells you how deep the effective substance should penetrate
- The type of inflammation, whether infectious or noncontagious
- The duration, i.e., chronicity
- The individual skin type (dry skin, sebostasis, or greasy skin)
- The localization (extensor sides versus flexures or intertriginous areas)

The intertriginous areas where skin touches skin, like in the anogenital area or the axilla, are not a good place for too fatty topicals. Here powders or pastes should be preferred (Fig. 4.7).

4.3.2 Basic Skin Barrier Therapy in Atopic Dermatitis

4.3.2.1 Skin Cleaning

Skin hygiene measures are discussed with respect to prevention. However, there are limited scientific studies with regard to evidence. In a European Round Table on "best practice for infant cleansing," an expert group discussed and reviewed the literature with regard to bathing and cleansing of newborns in the first year of life. Alkaline soaps have been found to have some disadvantages compared to liquid cleansers regarding skin surface pH and lipid content. Mild liquid cleaners for newborns should be used and preferably those which also contain some emollient. Bathing was regarded to be generally superior to washing also with regard to some emotional and psychological interactions between infants and parents (Blume-Peytavi et al. 2009).

In the USA, the "bleach bath" is popular for skin cleaning; small amounts of sodium hypochlorite are added to the tap water in the bathtub and induce an antimicrobial effect (Huang et al. 2009).

4.3.2.2 Hardness of Water

For skin cleaning procedures, the degree of hardness of water is of relevance. A study from the UK showed a significant dependence of atopic dermatitis prevalence and the degree of water hardness (McNally et al. 1998). With very hard water, decalcifying procedures are recommended (Gamble and Dellavalle 2011; Thomas et al. 2011).

4.3.2.3 Soaps and Detergents

The second problem is the selection of adequate soaps and detergents. For a long time, alkali soaps were not recommended or forbidden because of the irritative effect due to the alkalic nature of their constituents on the acid mantle of the skin surface (Marchionini and Hausknecht 1938).

However, in recent decades new detergents have been developed, better termed surfactants, which keep the acid pH and are also usable in hard water and available as liquid soaps (Braun-Falco and Korting 1991). Chemically, one can distinguish among syndets between anionic, nonionic, and amphoteric substances:

Anionic surfactants contain sulfates or sulfonates (sulfosuccinate) or carboxylate (sarcosinate) or alkyl phosphate.

Nonionic surfactants consist of polyglycol ethers or esters and fatty acid alkanolamides. Amphoteric syndets contain alkylbetaine among others (Braun-Falco and Korting 1991).

The debate about advantages and disadvantages of syndets versus soaps has been less intense over the last years. There is consensus that skin cleansing is an essential part of topical therapeutic management in skin diseases, also in atopic dermatitis. We are no longer "hydrophobic" in treating our patients (Blume-Peytavi et al. 2009; Gelmetti 2001). The removal of superficial microbial flora or epidermal proteins like crusts or dandruff represents a major factor in preventing further stimulation of immune reactions in the epidermis, also with respect to possible autoimmune reactions in severe atopic dermatitis (Valenta et al. 2000).

4.3.2.4 Oil Bath or Showering Oils

While many dermatologists forbade showering some decades ago, today, with the production of better detergents and refatting emollient-containing showering oils, there is no contraindication. However, it is clear that showering makes the skin drier than an oil bath. Therefore, in acute conditions or in very dry skin, we still recommend oil baths with adequate temperature (below 35 °C). There are different oil baths, namely, emulsion oil baths where the lipid part is emulgated in the form of small droplets in the aqueous face and spreading oil baths where the lipids are contained in the surface in a homogeneous way and spread over the body at the end of the bath.

It is important that after the bath or shower, patients do not rub themselves totally dry, but rather just take away the outer moisture and on the moist skin apply the necessary emollients, creams, or ointments in the humid skin (Table 4.9 shows a selection of available shower oils or oil baths in atopic dermatitis).

4.3.2.5 Sodium Chloride

Some authors recommend sodium chloride as an additive to baths together with oil for the

Table 4.9 Common showering oils or oil baths for atopic dermatitis

Name	Producer	Contents
Balneum hermal	Almirall Hermal	Soy oil
Balneum hermal F	Almirall Hermal	Peanut oil/paraffin
Balneum hermal Plus	Almirall Hermal	Soy oil/polidocanol
Balmandol	Galderma-Spirig	Almond oil
Cordes oil bath	Ichthyol Company	Soy oil
Eucerin Omega	Beiersdorf	Soy oil
Oleobal	Pierre Fabre	Soy oil/paraffin
Sulfo oil bath Cordes	Ichthyol Company	Soy oil/sulfonate

Table 4.10 Common basic dermatotherapeutics for atopic dermatitis

Brand name	Producer
Balneum Hermal Intensive Lotion	Almirall Hermal
Eucerin Dry Skin 3 %	Beiersdorf
Urea Lotion Eucerin	Beiersdorf
Lipikar	La Roche-Posay
Lipoderm Lotion	Galderma-Spirig
Toleriane	La Roche-Posay
Trixera	Avène
Eucerin anhydricum	Beiersdorf
Remederm Creme	Widmer
Dermatop Basic Creme/Ointment	Sanofi-Aventis
Excipial Lipolotio	Galderma
Allergika Lipocreme	Allergika
Physiogel	GSK-Stiefel

keratolytic and skin-softening effect. Salt concentrations up to 5 % are recommended. Sodium chloride bath oils in higher concentrations, sometimes also with addition of magnesium, should increase the effect of a balneotherapy mimicking the Dead Sea situation, also together with UV treatment (Dittmar et al. 1999; Ständer 1976) (see also Sect. 5.6).

4.3.3 Emollients Used for Basic Dermatotherapy

Basic dermatotherapy is the essence of every treatment of atopic dermatitis and should be performed over a long time (Loden et al. 1999a). In the acute flare, however, anti-inflammatory substances are needed, mostly glucocorticosteroids which then can be slowly reduced in the sense of a "tandem" therapy or interval therapy.

Most producers of corticosteroid-containing topicals also offer the corresponding "basic therapeutics" with the same vehicles but without the specific drug (Kantor et al. 1993).

The mixture of several substances in basic therapeutics is not a trivial matter; not everything can be mixed with everything. Pharmaceutical expertise is necessary since several mixtures can "break" and no longer be stable and homogeneous for the skin (Gloor and Gehring 2003; Schöpf et al. 1995). Table 4.10 shows a selection of common emulsions (lotion, cream).

4.3.4 Emollients with Specific Ingredients

Dry skin is a cardinal symptom of atopic dermatitis; therefore, adequate moisturizing of the upper layers of the epidermis is an absolute requirement. Under natural conditions, the skin itself produces the so-called natural moisturizing factors (NMF) consisting of low-molecular-weight substances like amino acids as degradation products of proteins. Low-molecular-weight compounds such as urea or glycerol may be added to emollients.

Urea is used in various conditions of dry skin or exaggerated keratinization as keratolytic (Wohlrab 1989, 1992; Wilhelm and Scholermann 1998) in concentrations up to 20 % and higher. In atopic dermatitis, usually 5 % urea is enough and better tolerated. Especially small children do not like urea because of a mild burning sensation. Glycerol and urea are used in creams and improve the hydration of stratum corneum considerably, thus adding to a protective effect. Care should be given when there is damaged skin because of burning sensation (Loden et al. 1999b).

By using emollients with urea, the consumption of anti-inflammatory substances, especially topical glucocorticosteroids, can be reduced significantly (Andersson et al. 1999; Gloor et al. 1997).

A variety of other ingredients are used not only for galenic reasons but also because of

Table 4.11 Emollients for basic skin care in atopic dermatitis

"Atopy ointment"	
Solutio acidi citrici 0.5 %	30.0
Glycerini	15.0
Unguentum Cordes	ad 100
"*Basic skin care cream*" of the German Pharmacopoeia	
Glycerol monostearate	4.0
Cetyl alcohol	6.0
Medium-chain triglycerides	7.5
Petrolatum album	25.5
Macrogol (100 glycerol monostearate)	7.5
Propylene glycol	10.0
Aqua purificata	ad 100.0
Lipophilic cream (according to Gehring)	
Triglycerol diisostearate	3.0
Isopropyl palmitate	2.4
Hydrophobic basic	24.6
Potassium sorbate	0.15
Acidum citricum	0.1
Magnesium sulfate heptahydrate	0.5
Glycerol 85 %	5.0
Aqua purificata ad 100.0	ad 100.0

specific effects such as antipruritic effects (see Sect. 5.5). A new topical emollient containing a unique lamellar matrix including palmitoyl ethanolamide—a cannabinoid agonist—was studied in a multinational multicenter prospective cohort study in over 2000 patients. There was a substantial relief of objective and subjective symptoms of atopic eczema after regular use of the cream (Eberlein et al. 2009a, b; Pflugshaupt 1992).

A well-accepted ointment for atopic dermatitis skin care is the so-called Atopikersalbe (see Table 4.11). If it is found too greasy, I use the well-known unguentum emulsificans aquosum (aqueous hydrophilic ointment of general prescription formulas of the German or European Pharmacopoeia) or a lipophilic cream according to Gehring (Gehring and Gloor 1996; Gehring et al. 1997).

4.3.5 Summary

Under the name "basic therapy," all procedures are comprised which are used to repair the disturbed skin barrier function. This also includes adequate skin cleaning measures as well as the application of emollients to restore lipids in the skin, be they used as shower oils or oil baths. One has to keep in mind that patients with atopic dermatitis are very individualistic also with regard to the selection of their skin care products. What is good for one patient may not be liked by the next one. Therefore, it is recommended to test skin care products possibly at different body sites prior to prescribing larger volumes. Certain ingredients with effects of natural moisturizing factors have proven helpful in adults, such as urea and glycerol.

4.4 Practical Tips in the Treatment of Atopic Eczema in the Acute Flare

4.4.1 Practical Management of an Acute Eczema Flare

In the management of atopic dermatitis, a stepwise procedure has proven practical (Fig. 4.8) which includes the acute treatment, the basic dermatotherapy of the disturbed skin barrier, and the special treatment of chronic, lichenified lesions. These steps can be used in an overlap and in parallel. As soon as there is improvement of the acute skin lesions, detection of individual provocation factors by using allergy diagnostics should be done (Darsow et al. 2010; Ring et al. 2012; Werfel et al. 2009).

The acute treatment procedures comprise:

- Anti-inflammatory treatment
- Antipruritic treatment
- Prevention of further skin damage

4.4.2 Antiinflammatory Treatment

In the focus of anti-inflammatory treatment of acute eczema flares are topical glucocorticosteroids (see Sect. 5.1) and topical calcineurin inhibitors (TCI). Rarely, systemic application of glucocorticosteroids (very short time!) is required

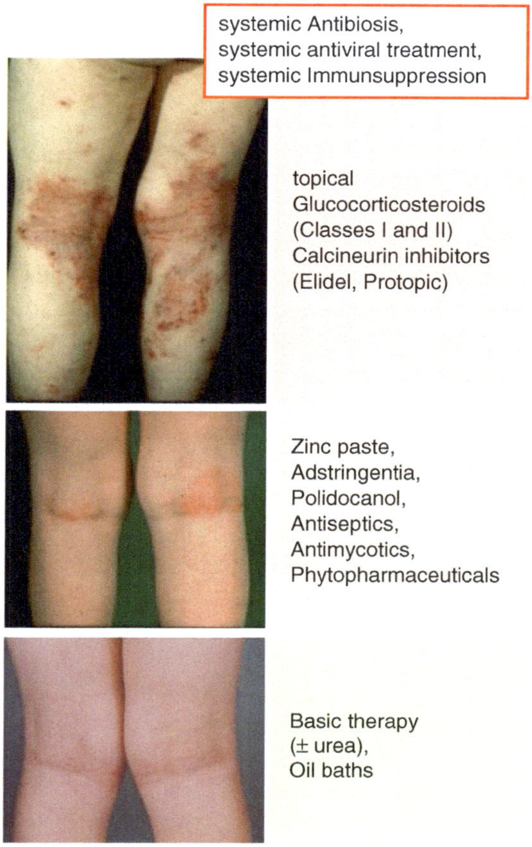

Fig. 4.8 Different stages of therapy of atopic dermatitis

(Heratizadeh et al. 2003). The correct choice of vehicle in the sense of adequate galenics is crucial (see Sect. 4.3).

4.4.3 Antipruritic Treatment

In order to fight the itch, moist preparations should be used which, however, may at the same time lead to further drying of the skin. Therefore, they should be combined with occlusion, i.e., as wet wraps (fat-moist in combination).

With this procedure, first, an ointment-covered textile is applied which then is covered with a moist layer in an occlusive bandage (tube bandage; this has the additional advantage to prevent direct scratching). If the whole body is affected, one can use the same principle with the so-called wet pyjama. Lukewarm baths with the use of bath oils can support the acute anti-inflammatory and antipruritic effects. Even lotio alba can be used with an antipruritic effect (Borelli 1995; Müseler et al. 1995). The most effective antipruritic treatment, however, is the application of topical glucocorticosteroids. Also TCI have a direct antipruritic effect.

Often also systemic antihistamines are used, mostly those with sedating side effects, sometimes as intravenous infusion (see Sect. 5.4).

This acute treatment with medium-strong glucocorticosteroid topicals usually brings rapid improvement of skin lesions.

4.4.4 In-patient Treatment

In the acute flare, patients can benefit greatly from a short inpatient therapy, since not only the adequate treatment procedures can be better performed, but also the change of environment often brings improvement (e.g., aeroallergens like house dust mites).

It is important that this phase of acute treatment is followed by consequent further treatment according to the stepwise management.

4.4.5 Amount of Topicals

One of the most common mistakes made by patients or inexperienced doctors is to prescribe and apply not enough emollients and specific topicals. Therefore, I usually ask the patients to bring me the empty tubes for the next visit, so I can immediately see how much has been really used.

A simple guide is the so-called fingertip rule: The amount of ointment on a fingertip of an adult corresponds to approx. 0.5 g ointment (tube opening 5 mm). This amount is good for an area of two adult palms (1 % of body surface).

This makes clear how much ointment has to be used with regard to body surface involved at different ages.

With the use of specific anti-inflammatory substances, one has to consider that penetration

Table 4.12 Absorption of topically applied drugs is different, depending on body sites

Body region	(Related to)
Volar forearm	1
Head	5
Face	13
Abdomen	2.5
Back	2.5
Legs	0.5
Genital area	40

of substances differs greatly between various body areas (Table 4.12).

Although it is actually simple, it is the topical dermatotherapy where most mistakes are made which explain very often the "unresponsiveness to treatment" in many patients. Therefore, educational programs also cover this aspect; special courses for dermatology or pediatric dermatology nurses, which then teach parents to correctly apply topical dermatotherapy, are offered in some countries (Ring et al. in prep.).

4.4.6 Summary

In the acute eczema flare, general management with using topical dermatotherapy (e.g., wet wraps) with the correct choice of the galenics is crucial. Topical glucocorticosteroids (mild to medium) are the strongest antipruritic agents, followed by topical calcineurin inhibitors. Most mistakes are made in topical dermatotherapy with regard to the way and the amount of ointment applied. The fingertip rule can help in practice to learn what amount of ointment is needed for which size of body surface involved.

5 Special Therapeutic Options and Substances in the Treatment of Atopic Eczema

5.1 Glucocorticosteroids

The introduction of topical glucocorticosteroids into dermatology may be regarded as the greatest progress in the treatment of numerous skin diseases in the second half of the twentieth century (Sulzberger and Witten 1952).

Only rarely, systemic glucocorticosteroids are necessary in atopic dermatitis. It is almost always possible to treat an acute flare (see above) with topical treatment, maybe supported by intravenous antihistamines.

Still today—in spite of increasing skeptical and critical attitude of many patients—topical glucocorticosteroids are in the focus of treatment of atopic dermatitis (Akdis et al. 2006; Darsow et al. 2010; Hoare et al. 2000; Ring et al. 2012; Werfel et al. 20a08b, 2009). In the physician's desk reference of Germany ("Rote Liste"), there are over 300 preparations under the heading "Dermatics/Corticosteroids" in various application forms, among them ca. 70 combination preparations with various galenic characteristics (systemic corticosteroids are not enlisted here).

5.1.1 Effects

The pharmacological effect of glucocorticosteroids is bound to specific molecular structures (Fig. 5.1). By introduction of halogen atoms (e.g., fluor or chlorine) in position 9 alpha, the biological activity is considerably increased, similarly in position 6 alpha. Furthermore, esters or acetonides lead to a stronger efficacy of topical glucocorticosteroids.

Glucocorticosteroids have numerous effects on the skin (Fig. 5.2). The steroid molecule after absorption is bound to a cytoplasmic receptor in the keratinocyte which then is included in the nucleus where it influences the transcription of messenger RNA. Steroids have both stimulating and inhibiting effects. The name derives from the best-known effect, namely, the mobilization of muscle glycogen and enhancement of neoglucogenesis from amino acids. In fatty tissue, glucocorticosteroids induce lipolysis; in various tissues, they induce an involution in the direction of atrophy, especially in lymphatic cells, bone, and skin. These effects are mainly due to an inhibition of DNA synthesis (Hatz 1998).

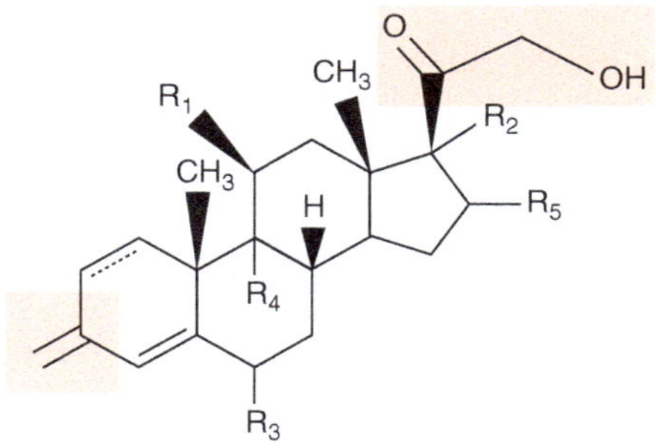

Fig. 5.1 Chemical structure of glucocorticosteroids

J. Ring, *Atopic Dermatitis: Eczema*, DOI 10.1007/978-3-319-22243-1_5

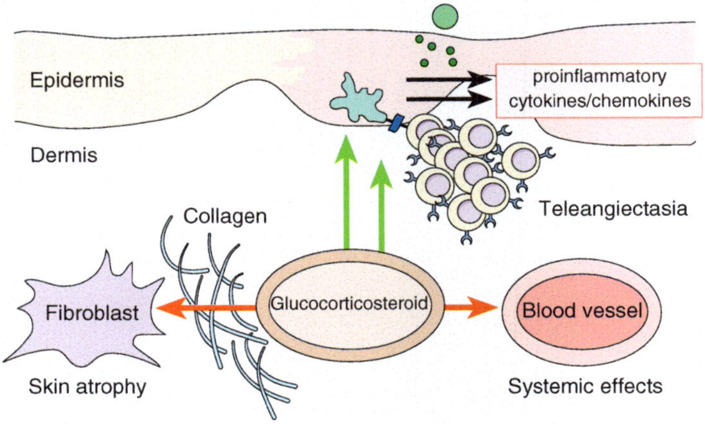

Fig. 5.2 Effects of glucocorticosteroids on the skin are intrinsically connected with undesired side effects

Via a gestagen-like effect, similar to progesteron, they also can induce sometimes serious psychologic alterations such as sleep loss, depression, euphoria, and nervosity.

Among the many variants of glucocorticosteroids, several substances have been developed with the aim to improve absorption efficacy while, on the other hand, minimizing side effects. Modifications include the hydroxylation, or adding further carbon side chains or adding halogenides. Methylprednisolone aceponate with double esterification increases the lipophilicity and thus the penetration into the epidermis. In several preclinical and clinical studies, this substance has shown to have a good efficacy safety profile (Luger 2010).

These differences in strength of efficacy have to be considered in the practical use. Table 5.1 shows a personal arbitrary classification for daily use. In my experience, only products from class 1 or 2 (mild to moderate) are necessary for atopic dermatitis; for other skin diseases, we very well need stronger preparations!

More important than the selection of the substance is the choice of the adequate galenics (see above Sect. 4.3). In the acute phase, topical glucocorticosteroids can be used twice daily; later on, the application once daily is enough (Turpenen 1991; Luger et al. 2004). In the acute phase, the application as wet wrap has proven helpful (Devillers et al. 2002; Hindley et al. 2006; Schnopp et al. 2002; Ring et al. 2012).

In therapy-resistant chronified lichenified lesions, occlusive treatment can be necessary. One should be careful with the application of glucocorticosteroids in intertriginous areas (axilla, anogenital area) because side effects will appear faster (e.g., striae distensae) (Furue et al. 2003).

5.1.2 Side Effects

5.1.2.1 Skin Atrophy

Systemic side effects of glucocorticosteroids are extremely rare in the treatment of atopic dermatitis (Table 5.2) (Bode 1980). However, patients continuously are confused by these phenomena through wrong information by newspapers and other patients. There seems to be sometimes a real "corticophobia" which takes away a lot of time in the daily physician/patient interaction.

More important are side effects of topical glucocorticosteroids on the skin (Table 5.3). Besides very rare cases of cortisone allergy, all these side effects more or less are directly connected to the pharmacological effect of the substance. The disturbance of the osteofollicular keratinization leads to the formation of comedones and steroid acne. The inhibition of proliferation and regeneration of epidermis induces atrophy; the degeneration of collagen and elastic tissue induces senile elastosis as well as the formation of telangiectasia, purpura,

Table 5.1 Classification of topical glucocorticosteroids according to their strength and side effects (Ring 2005)

Class	Substance
I (not halogenated)	Hydrocortisone, hydrocortisone butyrate, hydrocortisone acetate, budesonide, methylprednisolone aceponate, prednisolone, prednicarbate
II (weakly fluorinated)	Fluorcortinbutyl ester, clobetasone butyrate, fluticasone propionate, mometasone furoate
III (medium strength)	Betamethasone valerate, triamcinolone acetonide, flumethasone pivalate, flucortolone, dexamethasone
IV (strong)	Betamethasone propionate, fluocinolone acetonide, diflucortolone valerate
V (very strong)	Fluocinonide, halcinonide, clobetasol propionate

Table 5.2 Side effects of systemic glucocorticosteroids

Endocrinologic	Diabetes mellitus Catabolic metabolism Osteoporosis Disturbance of lipid metabolism Electrolyte disturbance Hypophyseal suppression (Cushing) Hypertension
Gastrointestinal	Gastritis, ulcus ventriculi
Immunosuppression	Weakened defense against infections
Neurologic	Myopathy (muscle weakness) Neuropathy Psychic alterations Behavioral change, sleep loss, nervosity, "withdrawal symptoms"
Ophthalmologic	Cataract Glaucoma
Hematologic	Thromboembolic complications

and ecchymosis as well as striae distensae (stripes of pregnancy) (Table 5.3 and Fig. 5.3).

Table 5.3 Side effects of topical glucocorticosteroids

Striae distensae
Atrophy (all skin layers) ("pseudo-cicatrices stellaires")
Embolia cutis (after intramuscular injection)
Increased light sensitivity
Cutis punctata linearis colli
Telangiectasia, rubeosis steroidica
Pigmentation alteration
Hypertrichosis
Purpura and ecchymoses
Acne
Hair loss
Disturbance of wound healing
Perioral rosacea-like dermatitis
Granuloma gluteale infantum (Fig. 5.4)
Contact allergy

5.1.2.2 Perioral Rosacea-Like Dermatitis

A special side effect of topical glucocorticoids is the so-called perioral rosacea-like dermatitis (perioral dermatitis) which occurs after the application of mostly halogenated glucocorticosteroids and—mostly in atopics—becomes manifest in the face as fine acute pointed papules and redness with burning sensation (little itch) (Fig. 5.5). Often the initial indication for the steroid treatment is no longer known, and the patients believe that the steroid is the only cure: Indeed, whenever the steroid is withdrawn, there is a rapid exacerbation which disappears immediately when the steroid is applied again. I explain to my patients—not quite scientifically—that in this phenomenon, "your skin is addicted to cortisone; we have to make a withdrawal procedure" (Fig. 5.6).

5.1.2.3 Ocular Complications

The risk of ophthalmic complications, especially glaucoma and cataract, in atopic dermatitis treated with topical glucocorticosteroids was studied in 88 patients with facial and eyelid involvement. There were one patient with transient ocular hypertension and one patient with optic disk cupping as well as seven patients with the diagnosis of cataract, two corticosteroid-induced and four age-related ones, and one in relation to atopic dermatitis itself. These patients also had used systemic corticosteroids. The authors concluded that topical application of glucocorticosteroids per se is not related neither to the

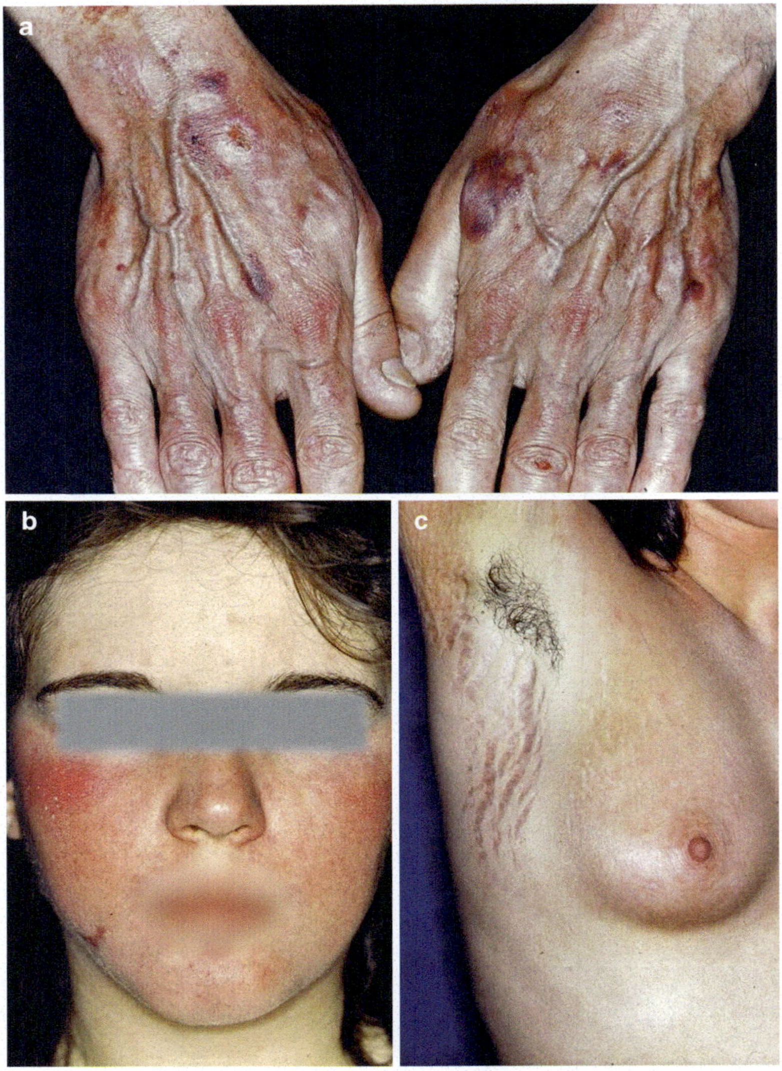

Fig. 5.3 Common side effects of topical corticosteroids in the skin. (**a**) Atrophy of the skin in atopic dermatitis. (**b**) Corticoderma after topical corticosteroids in atopic dermatitis. (**c**) Striae distensae after short-time application of topical corticosteroid

development of glaucoma nor of cataract; however, systemic glucocorticosteroids may lead to these complications (Haeck et al. 2011a and b).

5.1.2.4 Lipodystrophy

Furthermore, the rare but very unpleasant lipodystrophy after intermuscular injections of glucocorticosteroid crystal suspensions which can also lead to muscular atrophy has to be mentioned (Fig. 5.6).

5.1.3 Diminishing the Dose (Tapering)

Corticosteroid therapy never should be stopped abruptly since this might lead to a rebound of the skin disease. A slow dose reduction until the final stop is indicated. Either the efficacy strength of the steroid or the frequency of application (tandem therapy) can be decreased by choosing different classes of substances. This can be done by alternating the steroid application with basic

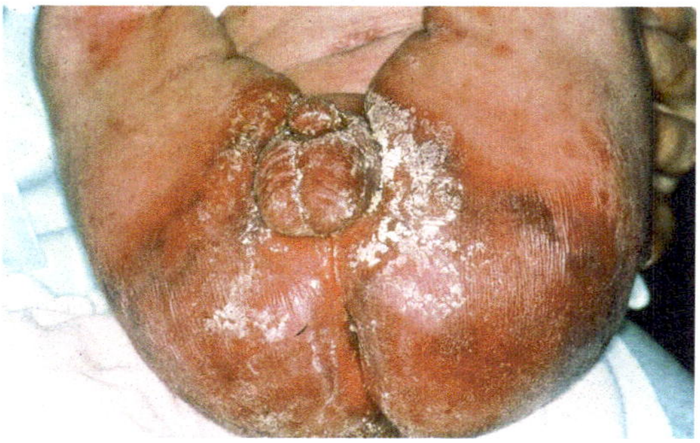

Fig. 5.4 Granuloma gluteale infantum in atopic dermatitis

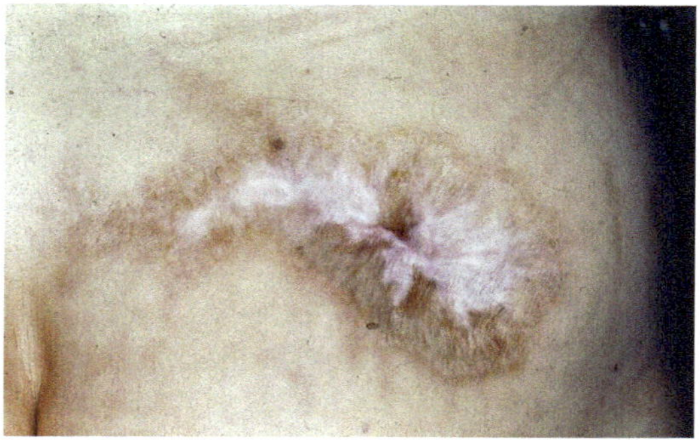

Fig. 5.6 Lipatrophy after intramuscular cortisone injection

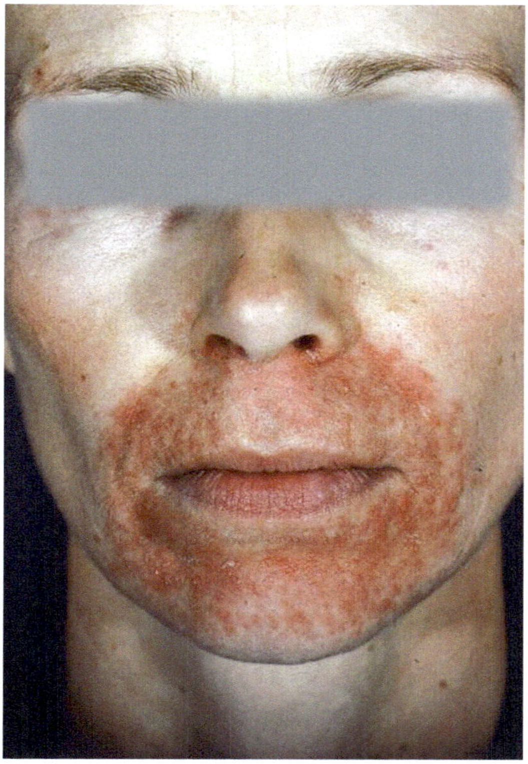

Fig. 5.5 Perioral rosacea-like dermatitis in atopic dermatitis

emollients in increasingly rarer steroid applications (4 days steroid, 3 days basic emollient until 2 days steroid, 5 days emollient or steroids only once a week). This regimen can be prolonged over longer time periods in order to prevent new exacerbations (Berth-Jones et al. 2003; Hanifin et al. 2002; Peserico et al. 2008). Similar principles have also been described for topical calcineurin inhibitors (see Sect. 5.2) and have been called "proactive therapy." For this regimen, it is helpful that many steroid producers also offer steroid-free skin care basic emollients with the same ingredients.

5.1.4 Combination Therapy

The use of combined glucocorticosteroids with antibiotics or antimycotics is seen critically; however, sometimes such a combination can be useful. What should be avoided is the uncritical "triple therapy" (corticosteroid, antibiotic, plus antimycotic) instead of performing adequate diagnosis!

Specific prescriptions (magistral prescriptions) with individual mixtures of certain substances are helpful, especially also with regard to the individual estimation by the patient. However, a good pharmacist has to guarantee the galenic compatibility of the final emulsion; not everything can be mixed with everything.

5.1.5 Summary

The introduction of glucocorticosteroids in dermatology was the greatest progress for eczema patients in the second half of the twentieth century (Fig. 5.8). Systemic glucocorticosteroids only rarely have to be given in atopic dermatitis. The selection of the substances depends on the strength of efficacy but more upon the galenic characteristics. For atopic dermatitis, mostly mild to moderate strength steroids are adequate. The application of topical glucocorticosteroids in the correct vehicle should be timely limited and ended via a "tandem therapy." Proactive strategies with once or twice weekly applications of the effective substance have proven helpful. The most important side effects of topical glucocorticosteroids include skin atrophy and the common manifestation of perioral rosacea-like dermatitis which occurs especially in young women after topical corticosteroids.

5.2 Topical Calcineurin Inhibitors

The introduction of topical calcineurin inhibitors (TCI) in the early 1990s can be regarded as major progress in the treatment of atopic dermatitis. At the moment, two topical TCI are available, the substance tacrolimus from the mushroom *Streptomyces tsukubaensis* (brand name Protopic) and the semisynthetic ascomycin derivative pimecrolimus (brand name Elidel). Those substances also are sometimes called macrolactams because of their similarity in structure with macrolide antibiotics (Fig. 5.7).

5.2.1 Pharmacological Effects

TCI have similar effects as cyclosporin A (see Sect. 5.8) with inhibition of T cells by binding to the cytosolic immunophilin (FK506 binding protein) and inhibiting calcineurin phosphatase (Fig. 5.8). Therefore, signal transduction and transcription of several proinflammatory cytokines in lymphocytes is inhibited (Bornhoevd et al. 2000; Wollenberg et al. 2001); furthermore, other inflammatory cells, like mast cells or basophil leukocytes, are inhibited. Contrary to glucocorticosteroids, TCI do not inhibit the proliferation of keratinocytes nor fibroblasts, i.e., they have no atrophy-inducing side effects (Reitamo et al. 1998).

In addition to the anti-inflammatory effects, TCI seem to have a direct effect on skin nerves and become manifest in a strong antipruritic activity independent of the anti-inflammatory effect (Meingassner et al. 1997; Stuetz et al. 2001).

Tacrolimus is also in systemic use for organ transplantation. Newer developments include rapamycin (sirolimus) as well as everolimus. Different to TCI, they act via a cytosolic protein mTOR (molecular target of rapamycin) and induce immunosuppressive effects in the nucleus (Fig. 5.8).

Numerous studies have shown the efficacy of tacrolimus and pimecrolimus in atopic dermatitis (Paller et al. 2001, 2005; Reitamo 2001, 2003; Reitamo et al. 2002, 2005, 2007; Ruzicka et al.

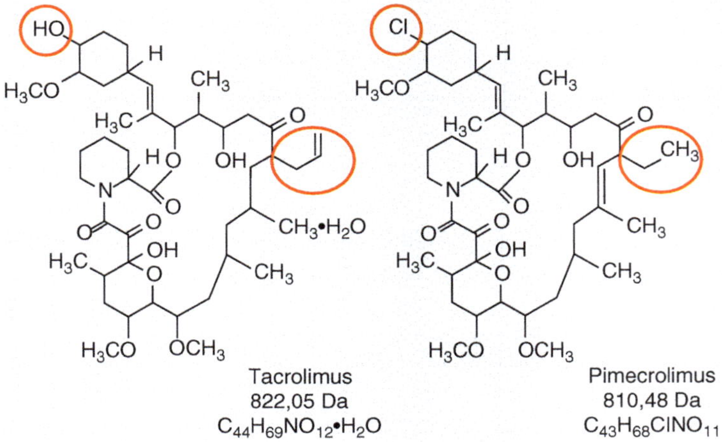

Fig. 5.7 Chemical structure of topical calcineurin inhibitors

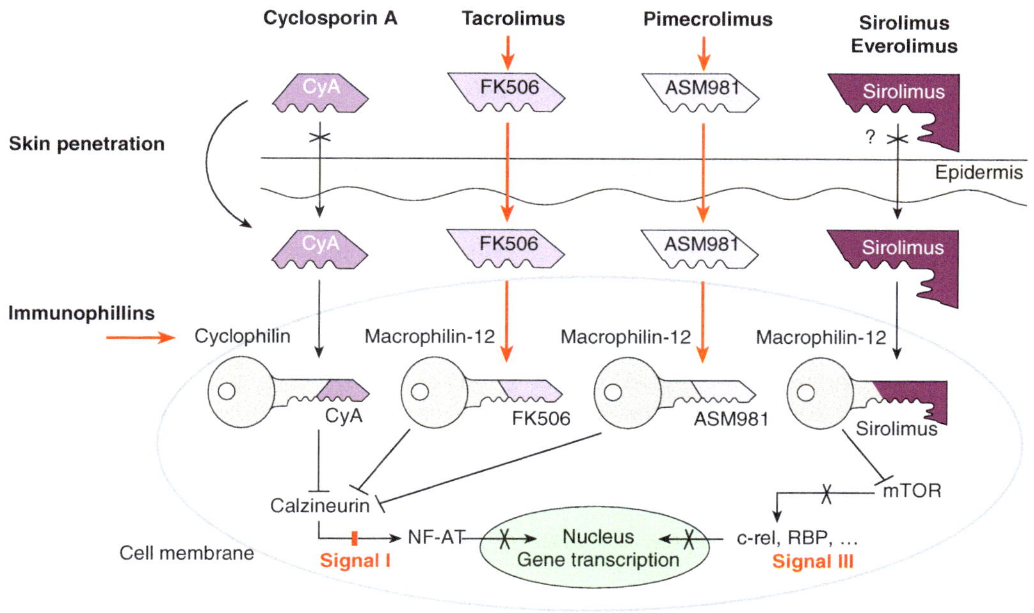

Fig. 5.8 Mechanism of actron of topical calcineurin inhibitors

1997; Luger et al. 2001). They are significantly effective compared to basic therapy; tacrolimus seems to be stronger than pimecrolimus (Paller et al. 2005). Overall, the efficacy is comparable to mild topical glucocorticosteroids of classes I and II. Tacrolimus is available in two concentrations (0.01 and 0.03 %) and in a relatively greasy ointment (Protopic). Pimecrolimus is available as 1 % cream and well accepted by the patients. For practical application of TCI, a similar procedure as used with glucocorticosteroids is helpful. One should not stop abruptly. From twice daily application, one goes down to once daily and finally in a way of interval therapy to twice or once weekly, which can be performed over longer time periods and has been called "proactive therapy"; for this procedure, tacrolimus has a special registration in Europe (Wollenberg et al. 2008).

Unfortunately, both preparations are only registered for children over 2 years, although according to the opinion of many experts, they are extremely helpful in infants, especially with facial involvement, because of their safety profile (Eichenfield et al. 2002; Lubbe 2003; Luger et al. 2015).

5.2.2 Side Effects

TCI have advantages compared to glucocorticosteroids since they do not show the well-known side effects of topical glucocorticoids. They even can be used in perioral rosacea-like dermatitis or pityriasis alba (Rigopolous et al. 2006).

Acute side effects consist in burning sensations after the first application (more common with tacrolimus), which mostly subside during prolonged treatment. Occasionally patients observe severe burning dysesthesia when they drink alcohol; the mechanism of this reaction is not clearly established (Milingou et al. 2004). Contrary to topical glucocorticosteroids, pimecrolimus does not deplete Langerhans cells in the epidermis and thus seems not to influence the local immune response. Therapy with TCI in children did not show inhibitory effects on antibody responses after vaccination (diphtheria, tetanus, measles, rubeola, or pneumococci). There is also no increased risk of skin infections after topical application of TCI (Alomar et al. 2004; Kapp et al. 2002; Meurer et al. 2002, 2004; Ring et al. 2009; Wahn et al. 2002; Sigurgeirsson et al. 2015). When correctly applied, percutaneous absorption and systemic effects can be neglected. Whenever measurable blood levels have been detected, they were below 1 μg/mL, with a detection rate of 0.5 μg/mL. However, patients with the rare Netherton syndrome seem to be an exception; here higher percutaneous absorption rates of tacrolimus have been found (Reitamo et al. 2001; Undre et al. 2009).

A major concern with the use of TCI is the risk of cancer induction, which on the basis of theoretical considerations has been mentioned by the Food and Drug Administration (FDA) of the USA in the spring of 2005 and led to the "black box warning" in the product information. The basis of this decision was an animal experimental study in hairless mice with well-known increased susceptibility to UV light effects and possible photocarcinogenicity, which was found for a higher (never commercially used) tacrolimus concentration in the sense of a shortened time until appearance of undefined "skin tumors" (Ring et al. 2005, 2008).

This model has been very controversially discussed; the study has not been reproduced by other groups. Therefore most expert committees or societies have recommended avoiding exaggerated sun exposure during a treatment with topical TCI (but also glucocorticosteroids).

In large and long-term observational and clinical studies of patients treated with TCI, no increased incidences of malignant tumors, lymphoma, melanoma, or nonmelanoma skin cancer have been observed (Arellano et al. 2007). In some studies, there were decreased prevalences of skin cancer in patients under TCI treatment, maybe due to better sun protection in this patient group (Luger et al. 2005; Ring et al. 2005).

There were no major serious adverse events in the study group. Furthermore, there was no influence of topical pimecrolimus on the development of normal immune responses after standard vaccination programs; thus, no clinically relevant systemic immunosuppressive effect was noted (Luger et al. 2015.)

In a prospective randomized open trial in over 2,000 infants, the efficacy and safety of pimecrolimus were investigated. Infants were attributed randomly to two groups at first appearance of atopic dermatitis: One group was treated with pimecrolimus 1 % cream as the first-line therapy, and the other group was treated with topical glucocorticosteroids as it used to be the standard some years ago. All children were observed over 5 years with regard to efficacy and safety. There was a similar and fast response to topical pimecrolimus therapy in infants treated with pimecrolimus compared to steroids. A rather high number of children never had to use topical steroids at all.

When disease was progressing, in the pimecrolimus group also topical steroids were used; in the steroid group, stronger preparations or systemic treatment was applied. There was no increased cancer rate (Sigurgeirsson et al. 2015).

5.2.3 Summary

The introduction of specific anti-inflammatory treatments like topical calcineurin inhibitors tacrolimus and pimecrolimus can be regarded as a major progress since they do not exert atrophy-inducing side effects like topical glucocorticosteroids. In addition, they have a specific antipruriginous effect. TCI are especially valuable in eczema treatment in problem areas like the face or the anogenital area. They seem to be weaker in efficacy than topical glucocorticosteroids. TCI can also be used in a proactive regimen over long time periods in order to prevent exacerbations.

5.3 Antimicrobial Therapy

One of the pathophysiological characteristics of atopic eczema with definite practical clinical relevance is the high density of bacterial or otherwise microbial colonization of the skin surface, even in clinically uninvolved skin (see Sect. 3.4). Apart from acute superinfections (e.g., impetiginized eczema, eczema herpeticum), the mere colonization of the skin surface with pathogenic germs may contribute via various mechanisms to the maintenance of inflammatory skin reactions.

In the treatment, one has to distinguish between general antiseptic therapy and specific antimicrobial treatment by antibiotics, antimycotics, or virostatics.

5.3.1 Antiseptics

Antiseptics are substances which kill microbes of any kind or inactivate them; chemically, they belong to quite different structural classes.

Table 5.4 enlists various antiseptic compounds which will be briefly discussed.

Chlorhexidine is a cationic bisbiguanide with a relatively low potential of allergic sensitization which shows good effects in a 1 % solution as chlorhexidine digluconate. It is useful for application in intertriginous areas and skin folds (Stalder et al. 1992).

Povidone-iodine can be used at large surfaces of infected or burnt skin; for eczema, it plays a minor role; however, it is used in small areas when they are eroded and superinfected.

Triclosan is effective in vitro against *S. aureus*, *Klebsiella*, and *Proteus* species and also has antimycotic activity. It exerts mild antibiotic effects which may give rise to the development of resistance. Triclosan can be mixed well in a water-in-oil emulsion and has anti-inflammatory effects. It can be used for a long-term treatment combined with adequate basic therapy (see Sect. 4.3).

Polyhexanide is a polymerized form of chlorhexidine which originally was used as surface disinfectant in the food industry. Its antimicrobial effect is due to disturbance of membranes and denaturation of microbial proteins. It is used for antisepsis in wound treatment; rare cases of allergies have been reported. It is also effective against methicillin-resistant *Staphylococcus aureus* (MRSA).

Octenidine is used for disinfection in surgery and as an antiseptic cleansing agent for oral hygiene with good compatibility. Until now, it is only available as solution.

Colorings have been used in topical antimicrobial therapy for decades; most of them are triphenylmethane dyes with broad antimicrobial activity (Brockow et al. 1999b). Due to difficulties to produce large amounts in adequate purity and decreasing commercial interest, colorings often are no longer offered by the producers. The most commonly used colorings are gentian violet (crystal violet, pyoctanin) which is used in

Table 5.4 Antiseptics in the treatment of atopic eczema

Substance	Chemistry	Characteristics
Chlorhexidine	Biguanide	Antibacterial, low toxicity
Povidone-iodine	PVP-iodine complex	Low sensitization potential, interaction with thyroid function
Triclosane	Trichloro-hydroxydiphenyl ether	Good antibacterial effect, low irritancy, and toxicity
Polyhexanide	Polyhexamethylene biguanide	Effective against MRSA, only available as solution and gel
Octenidine	Octenidine dihydrochloride	Effective against MRSA, good mucosal tolerance, only solution
Colorings Gentian violet	Methylrosanilinium chloride and para-dimethylamino-triphenylmethane, pyoctanin	Irritative effect in higher concentrations (>1 %), strong staining
Clioquinol	Di-iodohydroxyquinoline	Good in combination with topical steroids, yellow staining, low risk of allergy
Essential oils, e.g., tea tree oil	Farnesol	Good antimicrobial effect, high allergenicity
Potassium permanganate	KMnO4	Oxidative effects, to be used in bathtubs, staining effects
Sodium hypochlorite	"Bleach bath"	To be used in baths
Silver	Silver ions	Broad spectrum antiseptic low allergenicity, can be used in textiles

intertriginous areas in low concentrations (0.1–0.5 %). The red substance eosin can be used as 1 % solution in oozing eczema lesions. The disadvantage is the intense staining potential on skin and textiles, which has to be discussed with the patient before treatment.

Clioquinol is effective in combination with topical glucocorticosteroids, especially in combination with color therapy in nummular variants of eczema.

Essential oils have a high representation and popularity in the lay press. As a matter of fact, they contain natural antimicrobial substances with also anti-inflammatory properties. However, some of them have a rather high potential of allergenicity, especially tea tree oil (*Melaleuca alternifolia*).

Silver nitrate ($AgNO_3$) has been used for decades in wound treatment and in high dilution as an antiseptic.

5.3.2 Antimicrobial Textiles (Functional Textiles)

A new development can be seen in silver-coated textiles where the fiber—e.g., cotton—is coated with antiseptic substances, e.g., silver. Silver textiles have been used in atopic eczema and were able to significantly reduce colonization of the skin with *S. aureus*, leading to a marked improvement of eczematous skin lesions as measured in the SCORAD without additional therapy (Gauger et al. 2003) in a placebo-controlled trial.

Silver ions have a broad spectrum of antiseptic properties and do not induce development of resistance. Allergies against silver are almost unknown. One problem that has not quite been finally solved yet is an eventual absorption of silver ions in inflamed skin (Pluut et al. 2015). The acceptance of silver textiles from the side of the patients is very good (Gauger et al. 2006) (Fig. 5.9).

Apart from silver ions, also other antiseptic substances or detergents have been bound to textile fibers in order to produce antimicrobial textiles like benzalkonium chloride (Schnopp and Ring 2003; Jaeger et al., in prep).

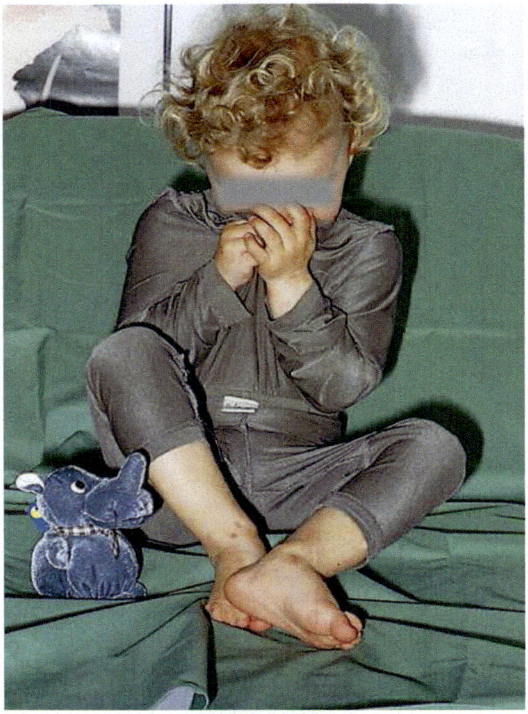

Fig. 5.9 Child with silver-coated textile

5.3.3 Antibiotic Therapy

5.3.3.1 Systemic Antibiotic Therapy

As long as there is only colonization of skin surface without clinical signs of an infection, there is no indication for systemic antibiotic therapy in eczema (Werfel et al. 2009). In impetiginized eczema, especially with large surfaces involved, a short-time systemic antibiotic has proven helpful, especially with cephalosporins of newer generations (cefuroxime, cefadroxil, cefotiam) or penicillinase-resistant penicilliums (oxacillin, flucloxacillin, dicloxacillin) (Boguniewicz et al. 2001; Ewing et al. 1998; Weinberg et al. 1992). In cases of penicillin allergy, macrolide substances or gyrase inhibitors or clindamycin can be used.

5.3.3.2 Topical Antibiotics

A topical antibiotic therapy is always connected with the possible risk of development of resistance and therefore has to be indicated. First antiseptic measures should be used. There is also the risk of a contact sensitization especially for neomycin, tetracycline, or polymyxin (Wilkinson 1998).

Fusidic acid is the substance of first choice when topical antibiosis is required; it inhibits staphylococci in low concentrations and is also active against MRSA (Hjorth et al. 1985; Ramsay et al. 1996). Unfortunately, there is an increasing resistance against fusidic acid to be observed. In impetiginized areas, especially in the face, a combination of fusidic acid with topical glucocorticosteroids can be used.

Mupirocin is used as a nasal ointment and effective against *S. aureus* carriers. It is used prophylactically (Lever et al. 1988).

Combinations of antibiotics with glucocorticosteroids are often used; however, it is questionable whether the antibiotic really brings additional effects. Most of clinical trials have not shown a significant advantage of combined topicals compared to the pure glucocorticosteroids (Korting 1995; Leung 2003).

In impetiginized eczema, the application of topical therapeutics is crucial. We recommend the procedure of "wet wraps" (see Sect. 4.4). An antiseptic substance like polyhexanide 0.2 % or chlorhexidine 0.5 % is applied in a wet wrap. This, together with a wet wrap of basic treatment or steroid, is placed on top and fixed by a commercially available tube bandage. Over this, a second dry tube bandage is fixed. The substances should remain for several hours, and the wet wraps should be continually moisturized (Abeck and Ring 2002).

5.3.4 Antimycotic Therapy

In seborrheic skin areas, sometimes patients have a predilection for eczema together with the growth of the opportunistic yeast *Malassezia furfur* (head and neck dermatitis). Here a therapy with antimycotics, e.g., ketoconazole, but also ciclopirox olamine is effective and leads to the improvement of eczematous skin lesions (Broberg and Faergemann 1995; Mayser et al. 2006; Scheynius et al. 2002). Systemic antimycotic therapy is rarely indicated. Some authors recommend combined antimycotic and antibacterial therapy in all forms of severe atopic dermatitis. It is natural that superinfection with *Candida albicans*, especially in intertriginous areas, or dermatophytes (*Trichophyton*) should be treated with antimycotics.

5.3.5 Antiviral Therapy

Herpes simplex infection in atopic eczema can give rise to the serious disease of eczema herpeticum (see Sect. 3.4). In these cases, systemic antiviral therapy, best with three times daily intravenous infusions of acyclovir 5 mg/m^2 or 15 mg/kg body weight, is the method of choice. In cases of relapses, long-term prophylaxis with valacyclovir is recommended.

Infections with molluscum contagiosum are not rare in atopic dermatitis and may give rise to involvement of large skin surfaces and special localizations (genital area), which makes treatment difficult. Careful removal and cryotherapy are the most commonly used treatment options.

5.3.6 Vaccination and Atopic Dermatitis

It is one of the most commonly asked questions whether patients with atopic dermatitis should be vaccinated like normal children. While this was a debate some decades ago, this question can now be answered clearly with "yes." There is not only no increased risk, but it is recommended to perform vaccination programs especially carefully in patients with atopic dermatitis since they are more at risk than other persons (James et al. 1995). The only caution which has to be observed is the time point of vaccination: One should not immunize during an acute eczema flare (see Chap. 6).

This also holds true for the new opportunities of vaccination against human papillomavirus (HPV); there have been single reports of exacerbation of eczema after vaccination with Gardasil and Cervarix, which, however, were spontaneously resolving.

Patients with atopic dermatitis have an increased risk after smallpox vaccination with scarification to develop eczema vaccinatum. That is why this classic vaccination against Variola vera was contraindicated in atopic eczema (see Sect. 3.4). With a newly developed vaccine using the modified virus Ankara (MVA) subcutaneously, it is possible to achieve immunogenicity with good compatibility also in patients with atopic eczema (Darsow et al., in prep.).

5.3.7 Summary

Antimicrobial strategies are important not only in the treatment of acute infections but also generally in the prophylaxis with regard to the high density of colonization of the skin surface with pathogenic germs in these patients. Generally antiseptics are used like triclosan in the acute treatment or clioquinol. Functional textiles coated with silver or other antiseptics represent an elegant method without using systemic or topical drugs ("textiles as drugs"). In severe cases, systemic antibiotic or antimycotic treatment in head and neck dermatitis can be used. The commonly discussed question whether patients with atopic dermatitis can be vaccinated like normals can be answered with a clear "yes." There are only considerations with regard to the time point. One should not vaccinate during an acute eczema flare. Patients with anaphylaxis to ovalbumin should be tested with the vaccine before treatment.

5.4 Antihistamines

Histamine is the best-known mediator substance of IgE-mediated allergic reactions (Dale and Laidlaw 1910). After its release from activated mast cells or basophil leukocytes, it exerts the well-known proinflammatory effects rapidly on the vessels, superficial skin nerves, and smooth muscles. When injected in the skin, the classic Lewis triad can be observed:

- Increase in capillary permeability of endothelial cells (plasma exudation, wheal formation)
- Increase of perfusion by vasodilatation (erythema)
- Axon reflex via superficial nerves (flare)

Together with these objectively visible effects goes the elicitation of the subjective symptom "itch." Therefore it was natural to use antihistamines for the treatment of itch.

5.4.1 Histamine Receptors

Histamine exerts its effects via four different specific receptors: the H1 and the H2 receptors are also expressed in the skin, while H3 receptors are located in the central nervous system and H4 receptors on various leukocytes (Church 1999; Gutzmer et al. 2002, 2009; Simons et al. 2000; Simons 2004).

For most allergic symptoms, H1 effects are important; H2 receptors play a role for the effect on the gastric mucosa (acid secretion) as well as on the heart. There are also H2 receptors in the skin, facilitating flush reactions (Ashida et al. 2001; Cowden et al. 2010).

H3 receptors in the central nervous system allow an autocrine inhibition of histaminergic neurons, leading to increased vigilance.

Bovet and Staub introduced antihistamines into the therapy of allergic diseases in 1937 (Bovet and Staub 1934). In the following, under the term antihistamines, mainly H1 antagonists are mentioned.

5.4.2 Generations of Antihistamines

In practice, one often reads about various generations of antihistamines (Table 5.5); classic antihistamines with the well-known sedating side effects are the first generation. They also exert anticholinergic and antiserotoninergic effects. On the other hand, also some tricyclic antidepressants have antihistamine effects. There is a certain overlap which can be used in strongly pruritic conditions (Frosch et al. 1984; Murota et al. 2010; Wahlgren et al. 1990).

The so-called second-generation non-sedating antihistamines came into use 25 years ago (Bieber and Ring 1987); they do not cross the blood-brain barrier and thus have no sedating effects in the central nervous system, at least in normal doses. Some of these substances also have other antiallergic effects by acting on inflammatory cells such

Table 5.5 Generations of antihistamines (H1 antagonists)

Classic sedating antihistamines	Newer, less sedating antihistamines	Metabolites of nonsedating antihistamines
Dimetinden	Terfenadine	Fexofenadine
Clemastine	Cetirizine	Levocetirizine
Diphenhydramine	Loratadine	Desloratadine
Alimemazine	Ebastine	
Bamipine	Mizolastine	
Cyproheptadine	Rupatadine	
Dexchlorpheniramine	Azelastine	
Hydroxyzine	Levocabastine	
Doxylamine		

as eosinophil migration (cetirizine) or mast cell activation (loratadine) or superoxide formation of leukocytes (loratadine and azelastine) (Purohit et al. 2001; Simons et al. 2000).

Under the term "third generation," substances comprise metabolites of well-known H1 antagonists which are no longer further metabolized in the liver or in the kidneys such as levocetirizine, desloratadine, and fexofenadine.

5.4.3 Effects of H1 Antagonists

Antihistamines are used all over the world as a standard treatment in the therapy of acute flares of atopic eczema; however, there is only limited evidence and only few well-controlled studies. This holds true especially for the older classical antihistamines with sedating properties like dimetinden, clemastine or doxylamine, and diphenhydramine. Maybe this can be explained by the fact that these substances have been introduced already 50 or 60 years ago before the era of randomized prospective controlled trials (Bovet and Staub 1934).

For the newer nonsedating antihistamines, there are a variety of studies which show positive effects against itch and atopic eczema (Hannuksela et al. 1993; Kawashima et al. 2003) as well as a high number of uncontrolled pilot studies (Klein and Clark 1999; La Rosa et al. 1994; Langeland et al. 1994; Murota et al. 2010; Ring et al. 2012).

5.4.3.1 Forms of Application

Usually antihistamines are applied systemically, most of them orally. There are only two preparations, namely, dimetinden and clemastine, which are available for intravenous injection. Apart from the topical application of medium-strength glucocorticosteroids in the correct galenics, the intravenous infusion of H1 antagonists is the standard therapy in treating pruritus and acute eczema flares in our department.

The sedating side effects can be neglected in the acute treatment of severe eczema flares in hospitalized patients or when applied in the evening.

Topical use of antihistamines as cream or gels for treating pruritus after insect stings is often advertised but probably only effective due to the cooling gel consistency of the vehicle. Due to these exsiccating properties of topical antihistamine preparations, they are not recommended in the treatment of atopic dermatitis.

5.4.3.2 Side Effects of Antihistamines

Classical H1 Antagonists

Here the sedating effects of classic H1 antagonists have to be mentioned first which also increase the side effects of other centrally active drugs or alcohol. Patients have to be informed about these side effects which become manifest in impaired speed of reactivity in traffic but also in occupational life when difficult machines have to be operated. I recall reports about severe traffic accidents by patients who continued a therapy with strongly sedating antihistamines (e.g., cyproheptadine, hydroxyzine) without or against medical advice. When an antihistamine therapy has to be continued over longer periods in everyday life, it is absolutely required to take a nonsedating antihistamine (fexofenadine) in the morning and sedating antihistamines (dimetinden) only in the evening (Behrendt and Ring 1990).

In small children, paradoxical reactions can occur if the sedating antihistamines stimulate an arousal reaction.

Due to the concomitant anticholinergic and antimuscarinic or antiserotoninergic effects, other side effects like difficulties in urination, attack of glaucoma, and dry mouth have to be considered, especially when other similarly acting drugs are given.

Second and Third Generations

The substances of the second or third generation are commonly called "nonsedating." There are marked individual differences which are at the moment not totally explained by pharmacology but also are not due to a simple placebo or nocebo effect (Traidl-Hoffmann et al. 2006).

Some companies circumvent the problem of sedation in some countries by the simple recommendation to take the tablets in the evening after dinner. According to my opinion, the least sedating H1 antagonists are terfenadine (Bieber and Ring 1987) and its metabolite fexofenadine as well as desloratadine, which are also registered in the USA and permitted for pilots of aeroplanes since they do not interfere with vigilance.

5.4.4 Cardiac Arrhythmia

Some antihistamines of the second generation (astemizole and terfenadine) were associated with severe cardiac arrhythmias, especially the prolongation of the QT time; this was due to increased levels of the substance with concomitant application of other drugs metabolized via cytochrome P450 enzymes (e.g., azole antimycotics, macrolide antibiotics) but also naturally occurring substances in grapefruit juice. These effects are no longer observed with the metabolite fexofenadine. Astemizole has been withdrawn from the market in many countries.

Several authors recommend increasing the dose of antihistamines when the effect is not sufficient up to a fourfold dose (Zuberbier et al. 2013). However, there may also be increased side effects.

5.4.5 Pregnancy

A special problem is the treatment of pregnant women. There are few convincing studies giving clear-cut evidence. For safety reasons, most companies write on their informations to avoid intake during pregnancy. We often advise patients then to take the antiemetics with antihistaminergic effects such as dimenhydrinate which have been proven safe for millions of pregnant women.

Also preparations of the first generation which are registered for infants, like doxylamine, dimetinden, and clemastine, can be used. Also no negative reports are published regarding loratadine and cetirizine.

5.4.6 Other Antiallergic Substances

Other antihistamines, i.e., antagonists of H2, H3, or H4 receptors, do not play a role in the treatment of atopic dermatitis at the moment. Drugs from the group of psychopharmaceuticals with simultaneous antihistaminergic properties can be helpful in some patients with severe atopic eczema in long-term treatment like opipramol or doxepin.

Also the mast cell blocker ketotifen with antihistamine properties can be used; its effect usually takes some weeks (Falk 1993; Iikura et al. 1992). Also topically applicable derivatives of cromoglycates which have been proven to be active in respiratory allergy can be used as mast cell stabilizers after oral application in patients with atopic eczema and concomitant food allergy. The oral application of cromoglycate as capsule or powder four times a day before the meals can show good effects.

The leukotriene antagonist montelukast is known in asthma therapy and has shown beneficial effects in pilot studies in atopic eczema (Yanase and David-Bajar 2001).

5.4.7 Summary

Antihistamines are the standard therapy in the treatment of itch all over the world; however, there are few controlled studies in atopic dermatitis. Topical antihistamines can be neglected in atopic eczema. The sedating side effects of classic antihistamines may be beneficial in the acute treatment of severe flares in hospitalized patients or when given in the evening. Although increased plasma histamine levels have been found in atopic eczema, histamine does not seem to be the critical mediator of the atopic itch sensation.

5.5 Other Antipruritic and Anti-inflammatory Substances

Itch is the central symptom of atopic dermatitis and represents a major problem for most patients and their families, impairing or destroying the quality of life. We all know the poster which went around the world with the introduction of pimecrolimus (Elidel), showing an infant with a T-shirt with the inscription "If I don't sleep, nobody sleeps!" as well as the pictures of bloody linen due to nightly scratch attacks.

5.5.1 Itch Sensation

Itch is the dysesthesia or unpleasant sensation which induces the urge to scratch. There is no better definition for this major symptom of allergic skin disease even 300 years after the first description by Hafenreffer (1660) (Ständer et al. 2015; Darsow et al. 1997b). When itch persists over a period of more than 6 weeks, it is called "chronic pruritus" (Yosipovitch and Bernard 2013). This condition occurs preferably in atopic eczema but also in a variety of other inflammatory skin diseases like psoriasis, scabies, and lichen planus or especially among the group of so-called prurigo diseases. In these conditions, often topical therapy is not enough, but systemic treatment strategies have to be considered with neuroactive medications like gabapentin and pregabalin (Yosipovitch and Bernard 2013) or antidepressants like sertraline, paroxetine, and mirtazapine (Ständer et al. 2015).

Chronic pruritus is not a rare condition. A cross-sectional observational study in 11,730 persons working in 144 companies in Germany showed a point preference of chronic pruritus of 16.8 %. There was an age dependence as this condition was more frequent in elderly patients (12.3 % in young adults aged 16–30 years, 20.3 % in persons aged 61–70 years) (Ständer et al. 2010).

In some cases of chronic pruritus, disturbances in iron metabolism have been suspected. If at all, the determination of ferritin may be helpful (Bharati and Yesudian 2008).

Itch and pain have in common that they only can be felt by the patient and not seen by other people. Thus they are difficult to be measured objectively. While patients with pain raise feelings of compassion immediately and everywhere, patients with itchy skin diseases are not taken seriously and often encounter the flippant sentence "just stop scratching!" This recommendation shows the complete ignorance about the dermatoneuropsychological mechanisms involved in pruritus (see Sect. 2.1).

5.5.2 Itch Research

While over many decades itch was regarded as the little brother of pain, this concept has been abandoned. Itch is mediated by a special subgroup of unmyelinated sensory C fibers and originates from the upper part of the dermis or the dermoepidermal junction. These fibers are sensitive to temperature but insensitive to mechanical stimulation. They express the vanillin receptor (TRPV1 = transient receptor potential vanilloid type 1), which is a nonselective ion channel expressed on keratinocytes and peripheral sensory C nerve fibers. Therefore also antagonists to this receptor, like PAC-14028, have shown to have an antipruritic effect in an atopic dermatitis model of mice (Yun et al. 2011).

These sensory nerves then transmit the sensation to dorsal route ganglia and from there via the spinal cord to the brain.

Recent imaging studies have shown that not only the thalamus is the major sensory organ, but

Table 5.6 Mediators of itch sensation (Buddenkotte and Steinhoff 2010; Yosipovitch and Bernard 2013; Ständer et al. 2015)

Histamine
Serotonin
Acetylcholine
Neuropeptides (e.g., substance P)
Cytokines
Interleukin-2
Interleukin-8
Interleukin-31
Neurotrophin-4
Nerve growth factor (NGF)
Tryptase
Kallikrein, cathepsin S
Platelet-activating factor
Prostaglandins
Leukotrienes
Opioid peptides

also areas of the anterior cingulate cortex, the insula, and secondary somatosensory cortex areas are activated, as well as centers of the limbic system. Notably, the most visible feature of cerebral activation patterns after itch-inducing stimulation is the activation of the motor areas for the scratch response (Darsow et al. 2000).

For a long time, the search for the classical itch mediator substance has been going on (Table 5.6).

Another clinical condition going along with extreme itch is cutaneous amyloidosis, where deposits of amyloid and apoptotic keratinocytes are found in the papillary dermis. In the rare variant of the familiar primary localized cutaneous amyloidosis (PLCA), it was found that the OSMR gene (oncostatin-M receptor beta) may play a major role since it involved, among others, interleukin-31, possibly then acting as major itch inducer (Tanaka et al. 2009 *neu*).

Unfortunately, itch research is far behind pain research. There are different qualities of itch. It is a well-known clinical experience regarding the morphology of skin lesions as well as the typology of scratch behavior. Using various questionnaires (Darsow et al. 1997a). With the Brest questionnaire the authors found significant differences in the quality of itch between atopic dermatitis, nonatopic eczema, urticaria, psoriasis, and scabies. There were also similarities that itch occurred more frequently over nighttime, following certain eliciting factors such as stress, dryness, and hot water. While application of cold was normally found to be beneficial in atopic dermatitis, the qualities of "stinging," "pincing," and "stabbing" were significantly more common than in the other dermatoses.

A major problem of pruritus research is its subjective character and the difficulty to be objectively measured. Usually visual analog scales (VAS) are used; however, they do not necessarily correlate well with the clinical appearance and intensity of the skin lesions (Darsow et al. 1997a). A new scale, the "5D itch scale," has been proposed, registering the five dimensions of duration, degree, direction, disability, and distribution of pruritus as a better outcome measure for clinical trials (Elman et al. 2010).

Therefore mechanical devices have been developed to measure the scratching behavior with the so-called itch watch (Felix and Schuster 1975).

Other so-called actigraphic methods have been developed and found suitable to assess pruritus over nighttime (Murray and Rees 2011).

The scratch response may considerably contribute to the pathophysiology of itch-induced skin damage, as has been shown by early "inhuman" studies in putting a limb into plaster or fixing a child in the bed so that it could not move (Engman et al. 1936) (see above).

In murine experiments with NC/Nga mice—atopic dermatitis induced by repeated application of house dust mite—the contribution of scratch behavior to the induced eczema was remarkable. In the light of modern findings regarding IgE autoantibodies against epidermal proteins possibly liberated from keratinocytes by the scratch trauma, these observations gain a new importance (Yamamoto et al. 2009).

There is a strong psychosomatic interaction in the itch sensation. Therefore also psychological processes have to be considered in evaluating patients suffering from chronic pruritus. Personality factors, life events, and psychological stress may have an important role as external stimuli. Therefore biopsychosocial models have been proposed to better understand the vicious cycle of the itch-scratch response (Verhoeven et al. 2008).

While everybody is full of compassion when a person suffers from pain, itch is often not understood by the surrounding; people laugh and say, "just scratch." In a cross-sectional study investigating the impairment in quality of life, 138 patients with chronic pain were compared to 73 patients with chronic pruritus with otherwise similar demographics. The authors used the health utility score as a measure of how much lifetime a person would be willing to give from his or her life expectancy to live without the condition and found that pruritus had a substantial impact on quality of life that may be comparable to that of pain (Kini et al. 2011).

A specially developed and validated pruritus-specific quality of life instrument, the ItchyQol, was developed (Desai et al. 2008).

In specially designed itch questionnaires (e.g., "Eppendorf Itch Questionnaire"), these differences can be measured (Darsow et al. 1997a, b).

With new imaging techniques like positron emission tomography (PET) or functional magnetic resonance imaging (fMRI), the activation of central nervous areas in the brain during itch can be visualized (Darsow et al. 2000; Pfab et al. 2010a) (Fig. 5.10). It is interesting that besides sensory areas, which transmit the itch sensation, and the motor areas, which mediate the scratch reaction, also areas of the limbic system are activated, which points to an involvement of emotional reaction patterns.

Everybody knows that looking at an individual who scratches vehemently may also induce a scratch response in observers such that there is anecdotal evidence of "contagious" itch. This susceptibility to visual effects seems to be increased in atopic dermatitis. In a study, healthy volunteers and eczema patients were asked to watch a five-minute movie showing individuals suffering from obvious itch and scratching. The study participants received either saline or histamine as itch-inducing stimulus on the volar side of the forearm. Patients with atopic dermatitis scratched more frequently and reported a higher severity of itch while watching the movie compared to controls (Papoiu et al. 2011). Pruritus can be so severe that inpatient therapy becomes necessary. The establishment of special "itch clinics" has been proposed (Naldi and Mercury 2010).

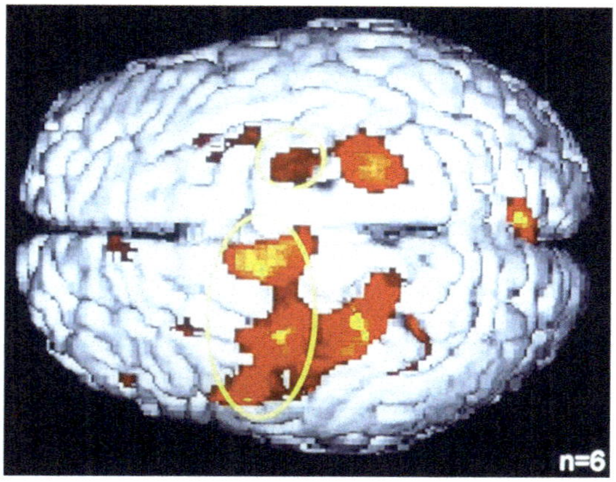

Fig. 5.10 Visualization of itch sensation in the brain in positron emission tomography (PET). Activation of motor areas in histamine-induced itch: gyrus precentralis and supplementary motor area (Darsow et al. 2000)

The psychosomatic involvement in pruritus is immense (Manenti and Vaglio 2005). Therefore application of psychopharmaceuticals may be indicated in severe conditions, starting from doxepin, which also has a combined histamine H1+H2 antagonistic effect, to tricyclic antidepressants (Hundley and Yosipovitch 2004) (Sect. 5.4.6).

5.5.3 Differences in Ethnic Populations

There may be differences in ethnic populations in itch perception on a global range with regard to various ethnic populations. This may be due to biologic factors like genetic predisposition to certain diseases, like amyloidosis or prurigo pigmentosa, which is more common in Asian individuals, or intrahepatic cholestasis of pregnancy, which seems to be more common in Latin America. Also genetic polymorphisms in the interleukin-31 receptor may play a role. In Africans, a common condition is chloroquine-induced itch and primary bilharziasis (Tey and Yosipovitch 2010).

Also the response to capsaicin, a substance known to destroy sensory nerves and usually inducing an initial burning sensation, is different between ethnic groups: African Americans do

Table 5.7 Antipruriginous agents

Topically applied substances	Systemically acting substances
Local anesthetics	Antihistamines
Glucocorticosteroids	Glucocorticosteroids
Calcineurin inhibitors	Opiates and opiate antagonists
Cannabinoid agonists	Antidepressants
Capsaicin	Anticonvulsants
Parasulfonates and others, e.g., bufexamac	Pain modulators Gabapentin, pregabalin

not suffer the same degree of acute hyperalgesia and neurogenic inflammation as people from Spain or East Asia (Tey 2010). Also psychosocial and lifestyle factors may be involved in the itch process.

Due to the multitude of qualities and elicitors but also mechanisms of the itch sensation, a variety of antipruritic strategies are available, partly to be applied topically, partly systemically, or reflecting central nervous involvement with behavioral techniques (see Sect. 5.4) (Table 5.7).

5.5.4 Topical Antipruriginous Agents

Glucocorticosteroids are the most potent antipruriginous topical agents (see Sect. 5.1) as well as topical calcineurin inhibitors (TCI) (see Sect. 5.2). Besides, a variety of other substances are used therapeutically in order to diminish or treat itch sensation.

5.5.4.1 Local Anesthetics

Since itch sensation is mediated via excitation of sensory nerve fibers in the skin, local anesthetics naturally have an effect especially after intradermal or subcutaneous injection. This is no acceptable method for larger skin areas. Yet, in treating very circumscribed, chronic lichenified, or pruriginous skin lesions, the intradermal injection of local anesthetics can be helpful.

The topical application of local anesthetics as a lotion, cream, or ointment (e.g., Emla) is of little use in treating eczema, except for small circumscribed areas which can occur in the condition of notalgia paresthetica. The topical application of local anesthetics is connected with a rather high risk of sensitization and development of contact allergy.

5.5.4.2 Polidocanol

Polidocanol is a polymerized local anesthetic from dodecyl alcohol and ethylene dioxide. This substance with a molecular weight of 600 D can penetrate especially into inflamed skin and reaches sensory nerves and thus exerts an antipruriginous effect (Freitag and Hoppner 1997).

Polidocanol is used either as lotion (5 %), suspension, or cream. In very dry skin, it can be combined with 3–5 % urea (Hauss et al. 1993). This treatment can be self-applied by the patients as often as they wish. Thus one can spare topical glucocorticosteroid use.

5.5.4.3 Cannabinoid agonists

Endogenous cannabinoids play a role in the epidermal differentiation; receptors can be found on keratinocytes, sensory nerve fibers, and inflammatory cells. With cannabinoid agonists, antipruriginous effects can be observed. In a larger study, by the edition of the cannabinoid agonist N-palmitoyl ethanolamine in a differentiated basic therapeutic vehicle, a good effect in atopic dermatitis has been observed (Eberlein et al. 2009b).

5.5.4.4 Capsaicin

The vanilloid alkaloid capsaicin binds to the receptor TRPV1 on sensory nerve fibers and keratinocytes and leads to an inactivation of sensory nerve fibers. Acutely after application, there is a burning painful sensation. Capsaicin, the effective substance in tabasco sauce, is better used in strongly itching chronic lesions or in pruritus on nonaltered skin than in atopic dermatitis. When used, one should carefully watch the concentration and start with lower doses from 0.025 % over 0.05 to 0.1 %. Capsaicin should not be used in intertriginous areas, in the face, or on mucous surfaces.

5.5.4.5 Tar Preparations

Coal tar is one of the oldest treatments going back into the history of dermatology. It is a not very well-defined mixture of more than 1000 substances, among them also high concentrations of polycyclic aromatic hydrocarbons (PAHs).

Crude coal tar is produced when coal is heated without oxygen. Liquor carbonis detergens is made by extracting pix lithanthracis 1:5 with alcohol.

In earlier times, tar treatment with wood, slate, or coal tar was standard, especially the coal tar extract (liquor carbonis detergens) or pure coal tar (pix lithanthracis). These preparations have an anti-inflammatory and antipruriginous effect without the mechanisms being known.

Tar is a mixture of many, partly still unknown substances which originate in the process of distillation. Tar products have antiproliferative, anti-inflammatory, and antimicrobial activities. Especially phenolic components seem to have antipruritic effects (Munkvad 1989). The use of tar preparations is controversial in many countries due to the carcinogenicity observed in animal experiments (Pion et al. 1995).

While there is animal data of carcinogenicity of coal tar, there is still a controversy with regard to the safety of its use in humans. Therefore a large historical cohort study was performed studying the late effects of coal tar treatment in eczema and psoriasis, the Radboud study (LATER study) in 14,009 patients suffering mostly from psoriasis or eczema. The study covered observational periods between 13 and 43 years after treatment and found no increased values neither for skin cancer nor non-skin malignancies (Roelofzen et al. 2010). This supports earlier studies from Larkö and Swanbeck (1982) or Hannuksela-Svaan et al. (2000). The authors concluded that coal tar can be maintained as a safe treatment in dermatological practice. We use pix lithanthracis rarely and only under hospital settings and prefer liquor carbonis detergens which can be mixed with emollients to produce acceptable preparations for the patients. There may be a far revival since it counteracts Th2 reactions via aryl hydrocarbon (AH) receptor activation and STAT6 dephosphorylation (van den Bogaard et al. 2013).

5.5.4.6 Sulfonates

Sulfonates differ from tar since they are neither phototoxic, mutagenic, teratogenic, nor cancerogenic (Colcha et al. 1994; Diezel et al. 1992; Warnecke and Wendt 1998). They are produced from slant oil and represent ammonium bituminosulfonates. Effective substances have a thiophen ring structure. Sulfonates are used also in folliculitis or furuncles to attract neutrophil leukocytes.

In atopic eczema, lotions or pastes can be used which have beneficial effects in chronic lichenified skin areas.

5.5.4.7 Adstringentia

By alteration of superficial proteins in the epidermis, adstringentia of natural or synthetic origin can have beneficial effects, going along with exsiccation and anti-inflammatory effects. Most commonly used are preparations from oak bark or synthetic tannins on the basis of gallic acid (Tannolact, Tannosynt). Lukewarm hand baths together with tannic acid have shown to be beneficial in dyshidrotic hand dermatitis, as well as seat baths in perianal or perigenital eczema.

5.5.4.8 Etheric Oils

Among etheric oils, especially menthol is the best-known antipruriginous agent; its effect is mediated via direct action on the cold receptor fibers, thus overlaying the itch sensation. However, menthol is only available in solution, mostly alcoholic, and thereby has a very strong exsiccating effect. It is mostly used in acute conditions such as after insect bites where there is a very localized application area.

5.5.4.9 Others

A variety of other substances are used topically against itch or against eczema. The nonsteroidal anti-inflammatory drug bufexamac was promoted for some years to be as active as corticoids. However, due to the rather strong sensitizing properties, it is no longer in wide use (Christiansen et al. 1977) and has been withdrawn in most countries.

Topical antihistamines which are used as gels for insect stings are not recommended for the treatment of atopic eczema. This also holds true for topical preparations of doxepin or acetylsalicylic acid.

5.5.5 Summary

Itch is the most important symptom of atopic eczema and is in the center of successful therapy. The order to children "stop scratching" does not make sense since itch is defined as the unpleasant sensation eliciting the urge to scratch. The most important antipruriginous strategy is topical anti-inflammatory treatment with glucocorticosteroids or calcineurin inhibitors. Besides, polidocanol in good galenic mixtures can have an antipruritic effect, equally cannabinoid agonist, tar, and sulfonate preparations as well as tannic acid which have been used in long-term treatment of lichenified areas and have been shown to spare topical corticosteroids.

5.6 UV Therapy

Phototherapy is a standard procedure in the treatment of many inflammatory skin diseases (Hönigsmann 2013). There are various modalities using different spectra of the UV irradiation (Bahvani et al. 2007; Hannuksela et al. 1985; Jekeler and Larkö 1991; Krutmann and Hönigsmann 1997; Reynolds et al. 2001):

- Heliotherapy (this is the exposure to natural sunlight)
- Broadband UVB (280–320 nm)
- Narrowband UVB (311–313 nm)
- UVA (320–400 nm)
- UVA1 (340–400 nm)
- Photochemotherapy using a combination of UV and psoralens, a photosensitizing agent (PUVA)
- Radiation with visible light or blue light

5.6.1 Heliotherapy

Heliotherapy uses the exposure to natural sunlight under controlled conditions. It is crucial to test the patient's photosensitivity (establishing the minimal erythema dose or checking Fitzpatrick's light sensitivity skin types).

Heliotherapy is especially performed using climate conditions such as different altitudes, either very low beyond sea level as on the Dead Sea in Israel (Simons et al., Harari et al. 2000) or at high altitude like in Davos, Switzerland (1560 m) (Vocks et al. 2002; Engst and Vocks 2000).

The patient is told to precisely watch the time of sun exposure, starting with very short periods of two or three minutes and slowly increasing the time.

5.6.2 UVB Radiation

UVB radiation is the standard treatment of psoriasis and many inflammatory skin diseases; it has also a very special effect upon pruritus, also on pruritus without skin alteration.

Studying the individual wavelength within the UV spectrum, it has been found that 311 nm seems to be most effective, which is called narrowband UV radiation (Krutmann and Hönigsmann 1997). It has been shown that phototherapy with UVB is able to stimulate the production of antimicrobial peptides in the epidermis (Gläser et al. 2009b).

5.6.3 UVA Radiation

Through the development of special lamps, the application of long-wave UV spectrum was possible, especially through the development of infrared filters which lower the typical heat induction.

The mechanisms of UV radiation-induced immunosuppression are complex, some of them obviously occurring as a result of the repair processes induced by damage to epidermal structures, especially DNA, but also changes in membrane phospholipids and trans-urocanic acid and tryptophan (Gibbs and Norval 2013). Since the group of Margaret Kripke has shown that UV radiation can suppress delayed-type immunity against transplanted tumors in mice (Fisher and Kripke 1977), photoimmunology has been developed as an exciting branch of research (Krutmann et al. 2012). In the epidermis, Langerhans cells (CD1d) and langerin-positive CD103-negative dendritic cells migrate to the draining lymph node and stimulate the production of regulatory T cells. In experimental studies, it has been found that there are obviously two peaks within the electromagnetic spectrum which show especially marked effects with regard to immunosuppression, namely, in the UVB range around 310 and in the UVA range around 370 nm (Gibbs and Norval 2013).

Especially within the long-wave spectrum of UVA, the UVA1 part (340–400 nm) has been first studied by Krutmann et al. (1992; 1998). Different doses of UVA1 are used (Dawe 2003). Krutmann in his first studies used the high dose of 130 J/cm^2; we prefer a medium dose (50–60 J/cm^2) which is more efficacious than the low dose (10–20 J/cm^2) and is tolerated well (Kowalzick et al. 1995; Schmidt et al. 1998).

Apart from atopic eczema, UVA1 is also used in localized scleroderma and granuloma anulare (Rombold et al. 2008). UVA1 has shown an inhibitory effect on mediator-secreting cells such as histamine from basophils or mast cells (Krönauer et al. 2003).

In our own study on 230 patients treated with low-dose, medium-dose, and high-dose UVA1 over 6 years, we could prove the good therapeutic effects in atopic eczema, scleroderma, lichen sclerosus et atrophicus, prurigo nodularis, and cutaneous T-cell lymphoma (Rombold et al. 2008). 84 % of 86 patients with atopic eczema showed moderate to marked improvement after 3 weeks of UVA1 radiation while low dose was considerably weaker (Kowalzick et al. 1995).

UVA1, besides anti-inflammatory effects, also seems to have specific antipruritic efficacy which is well accepted by the patients. We perform UVA1 treatment in a total of 15 sessions over 3 weeks with a slow increase of dose. UVA1 has its place in acute flares of eczema and is tolerated well (Von Kobyletzki et al. 1999).

5.6.4 Photochemotherapy

There is no doubt that the most effective type of UV therapy is, together with the use of photosensitizing substances, photochemotherapy, e.g., psoralens (with UVA, PUVA). However, this also is the treatment with most side effects; it should be preserved for severe cases and can be compared to systemic immunosuppression.

Systemic application of psoralens is nowadays used only rarely. The topical application in a bath (balneophotochemotherapy) or in a cream (cream PUVA) is now the method of choice (Krutmann and Hönigsmann 1997).

Psoralen is used in a concentration between 0.1 and 0.5 mg/l (methoxypsoralen 8-MOP) or 0.3 % meladinine in a lukewarm bath (32–35 °C over 20 min). Alternatively, psoralen can be incorporated in a cream (0.001 %) which is allowed to penetrate the skin over 30 min prior to UVA radiation. This method is preferably used in hand or foot eczema or in nummular variants.

5.6.5 Visible Light

New developments include the application of visible light, especially the spectrum of the blue light, sometimes called "light vaccine," which has been studied in pilot studies (Krutmann and Hönigsmann 1997, von Stebut et al., in prep).

Often UV therapy is combined with the use of salt baths (photosole therapy), trying to imitate the effects of climate therapy at the Dead Sea or at other seasides.

5.6.6 Extracorporeal Photopheresis

The method of extracorporeal photopheresis was introduced in the 1980s. Leukocytes are removed from the peripheral blood by cell apheresis and irradiated outside of the body with UV and 8-MOP (Knobler 1987). This method is real immunosuppression and preferably used in the treatment of cutaneous T-cell lymphomas, however, also in very severe cases of atopic eczema (Prinz et al. 1994).

5.6.7 Summary

Treatment with UV radiation is a standard regimen in the therapy of atopic eczema. Most commonly narrowband UVB (311 nm) or UVA1 wavelengths are used. When localized skin areas like the palms or soles are severely affected, also balneophototherapy or cream phototherapy (PUVA) can be helpful. Due to the unknown risk of long-term side effects, in childhood, this treatment should be reserved to very severe cases upon special indication (Ring et al. 2012).

In very severe cases of atopic eczema, extracorporeal photopheresis can be helpful.

5.7 Allergen-Specific Immunotherapy

While allergen-specific immunotherapy (ASIT), also called hyposensitization, has a standard place in the treatment of IgE-mediated allergies of airways and insect venom anaphylaxis (Ring 2005), it is surprising how relatively little we know about the effect of this causal treatment in atopic eczema. This is even more surprising when considering the clear-cut relevance of IgE-mediated sensitizations in many patients (see Sect. 3.3), as has been shown by the atopy patch test.

In certain recommendations for immunotherapy, atopic eczema may even be regarded as a contraindication for such a treatment; there is anecdotal evidence of acute flares of eczema after an immunotherapy injection when ASIT is performed against hay fever.

In animal experiments, it has been shown that it is possible to induce tolerance in a model of murine atopic dermatitis, either occurring spontaneously or after epicutaneous sensitization with ovalbumin. Tolerogenic dendritic cells were shown to successfully inhibit atopic dermatitis like skin lesions induced by repeated epicutaneous exposure to antigen (Katagiri et al. 2008).

5.7.1 Results of Clinical Trials

Reviews of the literature on ASIT for atopic dermatitis comprise open but also randomized and placebo-controlled studies (Bussmann et al. 2006; Darsow et al. 2005). Most of the studies showed a clear-cut effect of ASIT on the eczematous skin disease (Table 5.8).

The author performed a very simple placebo-controlled prospective trial in a pair of monozygous twins severely affected with eczema but also suffering from hay fever, after obtaining informed consent from the parents and the two girls. One was treated with grass pollen extract and the other one with saline placebo. After the first pollen season, one of the girls was significantly better than the other one (Fig. 5.11). So we decided to break the code and found out that the girl who had improved had been treated with the verum. Then also the sister was treated with true ASIT and also improved in the following year (Ring 1982b).

One of the most convincing studies has been performed by Werfel et al. in 89 patients where he could show a dose-dependent effect of subcutaneous ASIT with house dust mite allergen, regarding the improvement of atopic eczema as measured in SCORAD (Werfel et al. 2006). A variety of other studies have shown similar results (Czarnecka-Operacz and Silny 2006; Silny and Czarnecka-Operacz 2006; Grewe 2000; Zachariae et al. 1985).

Also sublingual application of allergen-specific immunotherapy (SLIT) can be effective (Pajno et al. 2007).

In pilot studies with house dust mite, also remarkable improvements of atopic eczema were seen (Bussmann et al. 2006).

Table 5.8 Allergen-specific immunotherapy (ASIT) in atopic dermatitis placebo-controlled studies (literature quoted in Darsow et al. 2005)

Authors	Number of patients	Method of ASIT duration	Outcome	Result
Kaufmann and Roth (1974)	16 Active 10 Placebo	Subcutaneous 2 Years	Clinical condition	Improvement Active 81 % Placebo 40 %
Warner et al. (1978)	27 Active 24 Placebo	Subcutaneous 1 Year	Clinical condition	Positive
Ring (1978)	Monozygous twins 10 Years	Subcutaneous 2 Years	Clinical condition Specific IgE, grass pollen	Positive
Glover and Atherton (1992)	13 Active 11 Placebo	Subcutaneous 8 + 6 Months	Clinical condition Specific and total IgE, skin prick test	Weak
Leroy et al. (1993)	24	Intradermal 4–8 Months	Clinical condition Specific IgE D. pteronyssinus	Positive
Petrova et al. (2001)	28 Active 39 Placebo 32 Control	Oral	Clinical and immunological results	Positive
Novak et al. (2012)	112 Active	Subcutaneous	Clinical condition (SCORAD)	Overall negative, positive in subgroup with SCORAD over 50

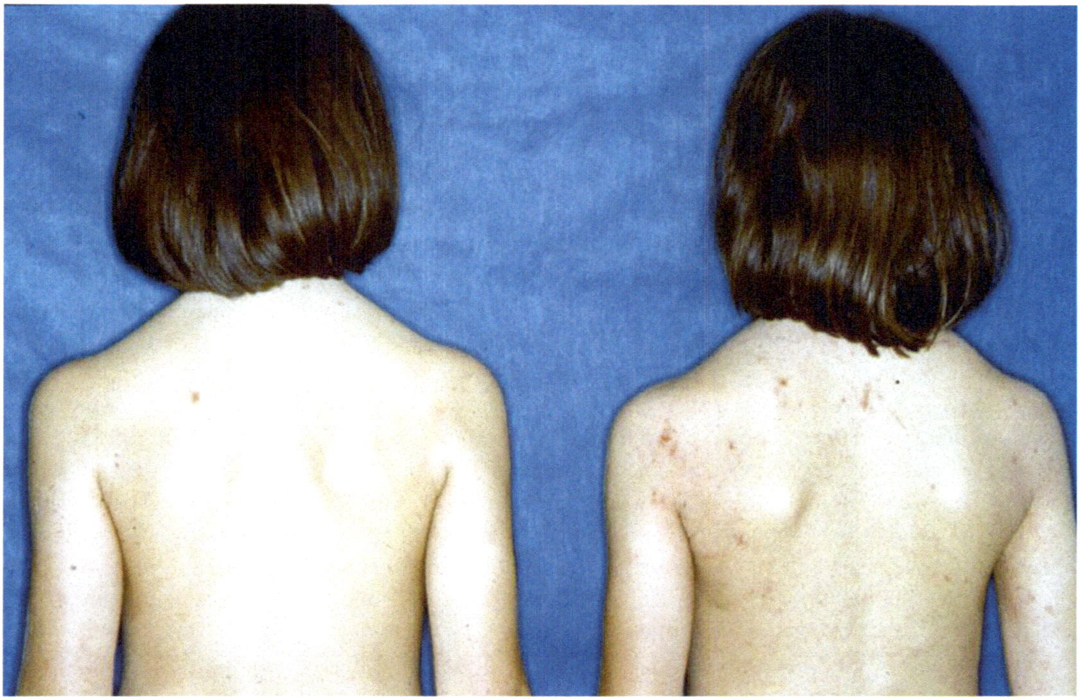

Fig. 5.11 Double-blind study with subcutaneous allergen-specific immunotherapy (ASIT) with grass pollen extract in homozygous twins with atopic dermatitis (left verum, right placebo) (Ring 1982b)

In a recent study by Novak et al., there was no overall difference in a group of 168 eczema patients. However, there was an interesting significant improvement in a subgroup analysis of patients with very severe atopic dermatitis, namely, a SCORAD over 15 (Novak et al. 2012).

Also rash protocols (3-day dose increase) and ultrarash (buildup in 1 day) have been shown to be effective in reducing eczema symptoms.

The major mechanism through which allergen-specific immunotherapy works is the induction of peripheral tolerance via T-regulatory cells (Treg) which supply the balance between Th1 and Th2 immune response reactivity patterns (Akdis et al. 2004).

50 years ago, the idea came that a complex of histamine and gamma globulin might affect plasma histamine levels in a beneficial way (Gelfand et al. 1963). In an animal experimental study, it was shown that this complex was able to regulate the Th1-Th2 balance in favor of Th1 cytokines (Nahm et al. 2008).

In a recent pilot study, a combined treatment of allergen-specific immunotherapy with house dust mites together with the application of the histamine-immunoglobulin complex led to significant clinical improvement of eczematous skin lesions (Nahm et al. 2008).

5.7.2 Practical Consequences

It makes sense to think about ASIT in selected cases of atopic dermatitis with clear-cut clinical relevance of IgE-mediated sensitization against aeroallergens. A special scheme has been developed as the so-called Davos immunotherapy where we use the allergen-pure conditions of the high altitude (no house dust mites) for the induction phase of dose increase in patients with house dust mite allergy and severe atopic eczema. This treatment often is not easy to perform under normal life conditions (Ring, Schupp et al., in prep.).

Since it could be shown that IgE-mediated sensitizations play a role in many patients in the elicitation and maintenance of eczematous skin lesions, several studies investigating the effects of allergen-specific immunotherapy (ASIT) have been performed in atopic eczema, most of them showing significant improvement. Therefore, in selected cases with clear-cut evidence for relevant IgE sensitization to aeroallergens, an allergen-specific immunotherapy may be helpful.

5.8 Systemic Immunosuppressive Therapy

The majority of patients with atopic dermatitis responds well to the above mentioned treatment strategies using mostly topical application of anti-inflammatory substances together with systemic antipruritic medication or antimicrobial therapy. However, there are very severe cases which do not respond and need systemic immunosuppression. In the following, some of the most important substances will be briefly discussed. It has to be mentioned that the level of evidence for these therapeutic strategies is limited due to a lack of large placebo-controlled clinical trials (Akhavan and Rudikoff 2003).

5.8.1 Glucocorticosteroids

Glucocorticosteroids are mainly used as topical preparations; however, in rare cases, they are also given systemically. It may be surprising that in large reviews on treatment habits among general practitioners, the systemic use of glucocorticosteroids is not so rare (Augustin et al. 2014). However, there is almost no controlled study with regard to the effect of systemic glucocorticosteroids. Recently, a study has been published as investigator-initiated double-blind randomized multicenter trial in adult patients with severe eczema (SCORAD over 40 and Dermatology Life Quality Index over 10); systemic prednisolone (0.5–0.8 mg/kg) was compared to cyclosporin (2.4–4.0 mg/kg). There were an unexpectedly high number of withdrawals in this severely affected group, so that finally only 38 patients were randomized and went into the study. Only in 1 out of 21 patients under prednisolone, compared to 6 out of 17 under cyclosporin, was stable remission achieved ($p < 0.03$). The authors concluded that cyclosporin is significantly more effective than prednisolone in treating severe adult eczema (Schmitt et al. 2010). I personally use systemic steroids for atopic eczema very rarely and only in special cases with acute dramatic flares for some days.

Systemic steroids may be given in pregnant women with severe eczema in order to avoid other immunosuppressives with their contraindications.

5.8.2 Cyclosporin A

Cyclosporin A was discovered in transplantation medicine, where it is meanwhile the classic immunosuppressive to prevent rejection after organ transplantation. It exerts its effects via binding to a cytosolic immunophilin similar to calcineurin inhibitors (see Sect. 5.2) but acts only systemically. In dermatology, cyclosporin A is used in various inflammatory diseases (Bourke et al. 1996; Schmitt et al. 2007b; Zurbriggen et al. 1999).

5.8.2.1 Dosage

Cyclosporin A is one of the most effective substances and is given at a dose of 2.5 mg/kg, slowly to be increased to 5 mg/kg body weight. One also can try a body weight-independent dosage of 150–300 mg/day. After marked improvement or stable remission, the dose is slowly reduced (0.5 mg/kg in 2- to 4-week intervals). Cyclosporin treatment has to be performed over longer time periods, since after withdrawal, severe "rebound" reactions can occur. Due to its side effects (see below), a maximal treatment duration of 2 years is recommended (Darsow et al. 2010; Ring et al. 2012).

Cyclosporin is also effective in children and adolescents (Bunikowski et al. 2001; Harper et al. 2000, 2002); however, the indication has to be put very strictly, and it should be reserved to severe cases.

5.8.2.2 Side Effects

The side effects of cyclosporin A include frequent gastrointestinal symptoms, headache, and especially disturbance of the renal function with resulting hypertonia. Therefore patients have to be checked intensively with regard to renal disease but also neoplasia, immunodeficiency, or hypertension prior to cyclosporin therapy. Under therapy, laboratory controls regarding urea and creatinine as well as electrolytes and differential blood counts have to be controlled.

Rare side effects include paresthesias, hypertrichosis lanuginosa, and hyperplasia of the gingiva.

Due to possible photocarcinogenicity or due to the actual immunosuppression, patients under cyclosporin A therapy should use sun protection.

Incompatibilities with other drugs such as antibiotics, antimycotics which are metabolized via cytochrome P450 have to be considered. Cyclosporin A acts by blocking T-cell activation and preventing the secretion of a variety of cytokines such as interleukin-2 (Kwiek and Novak 2010). Furthermore, cyclosporin A has an effect upon keratinocytes in preventing apoptosis and has a direct antipruritic effect by acting on mast cells. Possibly the place for cyclosporin is in the very severe eczema patients with IgE-mediated autoreactivity (see Sect. 3.3) (Kwiek and Novak 2010).

5.8.3 Azathioprine

Azathioprine is a purine analogue with a general effect on lymphocytes. It is usually used in order to spare steroids; however, it has a slow onset of action. It has been shown to be effective in atopic eczema (Murphy and Atherton 2002; Plötz et al. 2014). Prior to using azathioprine, one should measure the enzyme thiopurine methyltransferase (TPMT) since, when there are defects, rapid development of myelodepression can occur (Meggitt et al. 2006).

The therapeutic effect of azathioprine treatment only becomes visible after weeks or months. Regular controls of blood count and liver values are recommended. Side effects include nausea, leukopenia, and very rarely allergic reactions (Schmoeckel and von Liebe 1983).

5.8.4 Methotrexate

Methotrexate is an antimetabolite of folic acid and used as antineoplastic substance in the treatment of rheumatoid arthritis and psoriasis. It can also be used in severe cases of atopic eczema (Lyakhovitsky et al. 2010). In a randomized trial comparing methotrexate with azathioprine, it was found that methotrexate is equally effective as azathioprine (Schram et al. 2011).

Methotrexate can be given orally or parenterally. It is usually given once a week, starting with doses of 7.5 mg per week slowly increasing to 15 mg per week, followed by the application of folate (5 mg 1 day after the methotrexate application). We prefer the subcutaneous application which can be performed by the patient himself. Side effects include myelosuppression and hepatotoxicity, which has to be checked regularly. Methotrexate is contraindicated in pregnancy and during lactation.

5.8.5 Mycophenolate Mofetil

Mycophenolate mofetil is regularly used in organ transplantation but also more and more in inflammatory skin diseases such as autoimmune bullous disease and psoriasis. It also has been found effective in atopic eczema (Neuber et al. 2000). It is given in patients where cyclosporin A is contraindicated. Mycophenolate mofetil inhibits the inosine monophosphate dehydrogenase and thus the purine synthesis (Benez and Fierlbeck 2001; Grundmann-Kollmann et al. 1999; Hansen et al. 2000; Plötz et al. 2014). Under mycophenolate mofetil, blood count and liver, renal, and electrolyte values have to be controlled in 2-week intervals. In a controlled observer-blinded randomized trial, mycophenolate was compared to cyclosporin in patients with severe atopic dermatitis, showing that mycophenolate mofetil was as effective as cyclosporin A in maintenance therapy in patients with atopic dermatitis. However, the clinical improvement after mycophenolate took longer time in comparison to cyclosporin A (Haeck et al. 2011a, b).

5.8.6 Cyclophosphamide

Cyclophosphamide, which is widely used in hematological and collagen disease, should not be given in atopic dermatitis. It is an alkylating agent with special action on a subgroup of T cells, mainly regulatory T cells. It has been shown that several autoimmune diseases may be increased as is allergic contact dermatitis (Ikezawa et al. 2005).

5.8.7 Summary

Very severe cases of atopic eczema have to be treated with systemic immunosuppressives. Apart from cyclosporin A, azathioprine, mycophenolate mofetil, and methotrexate are in use. Several side effects have to be considered. The side effects of cyclosporin A include gastrointestinal complaints, headache, and severe disturbance of renal function with resulting hypertension.

5.9 New Therapeutic Options in Clinical Trials

5.9.1 Biologics

Biologics have been introduced in medicine 20 years ago, using the production of recombinant proteins with modern gene technology, thus allowing very specific actions on well-defined target structures. They comprise monoclonal antibodies against cytokines, monoclonal antibodies against specific receptors, soluble cytokines, and soluble receptors.

Also intravenous immunoglobulins or interferons may be called "biologics."

In the following, the most important biologics of possible relevance for atopic dermatitis will be discussed.

5.9.1.1 Anti-IgE

Since almost 20 years, the monoclonal antibody against human IgE (omalizumab) is available for the treatment of severe asthma (Milgrom et al. 2001; Buhl et al. 2002). It is a humanized IgG1 molecule and also has effects in allergic rhinitis, IgE-mediated food allergy (Leung et al. 2003), and recently chronic urticaria (Maurer et al. 2013). Omalizumab induces a marked and rapid decrease of serum IgE levels and has to be given in a dose according to the actual serum IgE concentration with good safety protile (Holgate et al. 2005; Cox et al. 2007).

There have been a variety of case reports with successful omalizumab treatment in atopic dermatitis (Forman and Garrett 2007; Vigo et al. 2006 neu; Caruso et al. 2010 neu, alle s. Caruso). We performed a pilot study in a total of 11 patients with severe atopic eczema and concomitant asthma who had been treated with systemic immunosuppressives and phototherapy without good effect before. In 6 of 11 patients, there was marked improvement (Belloni et al. 2007). These patients had serum IgE concentrations sometimes reaching 15,000 kU/L; therefore it was not possible to dose according to the recommendation of the producer, but we just use the typical dose used in asthma patients with 150 mg every 2 weeks.

It was interesting to see that under omalizumab, there was a marked change in the ratio of RNA from peripheral B lymphocytes with a strong increase of RNA for IgG4 versus IgE. We speculate that anti-IgE in severe atopic dermatitis may have another mechanism of action than just removing IgE from serum but may have a direct regulatory effect (Lim et al. 2007).

A controlled study by Stingl et al. showed no significant effect.

Recently we tried to combine anti-IgE with prior plasmapheresis removing excessively increased IgE values (Zink et al. 2015). In an ongoing study, it should be elucidated which biomarkers may possibly predict responders to anti-IgE treatment in atopic dermatitis (Thijs et al. 2015).

5.9.1.2 Anti-T Cell Strategies

Several biologics are used in order to target T-cell activation at different levels.

Alefacept is a fusion protein of lymphocyte function antigen LFA3 (CD58) which inhibits the costimulatory signals and induces T-cell apoptosis. In a pilot study, good effects have been seen in atopic eczema (Simon et al. 2008).

Efalizumab is a monoclonal antibody inhibiting T-cell recruitment and has been used in psoriasis effectively. It was also used in atopic dermatitis. However, due to some cases of progressive cerebral leukodystrophy, efalizumab is no longer available. In a study with 11 cases, only two showed mild improvement after efalizumab treatment (Ibler et al. 2010).

Another antibody is targeted against p40, a common structure in the cytokines interleukin-12 and interleukin-23 (ustekinumab), and is used in psoriasis (Papp et al. 2013); there are no convincing reports regarding its efficacy in eczema. Also Antagonists of TSLP (Tezepe lumab) have been tried (Lauffer and Ring 2016).

5.9.1.3 Anti-TNF Strategies

Tumor necrosis factor (TNF) is a central cytokine of delayed-type hypersensitivity which plays a major role in Th1-mediated immune reactions. Anti-TNF has shown remarkable effects in rheumatic diseases such as Crohn's disease, rheumatoid arthritis, and psoriasis.

There are several products available such as monoclonal antibodies against TNF (infliximab, golimumab, adalimumab) but also soluble receptor antagonists of the TNF receptor (etanercept).

There are some case reports describing mild to moderate effects (Cassano et al. 2006). However, there are a variety of serious side effects including allergic reactions as well as the development of sepsis (Bremmer et al. 2009).

With regard to the antagonistic behavior in immune reactivity between psoriasis and atopic dermatitis (see Chap. 3), the question arises whether treatments targeted to the Th1 part of the psoriatic inflammation really are desirable for the treatment of eczema. In a variety of patients suffering simultaneously from psoriasis and atopic dermatitis, we found that under infliximab, atopic dermatitis flared dramatically (Eyerich et al. 2011). We therefore feel that anti-TNF strategies are not a method of choice in the treatment of atopic dermatitis. In those patients affected by both psoriasis and eczema, the less specific strategy using cyclosporin A is recommended.

5.9.1.4 Anti-CD20

The monoclonal antibody against the B cell marker CD20 leads to a depletion of B cells in the peripheral blood and is used effectively in the treatment of hematologic diseases and autoimmune diseases such as pemphigus vulgaris. In a pilot study in some patients with severe atopic eczema, rituximab showed dramatic effects (Simon et al. 2008). We also saw similar effects but also severe side effects.

5.9.1.5 Anti-Interleukin-4/-Interleukin-13

Interleukin-4 and 13 are important cytokines in the production of immunoglobulin E from B lymphocytes and plasma cells as the characteristic Th2 cytokines. Monoclonal antibodies against IL-4 have been tried (pascolizumab). Pitrakinra is a recombinant variant of interleukin-4, inhibiting the IL-4 receptor, and is used as aerosol in patients with asthma.

Recent studies with anti-IL13 include Leprikizumab and Tralokinumab (Lauffer and Ring 2016).

Recently an antibody against the interleukin-4 receptor dupilumab has shown very promising results in the treatment of asthma and atopic eczema (Fajt and Wenzel 2014; Beck et al. 2015).

5.9.1.6 Anti-Interleukin-5

Interleukin-5 is the crucial cytokine in the recruitment, production, and activation of eosinophil granulocytes which represent a major characteristic of tissue inflammation both in asthma and in atopic dermatitis.

First clinical trials with a monoclonal antibody against IL-5 in asthma showed disappointing clinical results, although there was a clear-cut effect in the reduction of peripheral eosinophil counts. On the contrary, mepolizumab was highly effective in the rare group of patients with hypereosinophilic syndrome (HES) (Plötz et al. 2003; Rothenberg et al. 2008).

In a placebo-controlled study with only two injections of mepolizumab in atopic dermatitis, there was a significant but only moderate clinical effect (Oldhoff et al. 2005).

Future studies with a more prolonged therapy that compare different doses would be recommendable.

5.9.1.7 Anti-Interleukin-17 and Interleukin-22

For the treatment of psoriasis (Krueger et al. 2015), new monoclonal antibodies against interleukin-17 will soon be available (secukinumab) also against interleukin 22 (fezakinumab). Whether they also show an effect in atopic dermatitis remains to be studied.

5.9.1.8 Intravenous Immunoglobulins

The intravenous application of high doses of immunoglobulins has proven helpful in a variety of autoimmune diseases such as dermatomyositis and idiopathic thrombocytopenic purpura.

There are some case reports regarding the use of IVIg in atopic dermatitis (Paul et al. 2002) showing a transitory effect. Due to the high costs, this therapeutic option remains only for a limited number of patients.

5.9.1.9 Interferon

Recombinant interferon gamma has been shown in experimental studies to inhibit Th2 cytokine patterns and thus has been used in a clinical study in atopic dermatitis with controversial effects (Hanifin et al. 1993).

5.9.1.10 Summary

The progress through the introduction of biologics into medicine, which has been achieved in other diseases such as psoriasis, rheumatoid arthritis or Crohn's disease, or asthma, has not yet really reached atopic dermatitis. However, there are some reports of positive effects with certain agents in selected patients. The real breakthrough of biologics for atopic dermatitis has not yet been found; maybe the new results observed with anti-IL-4 receptor antagonist dupilumab are the most promising ones. Future studies are advisable.

5.9.2 Inhibition of Chemokines

More than 50 chemokines are known to act as mediators in the activation of various inflammatory cells. Chemokines act via specific receptors (CCR) and are grouped today under CCL (chemokine ligands). The most important chemokine for atopic dermatitis is the thymus and activation-dependent chemokine TARC (CCL17) binding to the chemokine receptor CCL4. It may be interesting to find specific antagonists of this receptor with regard to clinical effects in atopic dermatitis (Homey et al. 2006). A new chemokine antagonist tofacitinib is in clinical trials for psoriasis.

5.9.3 Inhibitors of Signal Transduction

Most cytokines act after intake into the cell and migration to the nucleus by binding to transcription factors such as NF-kB. Experimental studies using an inhibitor of NF-kB kinase IKK2 have shown an effect in asthma (Tudhope et al. 2007).

5.9.4 Toll-Like Receptor Agonists

Toll-like receptors (TLRs) are in the center of innate immunity (Sect. 3.3). In humans, 10 different TLRs are known, binding different microbial structures such as lipopolysaccharides, nucleotides, DNA, or RNA. On the basis of the hygiene hypothesis, describing immune stimulation in early childhood having a positive effect with regard to the development of atopic diseases, substances involved in the stimulation of TLRs have been investigated. Many of these studies are in the phase of animal experiments. They comprise substances from bacterial extracts such as from *Acinetobacter lwoffii*.

Also studies to increase Th1 response by microbial or parasitic antigens have to be mentioned here.

5.9.5 Induction of Antimicrobial Peptides (AMP)

Patients with atopic dermatitis have decreased epidermal defense reactions (see Chap. 3) and also decreased production of antimicrobial peptides (AMP) such as cathelicidin, LL37, and human beta defensin 2. The addition of vitamin D in vitro has shown to increase AMP production (Schauber et al. 2007; Schauber and Gallo 2008). Supplementation of vitamin D3 in patients with atopic dermatitis led to clinical improvement (Sidburi et al. 2000).

It may be of interest that the calcineurin inhibitor pimecrolimus also exerts effects on TLR2, leading to an increased expression of antimicrobial peptides in keratinocytes (Buchau et al. 2009).

Furthermore, it may be possible to apply synthetic antimicrobial substances or agents leading to increased production of AMP. The topical application of ceragenin (CSA-13) has antiviral activity and might be used in eczema herpeticum (Howell et al. 2007). The field of antimicrobial peptides and innate immunity in atopic dermatitis is promising (Harder et al. 2013).

5.9.6 Pre- and Probiotics

Probiotics such as lactobacillus mixtures have been used in atopic dermatitis and shown to lead to an improvement (Isolauri et al. 2000; Kalliomäki et al. 2001). Occasionally also a preventive effect of probiotics given during pregnancy could be observed (Isolauri et al. 2000). Other studies (Fölster-Holst et al. 2006b; Rosenfeldt et al. 2003), however, showed no significant effects. This coincides with our own experiences.

In a recent study in 800 infants, the effect of a prebiotic mixture of immunoactive oligosaccharides has been studied. There was a significant effect in a decreased occurrence of atopic dermatitis (Grüber 2012) (see also Chap. 6).

Whether the alteration of the intestinal or cutaneous microbiome will play a role in clinical practice is a matter of investigation (Penders et al. 2013).

5.9.7 Protein Kinase Inhibitors

On the basis of the surprising effects with protein kinase inhibitors in cancer therapy (e.g., imatinib), investigations were performed to apply specific kinase inhibitors in allergic inflammation.

5.9.8 Unsaturated Fatty Acids

There is a long tradition of hypothetical considerations that polyunsaturated fatty acids (PUFA) such as gamma linolenic acid and eicosapentaenoic acid may have beneficial effects on atopic inflammation and atopic eczema (Berth-Jones and Graham-Brown 1993; Buslau and Thaci 1996).

A prospective randomized trial performed by our group showed no significant effects over placebo (Ring and Kunz 1991). Maybe this therapeutic option could have a place in allergy prevention.

5.9.9 Phosphodiesterase Inhibitors

On the basis of studies showing a weakened reactivity of cyclic AMP and a decreased responsiveness to beta-adrenergic stimuli, an augmented phosphodiesterase activity has been postulated as a pathogenic factor in atopic dermatitis (Chan et al. 1993; Sidbury and Hanifin 2000).

Novel phosphodiesterase inhibitors like apremilast are under investigation (Moustafa 2014; Samrao et al. 2012; Papp et al. 2012). Topical preparations like crisaborole seem attractive with antipruritic activity (Furue et al. 2014)

5.9.10 Summary

A variety of scientifically interesting therapeutic approaches like interleukin 4R antagonists or PDE inhibitors are under experimental and clinical investigation. The future will show what will come to clinical practice.

5.10 Psychosomatic Strategies

The skin as expression organ of the soul has an eminent aesthetic function. Therefore it is not surprising that skin diseases not only become manifest in somatic complaints but often also lead to psychologic problems. The intensity of this psychosomatic interaction varies individually. One has always to consider that skin conditions have to be regarded both in a psychosomatic and in a somatopsychic way (Stangier 2001).

5.10.1 Exploration and Evaluation of Psychosomatic Involvement in the Disease

It is extremely important first to detect and evaluate together with the patient on how far psychological factors influence the skin disease toward exacerbation or eventually improvement. This requires an open conversation and motivation to self-perception. It is crucial not to give the impression that atopic dermatitis is a "psychological" disease. It has always to be stated that atopic dermatitis primarily is a skin disease which can be modulated through neural irritation and psychological influences but does not have per se a psychiatric cause! (See Sect. 3.5.)

This is especially important in the treatment of infants or small children where organic causes obviously are central; the induction of "feelings of guilt" in the mother or the father has to be absolutely avoided!

With increasing age, it is natural that the more severe the eczematous skin lesions are and the more often the frustrating experience of therapeutic failure has been observed, psychological alterations begin which have to be analyzed and discussed in a patient-doctor relation carried by mutual trust.

Note: There are many patients with very severe atopic eczema who are psychologically absolutely normal and benefit only little from psychosomatic or psychotherapeutic interventions.

Every human being has his/her everyday problems, stress, and emotional conflicts. It is a normal and "human" basis of patient-doctor interaction to also cover these aspects in the exploration of the history. This would need no special training. However—this cannot be denied—modern medicine is moving into a direction of utmost specialization in a way that residents in a university hospital call for a psychosomatic consultant with the note: "The patient is crying" Richter and Ahrens 1990. From my experience, I advise the parents of children with atopic dermatitis to know about psychosomatic interactions and try to realize and observe these psychodynamics of family situations with their impact on the skin disease of the offspring themselves (Egle et al. 2002). As shown above (Sect. 3.5), I also try to get the fathers more involved into the "family business" of every day and also into the care of the diseased skin of the child. At the same time, I try to motivate very stressed mothers to "relax" and not take everything so seriously.

The treatment of skin diseases always needs patience; good effects can never be forced (Prochazka 1994). Especially the basic therapy of the disturbed skin barrier function should not develop into a compulsory behavior in the form of a "skin hygiene ritual" which naturally will build up aversion in the child against parental authority.

5.10.2 Therapeutic Modalities

As soon as psychological components are recognized as relevant for the individual disease of a patient, the best possible therapeutic option has to be selected. This always has to be done on the basis of somatic general skin treatment. A cooperation between a dermatologist and psychologist or psychosomatic physician is absolutely essential (Ehlers et al. 1995)!

In Table 5.9, various opportunities of psychosomatic therapeutic options are enlisted, reaching from placebo treatment to psychoanalysis (Suárez et al. 2012).

Through the introduction of short-time analytic procedures with less time- and cost-associated sessions, also psychoanalytically oriented therapeutic options can make sense. However, it has to be mentioned that in the exploration of emotions, eczema flares may be triggered.

Rarely psychopharmaceuticals should be used, preferably those with also antihistaminergic components, thus having concomitant antipruritic effects (see Sect. 5.4). The well-known placebo effect is particularly notable in allergies and especially atopic dermatitis and may help to explain why so many anecdotal reports of effective "complementary" or "alternative" methods are reported (see Sect. 5.11).

From own experience with placebo-controlled clinical trials using new therapeutics, I know that it is the pure personal impact ("doctor's devotion to patients") of a physician which can have surprising effects in the treatment of atopic dermatitis. After many years, I receive Christmas postcards "Thank you, you have cured me!" from patients with severe atopic dermatitis who have been in the placebo group and experienced long-lasting significant improvement (Fig. 5.12).

Table 5.9 Therapeutic options in atopic dermatitis with psychosomatic involvement (in addition to classical dermatologic treatment)

Placebo treatment
Psychopharmaceuticals (sedatives, antihistamines, antidepressants)
Psychosomatic counseling
Behavioral therapy (cognitive behavioral stress management)
Family therapy
Relaxation techniques
Autogenic training
Biofeedback
Hypnosis
Psychotherapy/group psychotherapy
Psychoanalysis

The logical consequence from this is not a recommendation to prescribe placebos, but to intensify the personal involvement of a physician-patient interaction.

5.10.3 Behavioral Therapy

In atopic dermatitis, several behavioral therapeutical techniques have been used; they all comprise the classical stages (Young et al. 1986):

- Detection and characterization of problematic behavior
- Selection of relevant stimuli and consequences
- Intervention
- Evaluation of success

At the beginning, mostly relaxation techniques are used like the large muscle relaxation according to Jacobsen (1938). However, other methods like autogenic training and biofeedback are widely used (Stangier et al. 1996).

Recently a new technique of "mindfulness" in the coping with stress has also been used for atopic dermatitis (ongoing study).

These techniques have to be practiced with the patient; they cannot be learned on theoretical recommendation. Therefore this is a central part

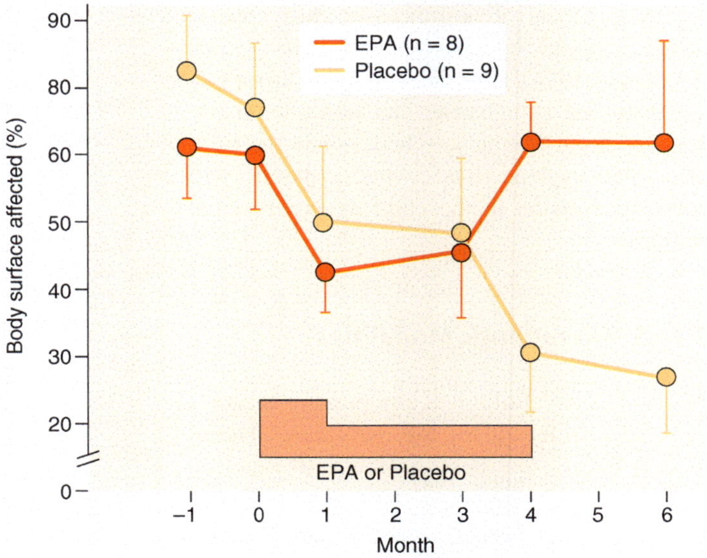

Fig. 5.12 Clinical improvement in patients with atopic eczema under treatment with eicosapentaenoic acid or placebo in a double-blind placebo-controlled clinical trial: at the end, placebo was better than verum (After Ring and Kunz (1991))

of educational programs in atopic dermatitis (Sect. 6.4).

Autogenic training as well as imagination techniques (e.g., cold imagination or the imagination of "healthy" environmental influences) may help in calming down the inflamed skin (Stangier et al. 1992).

Changes in behavior can be achieved via conditioning based on general principles of learning which have to be learned and practiced by the patient, leading to improvement (Table 5.10).

Practical techniques comprise recommendations for certain behaviors (Melin et al. 1986) focusing especially on scratching and the concomitant damage to the skin and maintenance of inflammation. This can be done by "distraction" techniques like using instruments for scratching (scratch cube) (Niebel 1990, 1995) the skin in respective situations. Sometimes already the recommendation to keep an "itch diary," where the patient makes a written note regarding the intensity of his itch sensations, can be helpful by the pure act of handwriting and distraction from scratching.

In the coping of the many burdens associated with this disease, many patients have lost hope and are additionally desperate when they often hear the term "incurable." This is where

Table 5.10 Techniques of behavioral therapy and conditioning

Classical	"Desensitization" (e.g., reciprocal inhibition with relaxation techniques after classification of a hierarchy of irritants) Flooding (exposure to an overwhelming dose of the stimulus) Assertiveness training (practicing the competence to express own feelings and wishes without hurting other individuals) Communication therapy of couples
Operant	Positive reinforcement Negative reinforcement Punishment Ignorance (e.g., "time-out") Oversatiation
Observational	Model learning from comparable situations
Cognitive	Development of new understanding of interactions Bibliotherapy Paradoxical communication

cognitive behavioral therapy starts (Beck 1999) which also acts against the peculiar "perfectionism" observed in many patients with atopic dermatitis. The sentence "the skin is no washing surface which has to be polished" often is helpful.

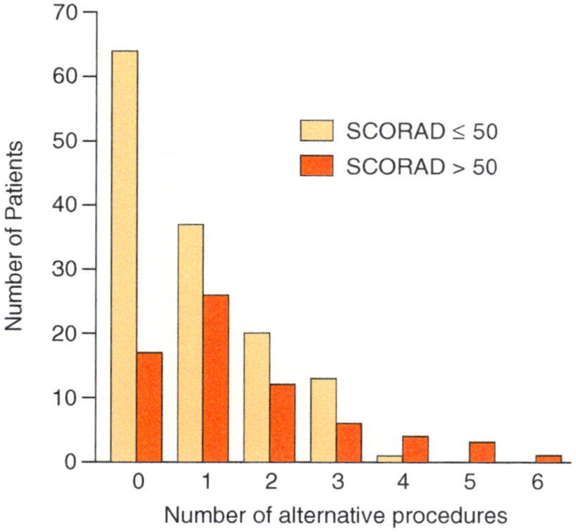

Fig. 5.13 Number of various "alternative" (unconventional) procedures used over a 3-month period by patients with atopic eczema ($n=204$) (From Schäfer et al. (2002))

Furthermore, the social competence which often is compromised in many patients with facial eczema has to be promoted. Always it has to be mentioned that patients with atopic dermatitis are not "neurotic" and do not have a psychiatric disease!

The understanding and practicing of cooperative communication improve the self-confidence of the patient. In this context, so-called role plays are helpful like they are used in programs for "eczema school." Wrong ways of thinking ("I am ugly"; "everybody is looking at me") can be overcome. Studies with volunteers wearing eyeglasses through which one could measure the direction of the gaze of the observer show clearly that patients suffering from facial dermatoses always believe that they are more and more intensively observed than is actually true with regard to the observing environment.

In a randomized controlled trial, a cognitive behavioral stress management program has been investigated in 28 patients with severe atopic dermatitis. A "public speaking" effort was the stimulus for acute stress. After undergoing cognitive behavioral stress management programs, the experimental group showed lower salivary cortisol levels under acute stress and remained calmer as measured by the cortisol-awakening response (Schut et al. 2013).

Hypnosis may be used in selected cases in order to relax fixed behavioral patterns and reflexes (Shenefelt 2000; Sokel et al. 1993, Willemsen in prep.).

A general experience which has to be told: It is so much easier to detect emotional conflicts and difficulties than to clear them.

5.10.4 Summary

Atopic dermatitis is primarily a skin disease, however, modulated via neural stimuli and reaction patterns and psychological influences. An intense exploration with regard to the influence of conflict situations or stress is helpful in many patients. On the basis of this, specific psychosomatic counseling can be recommended. The therapeutic options include behavioral therapy with different procedures which also can be included in eczema school programs.

5.11 Unconventional Methods

There are few fields in medicine where "alternative," "complementary," or "unconventional" methods have such a degree of popularity as in the management of atopic dermatitis (Fig. 5.13). Reports from the lay press about presumptuous "new miracle ointments or tablets" or "cures through bioscientific methods" (anonymous "cream from the other world," 1992) support this trend (Artik and Ruzicka 2003; Dorsch and Sitzmann 2001; Kukutsch 1997; Ruzicka 1998; Stiftung Warentest 1994; Fuhrmann et al. 2010; Nakano et al. 2015).

The increasing budgetary restraints in many countries give rise to a trend that "normal," scientifically oriented physicians also know unconventional methods if they are desired by the patient, in order to earn easy money, and thus support the routine office with science-oriented diagnostics and therapy. Some people repeat the old—but wrong—argument "who cures is right"; this sentence is not logical since it compares different categories similar to "who wins is beautiful"; correctly the sentence should be "Who cures does good; but whether he is right is another question."

The increasing specialization and introduction of technology into medicine, together with the acceleration and dwindling time physicians have for the individual patient and a deep longing for a harmonic world where illness and health of the whole human being are seen together, is growing in a romantic imagination of the unity of body and soul; man is part of nature and religion. Especially in Germany, this romanticism on the basis of the philosophical school of German idealism (Kant, Fichte, Schelling) has strong roots in all levels of the population. The hunt for the "blue flower" is still very attractive. Disease is seen as disturbance of the originally harmonic world, and biologic processes are interpreted philosophically or with religious content. There is an old experience: The "unconventional"/"alternative" medicine of today is the scientific medicine of the past century. Some of the thoughts are justified and interesting, but they are combined with totally outdated or obsolete methods.

When these diffuse irrational sentiments are combined with most modern technology (e.g., bioresonance), they become tricky and give the patient the wrong impression of a scientific basis ("pseudoscience").

Many patients with atopic dermatitis have used a variety of "unconventional" procedures before they come to the doctor (Augustin et al. 1999a; Schäfer et al. 2002). Partly this may be due to the frustration after repeated relapses of the skin disease and insufficient anti-inflammatory therapy or physician's care in this complex disease (Schmitt et al. 2008).

Table 5.11 enlists the most important "unconventional" procedures used widely in the management of eczema. As a matter of fact, in a survey in 2002, we found 120 different methods to be used, sometimes similar with very small differences but with very new names (Dorsch and Ring 2002). When people postulate that the science should have no hesitance to study these procedures, this is a difficult task.

Table 5.11 Most commonly used "alternative"/ "unconventional" procedures in allergy (alphabetical order!)

Acupuncture
Autologous blood injection
Autohomologous immunotherapy
Bach flower therapy
Bioresonance
Diet/curative fasting
Electroacupuncture
Hair mineral analyses
Homeopathy
Kinesiology
Neural therapy
Pendulum
Phytotherapy
Traditional Chinese medicine

According to Dorsch and Ring (2002)

Therefore we need plausibility criteria in sorting out various categories among the spectrum of "unconventional" procedures which may make sense or may be justified in certain patients (Table 5.12). It is noteworthy that sometimes so-called "unconventional" methods have interesting and plausible concepts and may lead to new therapeutic procedures which should be investigated with scientific methods (Kneipp 1984).

Many authors use the term "unconventional" or "complementary" for certain procedures which in fact present a meaningful addendum to classical dermatology therapy like:

- Psychosomatic counseling and relaxation techniques
- Dietary recommendations
- Climate therapy
- Phytotherapeutic procedures
- Physical therapy
- Sports therapy and ergotherapy
- Acupuncture (see below) (cum grano salis)

Contrary to these procedures, one can find a wide spectrum of methods which, according to current evidence, cannot be recommended since there is no evidence of efficacy, or the diagnostic reliability in controlled studies can be compared

Table 5.12 Unconventional procedures: categories of plausibility

New scientific procedure in the phase of clinical trials
Plausible concept founded on case reports; however, no exact studies are available
Procedure with little plausibility and lacking convincing case reports
Procedure lacking evidence of efficacy in spite of scientific studies
Procedure with such low plausibility or potential hazard that it is not advised to perform scientific studies
True quackery like fraud in mixing cortisone in presumptuous "cortisone-free" preparations

Table 5.13 Unconventional procedures which cannot be recommended according to current evidence

Autohomologous immunotherapy
Bach flower therapy
Bioresonance
Electroacupuncture
Kinesiology
Pendulum
Hair mineral analysis
Food-specific IgG for diagnostics and dietary recommendations

to throwing a dice (Table 5.13) (Dorsch and Ring 2002; Happle 1998; Oepen 1998; Schäfer et al. 2002). In the following, some procedures will be briefly discussed and evaluated. The practicing physician should at least know what his patients have read or even tried themselves. It makes no good impression when the doctor has to look up in the Internet what the patient is telling him; I help myself in these situations with the question "Well, how did this doctor actually do this?" Then the patient tells the story, and one can make at least a guess.

Table 5.14 Phytotherapeutic approaches in atopic dermatitis

Chamomile (*Matricariae flos*)
Marigold (*Calendulae flos*)
Hamamelis leaves and bark (*Hamamelidis folium et cortex*)
Oak bark (*Quercus cortex*)
Pansy herbs (*Violae tricoloris herba*)
Sage leaves (*Salvia folium*)
Bittersweet stalks (*Dulcamarae stipites*)
St. John's wort flowers (*Hyperici flos*)
Mahonia (*Mahonia aquifolium*)
Balloon vine (*Cardiospermum halicacabum*)
Evening primrose (*Oenothera biennis*)
Rockrose (*Cistus incanus*)

According to Reuter et al. (2010)

5.11.1 Evaluation of Some "Unconventional" Procedures

5.11.1.1 Acupuncture

Acupuncture comes from Chinese medicine and uses alterations of "energy streams" on the body surface and their alteration in illness through needle puncture. The needles have to be applied very precisely on certain classical "acupuncture points" and left there for several minutes. This is connected with pain; however, there should be no or minimal bleeding.

Acupuncture is used in school medicine in the therapy of pain. Regarding allergic reactions, acupuncture has been tried in experimental studies in hay fever (Langer and Hauswald 1992) with significant effects: skin test reactions and itch could be influenced by acupuncture (Pfab et al. 2010b). In this context, further studies are necessary; however, in single cases, acupuncture may be tried in atopic dermatitis (Yang 1997; Carlsson and Wallengren 2010). It has been found that in placebo-controlled clinical trials, under acupuncture, certain central nervous areas in the brain involved in the processing of the itch sensation may be downregulated (Pfab et al. 2012). Both placebo and nocebo responses can be documented in brain activation patterns (Napadow et al. 2015).

5.11.1.2 Phytotherapy and Traditional Chinese Medicine

Plant extracts have been used in medicine since early history, and many of today's pharmacological evidence-based drugs have been developed from plants. In dermatology, numerous plants are used against inflammation and for wound healing, but there is also vast literature on phytotherapy in atopic dermatitis (Table 5.14).

In the last years, the interest in East Asian medical concepts has increased considerably. Especially traditional Chinese medicine (TCM) has become very fashionable in the USA and Europe; these procedures have a strong connection with philosophical and religious concepts but use a variety of herbal extracts with considerable effects (Bedi and Shenefelt 2002). Significant improvements of eczema have been reported after the application of a mixture of ten different Chinese herbs in atopic eczema (Armstrong and Ernst 1999; Sheehan and Atherton 1992). Often it is impossible to select single substances in these mixtures and study them for their evidence. Recently a prospective randomized placebo-controlled trial reported significant effects of oral Xiaox-Iao-feng-sun (XFS), a mixture of 12 Chinese herbal preparations in atopic dermatitis (Cheng et al. 2011) from Taiwan.

It should be mentioned that these herbal extracts cannot be regarded generally as "safe": severe side reactions have been reported (Lord 1999) with hepatotoxicity and fatal consequences (Mostafa-Kara et al. 1992) as well as reversible dilated cardiomyopathy (Ferguson et al. 1997). In some herbal mixtures, potent glucocorticosteroids have been detected (O'Driscoll et al. 1992). These herbal mixtures should only be used under medical control and with knowledge of the content. Furthermore, plants can have very strong allergenic properties inducing allergic contact dermatitis also after systemic use (Hausen and Vieluf 1997). A similar degree of evidence can be found for Japanese phytotherapeutic measures (Campo medicine) (Kobayashi et al. 2004 *neu* in Reuter).

5.11.1.3 Homeopathy

Homeopathy was introduced into medicine by the German physician Samuel Hahnemann (1775–1843) who—in his time at the level of actual science—tried to understand and use pharmacological properties of a variety of substances (Hahnemann 1835). Unfortunately, the contact to scientific medicine with critical analysis and continuous methodological improvement has been lost over time in favor of a general characterization of "philosophy" (Weltanschauung). One factor comparable to scientific pharmacotherapy is the strong influence of a drug-producing lobby at the political level.

The basis of the homeopathy concept is the rule of "similarity" (similia similibus): Droplets, little balls (globuli), tablets, or injections are prepared with extreme dilutions of substances which are regarded to play a causal role in the disease. There is an inverse measurement of "potency" in that the higher the dilution, the more potent the preparation is believed to be. In some cases, even dilutions of 10^{23} are used, which means that, according to Loschmidt's number, there is no single molecule left in the solution (Weymayr and Heissmann 2012).

The concept of diluting effective substances is also used in allergen-specific immunotherapy (hyposensitization); however, in this case a clear-cut dose-response effect with increasing efficacy with increasing concentrations is applied.

There was marked publicity some years ago, when the group of a well-renowned scientist published in "Nature" that these extreme dilutions of allergens indeed were able to inhibit allergen-induced histamine release from peripheral basophil leukocytes (Benveniste et al. 1994). Also a clinical trial was performed with significant effects and published in "The Lancet" (Mayaux et al. 1988). The authors explained the effects of these dilutions by molecular vibrations thus leading to a "memory of water." As expected, these results could not be reproduced in any other lab. The editor of "Nature" ordered an external independent evaluation (the group consisted of a physicist, a statistician, and a magician) and found that the laboratory data were faked by a close female coworker trying to please the master!

It is extremely difficult to perform controlled studies with homeopathic regimens (Kleijnen et al. 1991); however, some studies showing positive effects in hay fever have been published (Wiesenauer et al. 1990); however, negative results are more common (Ernst and Barnes 1998).

We performed a randomized, placebo-controlled, double-blind clinical trial studying the effect of classic homeopathic therapy in atopic eczema and found no significant effect of homeopathy compared to placebo. However, both verum and placebo therapy led to marked improvement over the observational period of almost 1 year (Siebenwirth et al. 2009; Remy et al. 1995).

5.11.1.4 Cell Extracts and Thymus Factors

On the basis of good experiences with "fresh cell therapy" in the fifties of the twentieth century, also cellular extracts have been used in eczema as well as soluble supernatants of cell cultures, especially so-called thymus preparations. The best-known extracts are called thymosin or thymostimulin from calf thymus as well as thymopentin as a synthetic pentapeptide (Leung et al. 1990). The so-called transfer factor gained from stimulated leukocyte suspensions also has immunomodulating effects. All these procedures were more or less disappearing after the appearance of bovine spongiform encephalitis (BSE).

5.11.1.5 Bach Flower Therapy

The English physician Dr. Edward Bach introduced a therapeutical concept using leaves of flowers of different colors which are supposed to influence psychic conditions of humans by their vibrations. The concept has a strong resemblance to romantic medicine and philosophy and is very difficult to study under scientific conditions.

5.11.1.6 Anthroposophic Medicine

The concept of anthroposophic medicine is very complex and does not describe the effects of single substances or procedures, but rather represents a religious holistic concept with a specific emphasis on "natural" procedures and lifestyle. Antibiotics or vaccinations are avoided, the children should experience the natural course of infectious diseases.

However, it has to be mentioned that epidemiological trials studying children from anthroposophic families have shown that they develop less allergies than the normal population (Alm et al. 1999). Similar findings have been observed when studying farmers' children in alpine regions of Bavaria, Austria, and Switzerland where it was shown that farmers' children growing up on a farm and whose mother had worked in the stable during pregnancy develop less allergies (Riedler et al. 2001) (see Sect. 6.1).

5.11.1.7 Bioresonance

Bioresonance describes somatic electromagnetic vibrations which can be measured and which are disturbed in certain diseases and can be diagnosed and corrected by introduction of allergens both in a diagnostic and therapeutic use. Bioresonance can be regarded as a mixture of magic guru and modern high-tech medicine. There is no physical basis for this concept (Cap 1995); there has been no effect in placebo-controlled double-blind studies (Kofler et al. 1996; Pichler et al. 1996; Schöni et al. 1997; Wandtke et al. 1993; Wüthrich et al. 2006).

5.11.1.8 Electroacupuncture According to Voll

This procedure combines Chinese acupuncture with Western technology and uses energy streams of the patient altered through allergens. Again, in control studies, no diagnostic effect could be proven (Bresser 1993).

5.11.1.9 Kinesiology

The American physician Diamond developed the method of kinesiology ("touch for health"), assuming that muscular tension is an expression of the holistic energy field of a human individual and allows diagnostic information about possible disease elicitors. The examiner stands in front of the patient who has elevated his upper arm horizontally to press the arm down against resistance. As soon as he puts a vial with relevant allergen in front of the sternum, acute relaxation of the muscle occurs, and the arm drops down. We have tried this procedure in a double-blind placebo-controlled clinical trial; first of all, I had to include a coworker under a "hidden name" in the course of the master in order to learn the methodology and gain the "apostolic blessings" so that nobody could say we did not perform the method properly. Although there were single patients where surprisingly this effect could be observed, in the randomized clinical trial, the diagnostic reliability was even below that of throwing a dice (below 50 %) (Kunz et al. 2001).

5.11.2 General Recommendations for Dealing with "Alternative" Methods

When a patient asks for "alternative" therapies, we can safely state that scientific medicine always has a choice of several alternatives of scientifically well-based treatments. Also, new plausible therapeutic options may be used in a pilot study and then evaluated in a control trial. However, what is already investigated and rejected or absolutely not plausible should be avoided in the interest of the patient. As physicians, we are obliged to tell our patients the truth and treat them according to our knowledge and conscience. At the same time, we should never be arrogant or emotionally involved in quarreling with the patients or induce feelings of guilt. Physicians treating atopic dermatitis have to have a composure of utmost tolerance; however, tolerance is an attitude toward individual subjects, not against philosophical ideologies!

It is very helpful when patients are informed in a group as we do this in our eczema school program (see below) and discuss the controversies among themselves; there is always a patient who already has made very negative experience with some alternative methods and thus has a much higher authority than the doctor, who is regarded to be a "narrow-minded" supporter of "school medicine."

The physician can act as a moderator and does not appear to be the super teacher. In my contact with patients, I avoid academic debates; I say, "Lady (Sir)—this is a matter of religion, and I do not discuss religion with my patients."

5.11.3 Summary

There is almost no field in medicine where "alternative," "complementary," or "unconventional" methods are so popular as in the management of atopic dermatitis. Therefore it is important for the physician at least to know the name and the principle of the most commonly used procedures. When trying to categorize unconventional methods according to plausibility, there are a variety of procedures which may be recommended as a useful supplement to classical dermatologic therapy such as psychosomatic counseling, relaxation techniques, certain dietary recommendations, climate therapy, certain forms of phytotherapy, physical therapy, sports therapy, and—maybe to be better studied—acupuncture. On the contrary, there are procedures which, according to current knowledge, cannot be recommended. Double-blind trials with homeopathy have not shown significant improvements; similarly, negative results have been published from controlled trials to bioresonance and kinesiology. When talking to the patient about unconventional methods, the atmosphere should be calm and never lead to the induction of "feelings of guilt" in the patient.

Prevention

6

In addition to general activities to promote health, prevention recommendations comprise:

- Primary prevention
- Secondary prevention
- Tertiary prevention (Fig. 6.1)

6.1 Primary Prevention

The basis of rational recommendations for primary prevention of allergy or eczema is precise knowledge about causes and mechanisms of the development of these conditions as well as methods for the definition of possible risk groups (Von Hertzen and Haahtela 2010) (see Chaps. 1, 2, and 3).

6.1.1 Risk Groups

In all recommendations for primary prevention, it has to be distinguished between strategies involving the whole population and those which are only recommended for risk families (Wahn and von Mutius 2001).

The most simple way to define allergy risk is family history, i.e., children whose parents are suffering or have suffered from an atopic disease (one or both parents) are at greater risk. Measurable laboratory biomarkers from cord blood have been investigated but—in spite of progress in molecular genetics and experimental immunology—are not yet available for routine purposes such as T-cell subpopulations, phosphodiesterase concentrations in mononuclear cells, IgE or IgE receptor expression, filaggrin mutation, etc.

6.1.2 Allergy Development

Our knowledge regarding causal factors in allergy development is limited and comprises, apart from allergen exposure, anthropogenic and biogenic influences from the environment, which can act as modulators either in a protective or an enhancing sense (see Sect. 1.5). The avoidance of allergy-enhancing factors might make sense in primary prevention.

Current recommendations comprise avoidance strategies, preferably regarding nutrition, but also other environmental factors from indoor and outdoor air. An S3 guideline in Germany for primary allergy prevention has been recently actualized (Schäfer 2002; Schäfer et al. 2004a, b; Muche-Borowski et al. 2010).

Prevention strategies regarding nutrition and diet are covered under "hypoallergenic infant formula" and "nutrition."

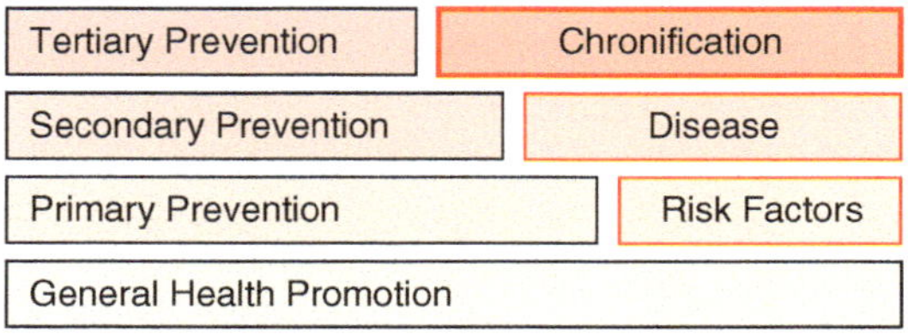

Fig. 6.1 Various levels of health promotion and prevention of disease

J. Ring, *Atopic Dermatitis: Eczema*, DOI 10.1007/978-3-319-22243-1_6

6.1.3 Avoidance Strategies and General Recommendations

6.1.3.1 Pet Keeping

While over decades the classical recommendation was to strictly avoid fur- and feather-bearing animals in the house, a variety of recent studies have brought new evidence in a more differentiated way. It has been shown that persons with extremely high contact to pets (maximal cat allergen exposure in indoor air corresponding to several cats) may develop protecting antibodies (quoted in Muche-Borowski et al. 2010; Schäfer et al. 2008).

Still the recommendation to avoid cats is actual. This may be different with regard to dogs. There are studies which show a decreased allergy prevalence in families where dogs are kept. Therefore, the strict recommendation to avoid dogs is no longer relevant. With regard to the mechanisms, it may be speculated that dogs with their natural "coprophilic" behavior can alter the microbiome in the family environment!

For the general population, there is no reason to restrict pet keeping with regard to primary allergy prevention. In this context, these strategies comprise allergies in general and are not specific for atopic dermatitis. There is, however, also no reason to keep pets for allergy prevention!

6.1.3.2 Farming Environment

One of the most exciting findings in the past has come from studies performed in the alpine regions of Bavaria, Austria, and Switzerland, where it has been found that living and growing up on a farm seemed to be protective with regard to the development of airway allergy (Riedler et al. 2001; von Mutius and Vercelli 2010; Alfvén et al. 2006; Illi et al. 2012). It was interesting that a special type of farming culture with traditional farming (cows and cultivation) was protective, as well as the number of different species kept on a farm seemed to be important in the sense of "diversity" as a protective element.

Particularly pronounced were the effects when the mother of a child had worked in the stable during pregnancy (Roduit et al. 2012; Ege et al. 2008a).

Regarding nutrition on the farm, see below.

6.1.3.3 Use of Parasite "Worms" in Atopy Prevention

According to the "jungle" or "hygiene" hypothesis, immunodeviation toward Th2 reaction pattern occurs when the natural stimulation of the immune system by parasitic infestation is lacking due to improved hygiene (Ring 1982a, b; Strachan 1989).

Therefore, people have tried to induce similar immunomodulating effects by applying worms or helminth substances in order to decrease Th2 reactions.

There are already clinical trials with parasites of the species *Trichuris* as well as *Necator americanus*. Most of the studies are still experimental; however, first clinical trials have not shown convincing effects (Bager et al. 2010).

A recently published study described a good therapeutic effect of a compound named IPBD WB1001 as a small molecule having shown to inhibit proinflammatory cytokines and T-cell migration. This compound was extracted from bacteria living in entomopathogenic nematodes (2-isopropyl-5-(E)-2-phenylethenyl-benzene-1,3-diol) (Bissonnette et al. 2011).

6.1.3.4 Aeroallergens

In the indoor air, where human beings spend most of their lifetime, it is advisable to produce a climate which does not favor mold growth, i.e., too high humidity and poor ventilation.

Exposure against house dust mites, especially in the bedroom, may play a role for allergic individuals; however, for primary prevention, reduction of mite exposure has not shown effective evidence.

6.1.3.5 Air Pollutants

The major air pollutant in the indoor air is derived from environmental tobacco smoke. Many studies have shown increased allergy and eczema prevalence rates in children passively exposed to tobacco smoke (Schäfer et al. 1997b; Krämer et al. 2004; Wang et al. 2008). Therefore, avoidance of smoking not only for the mother and during pregnancy but also generally for the family is one of the most important recommendations for primary allergy prevention.

In the outdoor air, pollutants derived from car traffic exhaust are most relevant, especially fine and ultrafine particles, which has been shown in children living close to a heavy traffic road (Kraemer et al. 2001; Morgenstern et al. 2008; Lee et al. 2008). Therefore, it is recommended to keep exposure against traffic exhaust as low as possible.

Apart from the alpine farmer's story, there is evidence from other studies that Western lifestyle is associated with increased allergy and eczema prevalence according to the hygiene hypothesis (Strachan 1989; Ring et al. 2001b) (see Sect. 1.4).

6.1.3.6 Vaccination and Immunomodulatory Strategies

One of the questions most often asked by mothers in daily practice is whether their children can be vaccinated. There are rumors that "natural infection," e.g., with measles virus, may be more protective and more "healthy" than the vaccination. There is a great deal of philosophical involvement in these debates. Once, a very nice and intelligent father of such a religious community told me that "there must be some reason for these childhood infectious diseases in evolution and some benefit for mankind." Not very politely, I answered "Yes, you are right, there is indeed a reason, namely there is a clear-cut effect against overpopulation."

Fact is that adequately performed vaccinations do not increase the allergy risk, neither for airway nor for skin atopy. Of course, vaccination should not be performed during an acute flare of the disease. Therefore, all children with atopic dermatitis can receive the normal vaccinations like other children! The second most asked question regarding egg allergy and vaccinations produced on eggs also can be answered clearly: "There is no contraindication for these vaccinations; in children with severe egg anaphylaxis it is recommended to test the vaccine prior to application."

The effect of immunomodulatory strategies such as application of pre- and probiotics will be covered below (see Sect. 6.1.4.6).

Furthermore, there is no evidence for a clear-cut association between application of antibiotics and development of atopic diseases (Muche-Borowski et al. 2010). Therefore, there is no need to avoid antibiotics when they are necessary.

Table 6.1 General avoidance of irritant factors

Skin-irritative clothing, wool, nylon, too vehement skin cleaning, too early use of potentially sensitizing jewelry, e.g., nickel ear piercing
Airways (dust, fog, air pollutants such as tobacco smoke, traffic exhaust, volatile organic compounds VOCs, etc.)
Nutrition (irritative or directly pharmacologically active compounds such as too hot spices, alcohol, etc.)
Psychosocial (unpleasant mental or emotional stress)

6.1.3.7 General Recommendations

General recommendations for primary prevention—also for secondary and tertiary prevention—comprise avoidance of irritants of all categories (see Table 6.1). This includes clothing, skin hygiene, jewelry, etc. (Frosch 1985; Schwanitz 1992; Langan et al. 2009). A recent study found that nylon clothing, dust, and shampoos may play a role as triggers of eczema flares in children (Langan et al. 2009).

An epidemiological trial had found an association between increased water hardness and eczema prevalence in the UK (McNally et al. 1998). However, the use of ion-coupled water softeners does not seem to have enough evidence to be recommended as a primary preventive strategy (Gamble and Dellavalle 2011).

6.1.3.8 Pharmacological Primary Prevention

Attempts to induce primary prevention with pharmacological substances such as histamine antagonists have not shown the desired effect as was found in the ETAC (Early Treatment of Atopic Child) study when the infants were treated with cetirizine at first signs of atopic dermatitis over 2 years (Diepgen et al. 2002).

6.1.3.9 Summary

Recommendations for primary prevention comprise dietary recommendations as well as avoidance strategies and general considerations. In the last years, these recommendations have been less rigid with regard to pet keeping: While cats should still be avoided, dog keeping does not seem to go along with an increased risk of allergy but may even have protective effects. However, there is no indication for the general population to keep pets for allergy prevention.

Indoor climate conditions of too high humidity allowing mold growth should be avoided. The most important recommendation with regard to air pollutants is avoidance of tobacco smoke in the indoor air and traffic exhaust in the outdoor air. There is no reason why atopic individuals should not be vaccinated like normal children. Interesting results from epidemiological trials such as in remote islands or alpine farm environments are very important for research but cannot be translated easily into practical prevention recommendations.

6.1.4 Nutrition and Dietary Recommendations

6.1.4.1 Breastfeeding

The longest-known and scientifically best investigated recommendation for primary allergy prevention starts at birth and includes strict breastfeeding from day 1. From epidemiological investigations as well as animal experimental studies, it is known that, in the first month of life, there is a special "window of opportunity" during which an organism can develop tolerance against environmental substances (Akdis et al. 2000; Blaser 2008; de Weck 1995; Wahn and von Mutius 2001; Høst et al. 2008; Burks et al. 2008).

Breastfeeding thus is the only "general antiallergic diet" which can be recommended; however, the effect is limited and does not last very long. Therefore, the recommendations comprise only the first 4 months of life (Muche-Borowski et al. 2010). Whether the positive effect of breast milk corresponds only to allergen avoidance, namely, of cow proteins, or whether there may be active protective factors in breast milk is a matter of speculation.

The fact that in breast milk also small amounts of allergenic proteins depending upon the maternal diet may be detected implies dietary recommendations for lactating mothers. In Scandinavian studies, a certain effect of oligoallergenic diet during lactation has been observed (Hattevig et al. 1999).

In the last years, the evidence regarding breastfeeding and prevention of eczema has been more and more controversially discussed. There are also studies which show increased rates of eczema in breastfed children, and meta-analyses have concluded that there was no convincing evidence of a protective effect of exclusive breastfeeding in eczema (Flohr et al. 2011).

6.1.4.2 Solid Food in the First Year of Life

With regard to the introduction of solid food, the recommendations have changed slightly: While previously introduction of solid food was recommended only after the sixth month, this has now been shortened to the fourth month of life. There is no evidence of a definite preventive effect of delayed introduction of solid food. Also a certain diversity of food groups—with special emphasis on yoghurt—seems to be helpful (Roduit et al. 2012).

6.1.4.3 General Recommendations

There is no general antiallergic diet. There have been studies showing that regular consumption of fish already in the first year of life may have a protective effect. Generally, Mediterranean diet with a high amount of polyunsaturated fatty acids may have beneficial effects (Chatzi et al. *Thorax* 2008 neu). This also holds true for dietary recommendations during pregnancy.

Generally also obesity seems to be a risk factor for asthma. Therefore, normal diet and avoidance of obesity is also recommended (Bouther and Sutherland 2007).

It is important that the diet in the first year of life contains all the necessary elements and vitamins and a certain degree of diversity according to general nutrition recommendations (Fig. 6.2). There is a shift in paradigm from strict avoidance to induction of tolerance by targeted application (Dutoit et al. 2008).

6.1.4.4 Nutrition During Pregnancy

For the time during pregnancy, recommendations are difficult and generally controversially discussed (see probiotics); there is limited evidence from prospective clinical trials.

Mostly nutrition for a pregnant woman is not easy and connected with a lot of problems. Therefore, it is important not to make it more

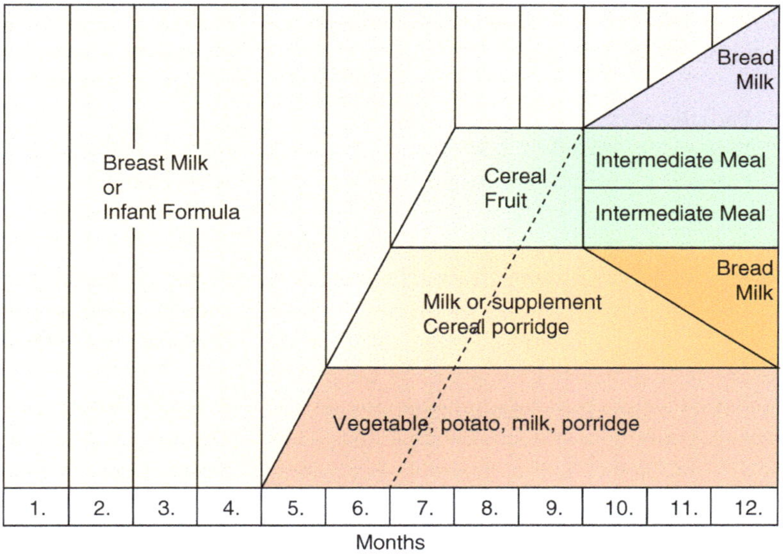

Fig. 6.2 Dietary schedule for healthy nutrition in the first year of life (With friendly permission of C. Kugler)

difficult. Most important is avoidance of smoking (see above) and too much calories (control of body weight), since obese pregnant women tend to give birth to overweight children. New studies have shown that increased body mass index is associated with higher prevalence of asthma (Warner 2009). There are no good studies with regard to atopic dermatitis.

Avoidance of overweight has therefore been included in current dietary recommendations for allergy prevention (Muche-Borowski et al. 2010).

Possible regular intake of fish—probably because of high amounts of polyunsaturated fatty acids—during pregnancy and lactation may have beneficial effects (Dunstan et al. 2004).

6.1.4.5 Hypoallergenic Formula

Whenever breastfeeding is not possible for one or another reason, there are a variety of "hypoallergenic" infant formulas which can be used as a supplement to cow's milk (Vandenplas et al. 1995).

The term "hypoallergenic" can only be used when certain requirements are fulfilled by law, i.e., among others a concentration of allergenic protein of less than 1 % in the original product in Germany. From the point of view of food technology, mostly hydrolysis is used to achieve these levels by either enzymatic digestion, ultra-high temperature, or ultrafiltration. Therefore, also the term "hydrolysate formula" is used. Apart from the chemical nature of the major ingredients of the original material, namely, casein or whey molecules, the intensity of the hydrolysis, which can lead to either partially or extensively hydrolyzed food, is crucial. Earlier mostly weak hydrolysates had been used for prevention, while extensively hydrolyzed formula are only given when there is already existing cow's milk allergy.

Among many studies with regard to the efficacy of hypoallergenic infant nutrition in allergy prevention, the GINI study (German Infant Nutritional Intervention) has yielded quite reliable results. More than 2000 newborns were investigated in a prospective randomized and double-blind study. Apart from a control group, one group was exclusively breastfed, and three groups received hydrolysate formula of different degrees. As parameters of outcome, the occurrence of atopic dermatitis, food allergy, or urticaria was observed (von Berg et al. 2003, 2008). The group with exclusive breastfeeding was not included in the final evaluation since for ethical reasons neither randomization nor blinding could be performed here. However, it is interesting that some of the extensively hydrolyzed formula had a similar allergy-preventive or even better effect than exclusive breastfeeding. The formula groups received are the following:

- Partially whey
- Extensively hydrolyzed whey
- Extensively hydrolyzed casein

In a careful analysis of the results, the authors came to the conclusion that there is a preventive effect of hypoallergenic infant formula which, however, does not seem to depend solely on the degree of hydrolysis or the nature of the protein but rather on the final total preparation and also the susceptibility of the infant (regarding family history of atopic dermatitis) (von Berg et al. 2003, 2008). In children with familial occurrence of allergy in general, however, and no atopic dermatitis in near first-grade relatives, hydrolyzed formula of all three groups showed a preventive effect with reduction in prevalence of atopic dermatitis by around 50 % compared to normal cow's milk baby formula.

However, when there was atopic eczema in the family, the weak and extensively hydrolyzed whey products were no longer effective, but only the extensively hydrolyzed casein product was able to reduce the incidence of atopic dermatitis by 50 %.

Apart from hypoallergenic products, there are allergen-free amino acid mixtures (e.g., Neocate) which can also be given as therapeutic nutrition (see Table 6.2).

Table 6.2 Therapeutic nutrition (extensively hydrolyzed or amino acid formulas, which can also be used in infants with existing cow's milk allergy)

Protein nature	Product
Whey hydrolysate	Alfaré (Nestle), Althera (Nestle) with lactose
	Aptamil Pepti
	Aptamil Pregomin (plus MCT fatty acids)
Free amino acids	Aptamil Pregomin AS
	Neonate infant (Nutritia)
	Neonate active (Nutritia)
	Neonate advance (Nutritia)
	Neonate junior (Nutritia)

6.1.4.6 Pre- and Probiotics

Preventive effects of probiotics are discussed controversially (Rosenfeldt et al. 2003) (see Sect. 5.9.6). Possible effects of prebiotic oligosaccharides have been reported in a controlled study (Grüber 2012).

There have been attempts to reduce allergy development by prophylactic intake of probiotics during pregnancy which, however, has not found enough evidence for general recommendation (Isolauri et al. 2000; Kalliomäki et al. 2001).

6.1.4.7 Summary

The longest and scientifically best investigated dietary recommendation for primary allergy prevention consists in exclusive breastfeeding over at least 4 months. Even this recommendation has been controversially discussed in the recent past with regard to atopic dermatitis.

When breastfeeding is not possible, application of hypoallergenic infant formula is recommended; partially hydrolyzed whey preparations as well as extensively hydrolyzed casein products have been shown in large clinical trials to yield the best effects. Eventually, regular intake of fish also as early as during pregnancy and lactation may have beneficial effects as well as a Mediterranean diet and a general diversity of foods. The role of introduction of solid food seems to be less important, and it can be started after the fourth month of life. Recent studies have shown that overweight is associated with a higher risk of asthma; therefore, avoidance of high-calory diets has also been included in recommendations for allergy prevention.

6.2 Secondary Prevention

Secondary prevention describes the detection of risk groups by early screening and the prevention or reduction of developing symptoms. In the case of allergy, this means screening for atopic sensitization and application of preventive measures only in these individuals. The general measures correspond to the above-discussed recommendations for primary prevention.

6.3 Tertiary Prevention: Rehabilitation

Tertiary prevention, also called rehabilitation, is one of the most important strategies in long-term management of allergic patients; it describes all activities after the first diagnosis and treatment in the acute phase in order to achieve as long as possible remission intervals, thus allowing participation in a normal active life in society and occupation. Among the total of rehabilitation costs of most insurance or government agencies, approx. 1–2 % regard allergic skin and airway diseases (Stachow 2002).

In many countries, there are legal conditions for outpatient or inpatient rehabilitation measures which also contain rules for standardization and quality control in the general management of patients with atopic dermatitis. In Central Europe, inpatient facilities specialized in allergic airway and skin diseases are available. In quality control and management programs, studies with regard to quality of life and patient satisfaction as well as days of work loss have been performed. For the indication "atopic dermatitis," similar to "allergic airway disease," there was an estimated reduction of costs of around 1000 € already in the first 6 months after an inpatient rehabilitation (Ring et al. 2010).

For adolescents, the question with regard to the choice of occupation is often a great problem in atopic individuals, especially when they suffer from hand eczema. An individual and adequate occupational counseling plays an important role for these adolescents. It needs to be evaluated and informed, but there should be no prohibited occupations. There are occupations with a high risk due to intensive contact with potent allergens such as baker, cook, or animal caretaker, or strongly irritative substances for the skin, such as hairdresser or car mechanic. In individuals with severe atopic dermatitis, one generally would advise to avoid occupations with great skin strain (Diepgen and Coenraads 2000; Frosch 1985).

Also counseling with regard to hobbies, pet keeping and vacation should be given. What is important is the individual and independent interaction with the informed patient with regard to basic therapeutic measures both in avoidance strategies with regard to specific and nonspecific irritants and active protection.

6.3.1 Socioeconomic Impact

There is a high degree of variability with regard to the yearly costs of atopic dermatitis when only doctor's visits or drug prescriptions are counted or when also the indirect costs for the patient are included.

In the outpatient sector, the introduction of an "office fee" for outpatients in Germany in January 2004 led to marked reduction in visits of patients with atopic dermatitis in the dermatologist's office. At the same time, there was a steep increase of "alternative," "unconventional" treatments as well as not evidence-based treatment of eczema with systemic glucocorticosteroids especially in patients with rare doctor visits (Schmitt et al. 2009a).

6.3.2 Summary

Rehabilitation is the most important aspect of tertiary prevention in atopic eczema where inpatient treatments are most successful. By adequate tertiary prevention already in the first year after an inpatient stay, direct and indirect illness costs can be reduced markedly.

6.4 Climate Therapy in Secondary and Tertiary Prevention

The term "climate therapy" describes a complex medical treatment which includes beneficial effects of certain climatic regions, but not exclusively these effects.

Already early sources of medical history in scriptures of Hippocrates and his disciples or from ancient China and Rome reveal that humans were seeking cure from chronic diseases in places with special climate characteristics. In the nineteenth century, these aspects were studied by scientific medicine especially for airway diseases. A special date is the year 1862 when the young physician from Southwest Germany who had to take refuge to Switzerland after the revolution of 1848, Alexander Spengler, came to Davos to take care of the population and later opened a sanatorium for lung diseases. Later the Dutch physician Holsboer intensified these treatments which became very popular all over the world and found their literature description in Thomas Mann's "The Magic Mountain" ("Der Zauberberg"). In 1953, climate therapy was started at the North Sea island of Norderney under Jo Hartung. The first German patient organization the "Hay Fever Association" (Heufieberbund), today "Deutscher Allergie- und Asthmabund" (daab), was founded in 1898 on the island of Helgoland, and this was not a coincidence!

Also in 1898, the German Hermann Burchard founded a special hospital for lung diseases in Davos-Wolfgang which was guided after the Second World War by Christian Virchow, a great-nephew of Rudolf Virchow as "high-altitude clinic for asthma patients." In 1961, Siegfried Borelli discovered, after early work of Alfred Marchionini (Marchionini and Borelli 1956), that the climate of Davos also had beneficial effects for certain skin diseases, especially atopic dermatitis (Borelli 1995).

In modern meteorology, climate describes the characteristic interplay and composure of atmospheric factors over a certain area together with the specific meteorological conditions of weather.

From this definition, it becomes clear that specific climates can only be found under very specific geographic and meteorologic conditions. These are areas on the seashore on the one hand and high altitude on the other hand. In between, daily weather changes contribute much more to the actual climate than a specific geographic characteristic (Halhuber 1959; Schuh and Nowak 2011; Skudlik et al. 1999).

Table 6.3 describes relevant geographic and meteorologic factors for determining a "climate." Apart from photoactinic factors with thermic-hygric effects, there is a complex interaction also with regard to oxygen concentrations as well as

Table 6.3 Factors influencing or determining a characteristic climate

Geographic factors	Meteorologic factors (weather)
Altitude above sea level	Solar irradiation
Distance to sea	Precipitation (fog, rain, snow)
Connection to high mountains and valleys	Air humidity
Composition of soil	Air temperature
Type of vegetation	Air pressure
Most frequent wind directions	Air movement (wind)
	Aerosol composition (natural, anthropogenic)

According to Vocks et al. (1994, 2002)

the ionization of the air and the composure of aerosol particles.

6.4.1 High-Altitude, North Sea and Dead Sea

Climate therapy tries to treat patients by using the exposure to physicochemical effects of the atmosphere with the aim to avoid noxious substances and, on the other hand, adapt to natural environmental irritants (Schuh and Nowak 2011; Fuchs and Hentschel 1959).

In various scientific investigations, influences of the Davos high-altitude climate on autonomic nervous system, immunologic reactivity, as well as general clinical parameters important for asthma or atopic dermatitis have been found (Borelli and Chlebarov 1966; Halhuber 1959; Humpeler et al. 1980; Schuh et al. 1989).

In the healthy climate of Davos, the low allergen content of air, especially the absence of house dust mites, has special importance for atopic dermatitis (Petermann et al. 2004; Schultze-Werninghaus 2006) (see Sect. 4.1).

Similar climate effects have been described on North Sea islands (except for house dust mites) and to a lesser extent on other seashores. Experiences with the climate therapy on the Dead Sea in Israel report beneficial effects in psoriasis and to a minor extent on eczema, mostly due to the increased long-wave UV radiation and the high salt content of the water (Harari et al. 2000).

The protected high-altitude situation in Davos also is characterized by a relatively low occurrence of wind, which is accepted well by most patients. Too strong gusty winds may irritate the skin and the airways.

Climate therapy can either be performed in an acute exacerbation of eczema or as inpatient rehabilitation (Breuer and Kapp 2006; Buhles et al. 2003; Farin et al. 2003; Menz et al. 2007; Nürnberg 2005; Skudlik et al. 2009; Stachow 2002).

Scientific investigations with regard to the itch sensation showed an interesting dependence of itch intensity on meteorologic changes: Especially when the weather changed, and before a change of air humidity, many patients suffer from more intense itch sensations (Vocks et al. 2002).

Of practical importance is the fact that under climate therapy conditions, a significant steroid-sparing effect can be observed. After a short phase of adaptation with occasional and reversible flares in the first days, most patients experience improvement and long-lasting stabilization without strong systemic or topical therapeutics (Drzimalla et al. 1999; Engst and Vocks 2000).

In many patients, adequate allergy diagnostics (see Sect. 4.1) are only possible under the conditions of climate therapy, since under normal conditions at home, they either suffer from generalized eczema, and the skin cannot be tested, or they have to be treated with systemic or topical anti-inflammatory substances not allowing allergy testing.

A randomized comparative study of rehabilitation measures in the Netherlands compared the high-altitude situation in Davos with similar treatment in the Netherlands in asthma and showed significant improvement by high-altitude climate therapy (Grootendorst et al. 2001).

Of course, climate never can act alone but always in connection with classic dermatologic as well as general treatment, including psychosomatic counseling, dietary recommendations, sports and ergotherapy, etc. For the severe patients, it is easier when they have adequate time and the right ambient to learn and accept the conditions of their disease and gain motivation to change certain factors in their lifestyle. Therefore, also educational programs are often easier and more effective under these conditions than in the normal life at home (Premerlani et al. 2006; Scheewe et al. 1997).

A climate therapeutic intervention should cover a period of 4 weeks, better 6 weeks. It is sad that in our more and more hectic times, with acceleration of daily life, many patients cannot afford this period.

6.4.2 Summary

Climate therapy describes a complex treatment schedule in areas with specific characteristic geographic and meteorologic conditions for atopic dermatitis, in Central Europe particularly North Sea islands as well as high altitudes. Numerous investigations described influences especially in the Davos high-altitude climate on autonomic nervous system, immune reactions, as well as allergologic parameters in atopic dermatitis. Acute inpatients stays as well as inpatient rehabilitation measures under climate therapy conditions lead to improvement in many patients with severe atopic dermatitis, often lasting over years and sometimes decisively changing the progression of the disease toward improvement. In some patients, adequate allergy diagnostics is only possible under allergen-poor climate therapeutical conditions.

6.5 Educational Programs ("Eczema School")

From the manifold illustrations and texts with regard to clinical symptomatology and multiple causes and trigger factors as well as diagnostic therapeutic and preventive recommendations, it becomes clear that it is not possible to give all this information in the average daily office (Hurrelmann et al. 1998, 2003; Lob-Corzilius and Petermann 1997; Petermann and Warschburger 1999; Gebert et al. 1998).

6.5.1 Development of "Eczema Schools"

Therefore at the end of the 1980s, several groups started to develop educational programs for certain diseases which started as group sessions mostly devoted to giving information. In 1993, the German Ministry of Health started a project to improve the care and prevention of atopic eczema in children (Ring 1998) trying to learn from already existing "asthma school" (Szczepanski et al. 1996). On the basis of this expertise, the development of an educational program was started in a national consensus and in an interdisciplinary setting including psychological, pedagogic, and also nutritional aspects. From this project, the "working group eczema school" ("Arbeitsgemeinschaft Neurodermitisschulung" AGNES 2005) developed as an institution to guarantee permanent quality control and standardization of this program (Diepgen et al. 2003; Gieler et al. 2001; Staab et al. 2006; Werfel et al. 2008c; Ring 1998).

6.5.2 Contents

The contents of this "eczema school" comprise not only information on structure and function of the skin, disturbances in skin barrier, and immune mechanisms in atopic dermatitis but also knowledge on individual provocation factors and their avoidance. In addition, psychological aspects of symptom perception, together with relaxation techniques and role plays for coping with emotional aspects, are trained (Premerlani et al. 2006). Furthermore, family dynamic aspects and psychosocial aspects are covered (Gebert et al. 1998; Warschburger et al. 2004). Special emphasis is given on psychosomatic aspects and relaxation techniques. Recently, new programs for stress reduction via "mindfulness" training are investigated. Finally, the various therapeutic options including unconventional procedures are covered (Gieler et al. 2001).

6.5.3 Evaluation

This complex intervention program "eczema school" was then studied in a prospective randomized trial with a waiting control loop in over 1000 patients and found to be significantly effective (Staab et al. 2006). It was of particular interest that not only the parameters of quality of life and psychological well-being or coping with illness-induced stress showed improvement but also the very simple real intensity of eczematous skin lesion as measured in the scoring system SCORAD!

6.5.4 Practical Performance

The eczema school is offered in six consequent 2 h sessions (e.g., every Wednesday evening from 7.00 to 9.00 pm) for maximally 6–12 parents of six children. It is essential that there is an interdisciplinary approach: At least one physician—dermatologist, pediatrician, or allergist—a psychologist or psychosomatic physician, and a nutrition expert have to work together in order to guarantee the quality and get reimbursement from insurances. The inclusion of a specially trained nurse is optional.

6.5.5 Qualification of Trainers

In order to guarantee the quality of the program, only individuals with a certificate as "eczema trainer" are allowed to do the school. It has to be learned that not every physician is also a good teacher. In Germany, there are specialized "eczema academies" which are entitled to offer "train-the-trainer seminars" for physicians, psychologists, and nutritional experts. In a program of 40 h, including practical exercises, a hospitation in an already existing eczema school and a final supervision (personal or video) have to be documented before the individual is accepted as an "eczema trainer." This model of eczema school is now spread all over Germany and has become so successful that it has been copied by many other countries.

6.5.6 Music Therapy

In the context of educational programs, also music therapy has been used, together with melodies and rhythms—depending on the life events and the actual situation—and with improvisation, singing, and instrumental performance, emotions of the patients are registered and evaluated in the group session. This interpersonal perception, together with the physical expression, allows the patient a very special and facilitated communication—often without words.

In music therapy, one can differentiate between:

- Receptive music therapy for relaxation and calming down
- Active music therapy with the aim of musical improvisation in order to facilitate communication and own musical activities which help the patient to cope with difficult life situations (Münch 2006)

6.5.7 Summary

In the 1990s, in a national consensus supported by the German Ministry of Health, an interdisciplinary educational program for atopic eczema was developed which comprises six consequent 2 h sessions for maximally 6–12 parents of six children. The educational program is interdisciplinary in nature with a physician (dermatologist, pediatrician, or allergist), a psychologist, and a nutritionist together with an optional specialized nurse. This educational program "eczema school" was studied in a prospective controlled randomized trial and found to be significantly effective both for improving quality of life and also for improving actual eczematous skin lesions. In Germany, this program is reimbursed by the insurances. In order to guarantee the standardization and quality control, train-the-trainer seminars in order to get the qualification "eczema trainer" are offered in various "eczema academies" in Germany in a standardized fashion. Music therapy may be of additional help in these programs.

7 Concluding Remarks: How to Live with Atopic Dermatitis

The many informations and commentaries in this book, starting from the clinical morphology via pathophysiology, diagnostics, therapy, and prevention, make clear that atopic dermatitis is a very complex illness which cannot be treated well in a quick physician-patient contact and by writing a prescription for a cream or an injection.

In spite of clear-cut psychosomatic interactions with deteriorations of skin lesions in specific stress situations, it has to be stated that atopic dermatitis is no "psychiatric" disease, but a skin disease which can be modulated by psychological influences—negatively and positively! The development of atopic eczema is never the product of "guilt"—neither of the patient nor of the mother or father—rather it is a complex interplay of genetic predisposition and environmentally induced factors.

Although patients may be very severely affected, it is possible in most cases to improve the disease in a way that a normal and enjoyable life is possible. To achieve this, the efforts not only of the patient but also of his environment, in family and occupation, and a continuous activity and observation of various aspects are necessary. These include strategies for daily skin care and avoidance of noxious influences. Psychological influences neither should be overestimated, however, also not be neglected. It may happen that a short eczema flare can start in a period of extreme happiness.

It should be stressed that patients with atopic dermatitis—similar to those with atopic airway disease—are not helpless victims of their destiny. Even if the genetic predisposition cannot be changed at this time, and the patients will have the tendency to hypersensitivity of the skin organ and possible development of eczema, I do not like the term "incurable" for this illness. The excruciating eczematous skin lesions can be very well treated—and this can be done in any case of flare. Furthermore there is hope for future more targeted therapies with prologics and small molecular on the way through clinical trials!

The basis of a good prognosis for a relatively normal life is a confidential cooperation between the patient and a physician with special experience in this disease and who can give the patient, even in difficult times, the joy of life and the capability to work with adequate therapeutic strategies.

I tell my patients:

"You will be your own skin doctor; you will know what cream to apply at which time to which area of your body and in which concentration and what you should take systemically in order to be symptom-free. For possible catastrophes, I feel responsible and you can come back to me, we will deal with those!"

J. Ring, *Atopic Dermatitis: Eczema*, DOI 10.1007/978-3-319-22243-1_7

References

Abeck D, Ring J, editors. Atopisches Ekzem im Kindesalter. Neurodermitis – das zeitgemäße Management. Darmstadt: Steinkopff; 2002.

Abels C, Brocks E. Therapie des atopischen Ekzems. Hautarzt. 2006;57:711–25.

Adachi J, Endo K, Fukuzumi T, Tanigawa N, Aoki T. Increasing incidence of streptococcal impetigo in atopic dermatitis. J Dermatol Sci. 1998;17:45–53.

Ader R, Felton D, Cohen N, editors. Psychoneuroimmunology. 3rd ed. London: Academic Press; 1991.

Aetios von Amida. Aetii medici Graeci contractae ex veteribus medicinae tetrabiblos. Basel; 1542.

Ahmad-Nejad P, Mrabet-Dahbi S, Breuer K, Klotz M, Werfel T, Herz U, et al. The toll-like receptor 2 R753Q polymorphism defines a subgroup of patients with atopic dermatitis having severe phenotype. J Allergy Clin Immunol. 2004;113:565–7.

Akdis M, Akdis C. IgE class switching and cellular memory. Nat Immunol. 2012;13:312–4.

Akdis M, Simon HU, Weigl L, Kreyden O, Blaser K, Akdis CA. Skin homing (cutaneous lymphocyte-associated antigen-positive) CD8+ T cells respond to superantigen and contribute to eosinophilia and IgE production in atopic dermatitis. J Immunol. 1999;163:466–75.

Akdis C, Akdis M, Trautmann A, Blaser K. Immune regulation in atopic dermatitis. Curr Opin Immunol. 2000;12:641–6.

Akdis CA, Blaser K, Akdis M. Genes of tolerance. Allergy. 2004;59:897–913.

Akdis CA, Akdis M, Bieber T, Bindslev-Jensen C, Boguniewicz M, Eigenmann P, Hamid Q, Kapp A, Leung DY, Lipozencic J, Luger TA, Muraro A, Novak N, Platts-Mills TA, Rosenwasser L, Scheynius A, Simons FE, Spergel J, Turjanmaa K, Wahn U, Weidinger S, Werfel T, Zuberbier T, European Academy of Allergology and Clinical Immunology/American Academy of Allergy, Asthma and Immunology. Diagnosis and treatment of atopic dermatitis in children and adults: European Academy of Allergology and Clinical Immunology/American Academy of Allergy, Asthma and Immunology/PRACTALL Consensus Report. J Allergy Clin Immunol. 2006;118:152–69. Review. Erratum J Allergy Clin Immunol 2006;118:724.

Akhavan A, Rudikoff D. The treatment of atopic dermatitis with immunosuppressive agents. Clin Dermatol. 2003;21:225–40.

Akira S, Uematsu S, Takeuchi O. Pathogen recognition and innate immunity. Cell. 2006;124:783–801.

Alessandrini F, Schulz H, Takenaka S, et al. Effects of ultrafine carbon particle inhalation on allergic inflammation of the lung. J Allergy Clin Immunol. 2006;117:824–30.

Alexander F. Psychosomatische Medizin. Berlin: De Gruyter; 1971.

Alfvén T, Braun-Fahrländer C, Brunekreef B, von Mutius E, Riedler J, Scheynius A, et al. Allergic disease and atopic sensitization in children related to farming and anthroposophic lifestyle – the PARSIFAL Study. Allergy. 2006;61:414–21.

Alm JS, Swartz J, Lilja G, Scheynius A, Pershagen G. Atopy in children of families with an anthroposophic lifestyle. Lancet. 1999;353:1485–8.

Alomar A, Berth-Jones J, Bos JD, et al. The role of topical calcineurin inhibitors in atopic dermatitis. Br J Dermatol. 2004;151 Suppl 70:3–27.

Aly R. Bacteriology of atopic dermatitis. Acta Dermatol Venereol Suppl. 1980;92:16–8.

Aly R, Maibach HI, Shinefield HR. Microbial flora of atopic dermatitis. Arch Dermatol. 1977;113:780–2.

Amon U, Menz U, Wolff HH. Investigations on plasma levels of mast cell mediators in acute atopic dermatitis. J Dermatol Sci. 1994;7:63–7.

Andersson AC, Lindberg M, Loden M. The effect of two urea-containing creams on dry eczematous skin in atopic patients. I. Expert, patient and instrumental evaluation. J Dermatolog Treat. 1999;10(3):165–9.

Anonymous. Alphaderm ("Crème aus dem Jenseits"). Erhältlich bei: Commings, POB 1143, D-33748 Schloss Holte-Stukenbrok; 1992.

Arbeitsgemeinschaft Neurodermitisschulung, 2005: Qualitätsmanagement in der Neurodermitisschulung von Kindern und Jugendlichen sowie ihren Eltern (über: www.neurodermitisschulung.de).

Arellano FM, Wentoworth CE, Arana A, Fernandez C, Paul CF. Risk of lymphoma following exposure to calcineurin inhibitors and topical steroids in patients with atopic dermatitis. J Invest Dermatol. 2007;127:808–16.

J. Ring, *Atopic Dermatitis: Eczema*, DOI 10.1007/978-3-319-22243-1

Armstrong NC, Ernst E. The treatment of eczema with Chinese herbs: a systematic review of randomized clinical trials. Br J Clin Pharmacol. 1999;48:262–4.

Arshad SH. Exposure to indoor allergens in the development of asthma and allergy. Curr Allergy Asthma Rep. 2003;3:115–20.

Artik S, Ruzicka T. Complementary therapy for atopic eczema and other allergic skin diseases. Dermatol Ther. 2003;16:150–63.

Asher M, Montefort S, Björkstén B, et al. Group IPTS. Worldwide time trends in the prevalence of symptoms of asthma, allergic rhinoconjunctivitis, and eczema in childhood: ISAAC phases one and tree repeat multicountry cross-sectional surveys. Lancet. 2006;368:733–43.

Ashida Y, Denda M, Hirao T. Histamine H1 and H2 receptor antagonists accelerate skin barrier repair and prevent epidermal hyperplasia induced by barrier disruption in a dry environment. J Invest Dermatol. 2001;116:261–5.

Atherton DJ, Sewell M, Soothill JF, Wells RS, Chilvers CE. A double-blind controlled crossover trail of an antigen-avoidance diet in atopic eczema. Lancet. 1978;1:401–3.

Augustin M, Mrowietz U, Bonnekoh B, et al. Topical long-term therapy with vitamin D_3 analogues, corticosteroids and their two compound formulations. JDDG. 2014;12:667–82.

Augustin M, Zschocke I, Buhrke U. Attitudes and prior experience with respect to alternative medicine among dermatological patients: the Freiburg questionnaire on attitudes to naturopathy (FAN). Forsch Komplementarmed. 1999a;6:26–9.

Augustin M, Zschocke I, Lange S, Seidenglanz K, Amon U. Lebensqualität bei Hauterkrankungen: Vergleich verschiedener Lebensqualitäts-Fragebögen bei Psoriasis und atopischer Dermatitis. Hautarzt. 1999b;50:715–22.

Augustin M, Zschocke I, Seidenglanz K, Lange S, Schiffler A, Amon U. Validation and clinical results of the FLQA-d, a Quality of Life Questionnaire for patients with chronic skin disease. Dermatol Psychosom. 2000;1–7.

Bae JM, Choi YY, Park CO, Chung KY, Lee KH. Efficacy of allergen-specific immunotherapy for atopic dermatitis: a systematic review and meta-analysis of randomized controlled trials. J Allergy Clin Immunol. 2013;132:110–7.

Bager P, Arnved J, Rønborg S, Wohlfahrt J, Poulsen LK, Westergaard T, Petersen HW, Kristensen B, Thamsborg S, Roepstorff A, Kapel C, Melbye M. Trichuris suis ova therapy for allergic rhinitis: a randomized, double-blind, placebo-controlled clinical trial. J Allergy Clin Immunol. 2010;125:123–30.

Bair B, Dodd J, Heidelberg K, Krach K. Cataracts in atopic dermatitis: a case presentation and review of the literature. Arch Dermatol. 2011;147:585–9.

Bandmann HJ. Ekzem und ekzematoide Dermatitiden im Kindesalter. In: Miescher G, Storck H, editors. Handbuch der Haut- und Geschlechtskrankheiten 8I. Johansson), Ergänzungswerk v. A. Marchionini. Bd II/1, Entzündliche Dermatosen. Berlin: Springer; 1962. p. 320–68.

Bannister MJ, Freeman S. Adult-onset atopic dermatitis. Australas J Dermatol. 2000;41:225–8.

Barbarot S, Bernier C, Deleuran M, De Raeve L, Eichenfield L, El Hachem M, et al. Therapeutic patient education in children with atopic dermatitis: position paper on objectives and recommendations. Pediatr Dermatol. 2013;30:199–206.

Bard S, Paravisini A, Avilés-Izquierdo JA, Fernandez-Cruz E, Sánchez-Ramón S. Eczematous dermatitis in the setting of hyper-IgE syndrome successfully treated with omalizumab. Arch Dermatol. 2008;144:1662–3.

Bauer CP. Hypoallergene Babynahrung und Atopieprävention. In: Behr-Völtzer C, Hamm M, Vieluf D, Ring J, editors. Diät bei Nahrungsmittelallergien und –intoleranzen. 4th ed. Munich: Urban & Vogel; 2008. p. 59–65.

Bauer CP. Hausstaubmilbenallergie-Aspekte zur Sensibilisierung und Allergenreduktion. Pädiatr Allergologie Klin Prax. 1985;1:6–13.

Baur X, Aschauer H, Dewair M, et al. Relationship between primary structures and allergenicity of asthma-inducing insect proteins (chironomid hemoglobines). Chest. 1982;82:254–9.

Baurecht H, Irvine AD, Novak N, et al. Toward a major risk factor for atopic eczema: meta-analysis of filaggrin polymorphism data. J Allergy Clin Immunol. 2007;120:1406–12.

Beck J. Praxis der kognitiven Therapie. Weinheim: Psychologische Verlags Union; 1999.

Beck LA, Thaci D, Hamilton JD, Graham NM, Bieber T, Rocklin R, et al. Dupilumab treatment in adults with moderate-to-severe atopic dermatitis. N Engl J Med. 2014;371:130–9.

Becker D, Langer E, Seemann M, Seemann G, Fell I, Saloga J, Grabbe S, von Stebut E. Clinical efficacy of blue light full body irradiation as treatment option for severe atopic dermatitis. PLoS One. 2011;6:e20566.

Bedi M, Shenefelt P. Herbal therapy in dermatology. Arch Dermatol. 2002;138:232–42.

Beetham WP. Atopic cataracts. Arch Ophth. 1940;24:21–37.

Behne MJ, Barry NP, Hanson KM, Aronchik I, Clegg RW, Gratton E, Feingold K, Holleran WM, Elias PM, Mauro TM. Neonatal development of the stratum corneum pH gradient: localization and mechanisms leading to emergence of optimal barrier function. J Invest Dermatol. 2003;120(6):998–1006.

Behrendt H, Becker WM. Localization, release and bioavailability of pollen allergens: the influence of environmental factors. Curr Opin Immunol. 2001;13:709–15.

Behrendt H, Ring J. Histamine, antihistamines and atopic eczema. Clin Exp Allergy. 1990;20 Suppl 4:25–30.

Behrendt H, Ring J. Genetik und Umwelteinflüsse in der. In: Heppt W, Bachert C, editors. Epidemiologie von Allergien. Stuttgart: Thieme; 2011. p. 1–12.

Behrendt H, Krämer U, Dolgner R, Hinrichs J, Willer H, Hagenbeck H, Schlipköter HW. Elevated levels of total serum IgE in East German children: atopy, parasites, or pollutants? Allergo J. 1993;2:31–40.

Behrendt H, et al. Der Rat von Sachverständigen für Umweltfragen (SRU). Sondergutachten: Umwelt und Gesundheit. Stuttgart: Metzler-Peschel; 1999.

Behrens T, Taeger D, Maziak W, Duhme H, Rzehak P, Weiland SK, Keil U. Self-reported traffic density and atopic disease in children. Results of the ISAAC Phase III survey in Muenster, Germany. Pediatr Allergy Immunol. 2004;15:331–9.

Behr-Völtzer C, Hamm M, Vieluf D, Ring J, editors. Diät bei Nahrungsmittelallergien und –intoleranzen. 4th ed. Munich: Urban und Vogel; 2008.

Belloni B, Ziai M, Lim A, Lemercier B, Sbornik M, Weidinger S, Andres C, Schnopp C, Ring J, Hein R, Ollert M, Mempel M. Low-dose anti-IgE therapy in patients with atopic eczema with high serum IgE levels. J Allergy Clin Immunol. 2007;120:1223–5.

Benez A, Fierlbeck G. Successful long-term treatment of severe atopic dermatitis with mycophe-nolatemofetil. Br J Dermatol. 2001;144(3):638–9.

Benveniste J, Ducot B, Spira A. Memory of water revisited. Nature. 1994;370:322.

Benveniste J, Arnoux B, editors. Platelet-activating factor and structurally related ether-lipids. Inserm Symp 23. Amsterdam: Elsevier; 1981.

Bergmann KC, Ring J, editors. History of allergy. Basel: Karger; 2014.

Bergmann RL, Bergmann KE, Lau-Schadendorf S, et al. Atopic diseases in infancy. The German multicenter atopy study (MAS-90). Pediatr Allergy Immunol. 1994;5:19–25.

Bergstresser PR, Takashima A, editors. Gamma-delta T cells. Chemical Immunology 1979. Basel: Karger; 2001.

Bernard A. Eczéma et gastrite hypertrophique. J Sc Méd Lille. 1953;71:219–22.

Berth-Jones J, Graham-Brown RA. Placebo-controlled trial of essential fatty acid supplementation in atopic dermatitis. Lancet. 1993;341:1557–60.

Berth-Jones J, Damstra RJ, Golsch S, Livden JK, Van Hooteghem O, Allegra F, Parker CA. Twice weekly fluticasone propionate added to emollient maintenance treatment to reduce risk of relapse in atopic dermatitis randomized double blind, parallel group study. BMJ. 2003;326:1367.

Besnier E. Première note et observations preliminaries pour servir d'introduction à l'étude diathésique. Ann Dermatol Syphiligr. 1892;4:634.

Besnier E. La Practique Dermatologique, Vol 2; 1901. p. 3

Beyer K, Wahn U. Is atopic dermatitis predictable? Pediatr Allergy Immunol. 1999;10:7–10.

Bharati A, Yesudian PD. Positivity of iron studies in pruritus of unknown origin. J Eur Acad Dermatol Venereol. 2008;22:616–8.

Bhavani Meduri N, Vanderriff T, Rasmussen H, Jacobe H. Phototherapy in the management of atopic dermatitis: a systemic review. Photodermatol Photoimmunol Photomed. 2007;23:106–22.

Bieber T. Atopic dermatitis. N Engl J Med. 2008;358:1483–94.

Bieber T. Atopic dermatitis 2.0: from the clinical phenotype to the molecular taxonomy and stratified medicine. Allergy. 2012;67:1475–82.

Bieber T. Many ways lead to Rome – a glance at the multiple immunological pathways underlying atopic dermatitis. Allergy. 2013;68:957–8.

Bieber T, Leung DM, editors. Atopic dermatitis. New York: Marcel Dekker; 2002.

Bieber T, Ring J. Terfenadin und Kraftfahrzeugführung. Eine placebokontrollierte Doppelblindstudie zum Einfluss verschiedener Antihistaminika auf das Fahrverhalten. Med Klin. 1987;82:683–6.

Bieber T, Rieger A, Neuchrist C, Prinz JC, Rieber EP, Boltz-Nitulescu G, Scheiner O, Kraft D, Ring J, Stingl G. Induction of FCeR2/CD23 on human epidermal Langerhans-cells by human recombinant IL4 and IFN. J Exp Med. 1992;170:309–14.

Bieber T, de la Salle H, Wollenberg A, Hakimi J, Chizzonite R, Ring J, Hanau D, de la Salle C. Human Langerhans cells express the high affinity receptor for IgE (FCeR1). J Exp Med. 1995;175:1285–90.

Biedermann T. Dissecting the role of infections in atopic dermatitis. Acta Derm Venereol. 2006;86:99–109. Review.

Bienenstock J, Kunze W, Forsythe P. Microbiota and the gut-brain axis. Nutr Rev. 2015;73 Suppl 1:28–31. doi:10.1093/nutrit/nuv019.

Bindslev-Jensen C, Ballmer-Weber BK, Bengtsson U, et al. Standardization of food challenges in patients with immediate reactions to foods – position paper from the European Academy of Allergology and Clinical Immunology. Allergy. 2004;59:690–7.

Bisgaard H, Simpson A, Palmer CN, Bønnelykke K, Mclean I, Mukhopadhyay S, et al. Gene-environment interaction in the onset of eczema in infancy: filaggrin loss-of-function mutations enhanced by neonatal cat exposure. PLoS Med. 2008;5, e131.

Bissonnette R, Poulin Y, Zhou Y, Tan J, Hong HC, Webster J, Ip W, Tang L, Lyle M. Efficacy and safety of topical WBI-1001 in patients with mild to severe atopic dermatitis: results from a 12-week, multicentre, randomized, placebo-controlled double-blind trial. Br J Dermatol. 2011;166:853–60.

Björksten B. Allergy priming in early life. Lancet. 1999;353:167–8.

Björksten B, Sepp E, Julge K, Voor T, Mikelsaar M. Allergy development and the intestinal microflora during the first year of life. J Allergy Clin Immunol. 2001;108:516–20.

Blaser K, editor. T cell regulation in allergy, asthma and atopic skin disease. Basel: Karger; 2008.

Blumenthal F, Jaffe K. Ekzem und Idiosynkrasie. Berlin: Karger; 1933.

Blume-Peytavi U, Cork MJ, Faergemann J, Szczapa J, Vanaclocha F, Gelmetti C. Bathing and cleansing in newborns from day 1 to first year of life: recommendations from a European round table meeting. J Eur Acad Dermatol Venereol. 2009;23:751–9.

Bockelbrink A, Heinrich J, Schäfer I, Zutavern A, Borte M, Herbarth O, Schaaf B, von Berg A, Schäfer T, for the LISA Study Group. Atopic eczema in children: another harmful sequel of divorce. Allergy. 2006;61:1397–402.

Bode HH. Dwarfism following long-term topical corticosteroid therapy. JAMA. 1980;244:813–4.

Bode U, Ring J, Neubert U. Intrakutantestungen und bakteriologische Untersuchungen bei Patienten mit atopischem Ekzem. Allergologie. 1982;5:259–61.

Boehncke WH, Zollner TM. Die Rolle bakterieller Superantigene in der Pathophysiologie der Haut. Hautarzt. 1999;50:91–7.

Boettger MK, Bär K-J, Dohrmann A, Müller H, Mertins L, Brockmeyer NH, Agelink MW. Increased vagal modulation in atopic dermatitis. J Dermatol Sci. 2009;53:55–9.

Boguniewicz M, Sampson H, Leung SB, Harbeck R, Leung DYM. Effects of cefuroxime axetil on Staphylococcus aureus colonization and superantigen production in atopic dermatitis. J Allergy Clin Immunol. 2001;108:651–2.

Boos AC, Hagl B, Schlesinger A, Halm BE, Ballenberger N, Pinarci M, Heinz V, Kreilinger D, Spielberger BD, Schimke-Marques LF, Sawalle-Belohradsky J, Belohradsky BH, Przybilla B, Schaub B, Wollenberg A, Renner ED. Atopic dermatitis, STAT3- and DOCK8-hyper-IgE syndromes differ in IgE-based sensitization pattern. Allergy. 2014;69:943–53.

Borelli S. Untersuchungen zur Psychosomatik des Neurodermitikers. Hautarzt. 1950;1:250–6.

Borelli S. Probleme der Klimatherapie bei Dermatosen. MünchMed Wschr. 1969;35:1709–17.

Borelli S. Climate therapy of skin diseases. Ther Umsch. 1972;29:610–6.

Borelli S. Die Dermatologische Klinik und Poliklinik am Biederstein der Technischen Universität München und die Deutsche Klinik Alexanderhaus Davos. Munich: Lindner; 1995.

Borelli S, Chlebarov S. Änderungen der Histamin-Reagibilität der Haut nach Hochgebirgs-Klimabehandlung. Münch MedWschr. 1966;11:592–6.

BorelliS, SchnyderUW. Neurodermitisconstitutionalissive atopica. II. Ätiologie, Pathophysiologie, Pathogenese, Therapie. In: Miescher G, Storck H, editors. Handbuch der Haut- und Geschlechtskrankheiten, Entzündliche Dermatosen I, vol. 2/1. Berlin/Göttingen/Heidelberg: Springer; 1962. p. 254–319.

Borelli S, Michailov P, Ene-Popescu C. Die Veränderungen der allergisch-mediatorischen Reaktivität bei Neurodermitis-constitutionalis-Kranken nach Höhenklimatherapie. Hautarzt. 1967;18:456–8.

Bork K, Hoede N. Juvenile papulöse Dermatitis. Hautarzt. 1978;290:216–9.

Bornhoevd EC, Schuller E, Bieber T, Wollenberg A. Immunsuppressive Makrolide und ihr Einsatz in der Dermatologie. Hautarzt. 2000;51:646–54.

Bos JD. Atopiform dermatitis. Br J Dermatol. 2002;147:426–9.

Bos JD, Van Leent EJ, Sillevis Smitt JH. The millennium criteria for the diagnosis of atopic dermatitis. Exp Dermatol. 1998;7:132–9.

Bosse KA. Psychosomatische Gesichtspunkte bei der Betreuung atopischer Ekzematiker. Z Hautkr. 1990;65:543–5.

Bosse KA, Gieler U, editors. Seelische Faktoren bei Hautkrankheiten. Bern: Huber; 1987.

Bourke JF, Berth-Jones J, Holder J, Graham-Brown RA. A new microemulsion formulation of cyclo-sporin (Neoral) is effective in the treatment of cyclosporin-resistant dermatoses. Br J Dermatol. 1996;134: 777–9.

Beuther DA, Sutherland ER. Overweight, obesity, and incident asthma: a meta-analysis of prospective epidemiological studies. Am J Respir Crit Care Med. 2007;175:822–8.

Boralevi F, Saint Aroman M, Delarue A, Raudsepp H, Kaszuba A, Bylaite M, Tiplica GS. Long-term emollient therapy improves xerosis in children with atopic dermatitis. J Eur Acad Dermatol Venereol. 2014;28:1456–62.

Bovet D, Staub AM. Action protectrice des éthers-phénoliques au cours de l'intoxication histaminique. C R Soc Biol Paris. 1934;124:547–9.

Bozek A, Fisher A, Filipowska B, Mazur B, Jarzab J. Clinical features and immunological markers of atopic dermatitis in elderly patients. Int Arch Allergy Immunol. 2012;157:372–8.

Bradley M, Soderhall C, Wahlgren CF, Luthman H, Nordenskjold M, Kockum I. The Wiskott-Aldrich syndrome gene as a candidate gene for atopic dermatitis. Acta Derm Venereol. 2001;81:340–2.

Braun-Fahrländer C, Riedler J, Herz U, et al. Environmental exposure to endotoxin and its relation to asthma in school-age children. N Engl J Med. 2002;347:869–77.

Braun-Fahrländer C, Gassner M, Grize L, et al., SCARPOL TEAM. No further increase in asthma, hay fever and atopic sensitisation in adolescents living in Switzerland. Eur Respir J. 2004;23:407–13.

Braun-Falco O, Korting HC. Syndets in the treatment of atopic eczema. In: Ruzicka T, Ring J, Przybilla B, editors. Handbook of atopic eczema. Berlin/Heidelberg/New York: Springer; 1991. p. 356–63.

Braun-Falco O, Ring J. Zur Therapie des atopischen Ekzems. Hautarzt. 1984;35:447–54.

Braun-Falco O, Ryckmanns F, Heilgemeir GP, Ring J. Zum Syndrom: Unkämmbare Haare. Hautarzt. 1982;33:366–72.

Breit R. Neurodermitis (Dermatitis atopica) im Kindesalter. Z Hautkrankh. 1997;2(Suppl):72–82.

Bremmer MS, Bremmer SF, Baig-Lewis S, Simpson EL. Are biologics safe in the treatment of atopic dermatitis? J Am Acad Dermatol. 2009;61:666–76.

Brenninkmeijer EE, Schram ME, Leeflang MM, Bos JD, Spuls PI. Diagnostic criteria for atopic dermatitis: a systematic review. Br J Dermatol. 2008;158:754–65.

Bresser H. Allergietestung mittels Elektroakupunktur nach Dr. Voll Hautarzt. 1993;46:408–9.

Breuer K, Kapp A. Stationäre medizinische Rehabilitation bei erwachsenen Patienten mit atopischer Dermatitis. Hautarzt. 2006;57:592–602.

Broberg A, Augustsson A. Atopic dermatitis and melanocytic naevi. Br J Dermatol. 2000;142:306–9.

Broberg A, Faergemann J. Topical antimycotic treatment of atopic dermatitis in the head/neck area. A double-blind randomized study. Acta Derm Venereol. 1995;75:46–9.

Brockow K, Ring J. Nahrungsmittel als Auslöser einer Anaphylaxie. Allergologie. 2008;31:286–92.

Brockow K, Abeck D, Ring J. Die systemische Therapie im Behandlungskonzept des atopischen Ekzems. Hautarzt. 1999a;50:323–9.

Brockow K, Grabenhorst P, Abeck D, et al. Effect of gentian violet, corticosteroid and tar preparations in Staphylococcus-aureus-colonized atopic eczema. Dermatology. 1999b;199:231–6.

Brocq L. L'eczéma considéré comme une réaction cutaneé. Ann Dermatol Syph. 1903;4:172.

Brocq L. Conception générale des dermatoses, nouvelle note sur leur classification. Ann Dermatol Syphilol. 1927;8:65.

Bruijnzeel-Koomen CA, Mudde GC, Bruijnzeel PL. The presence of IgE molecules on epidermal Langerhans cells in atopic dermatitis and their significance for its pathogenesis. Allerg Immunol (Paris). 1989;90 Suppl 1:51–6.

Bruijnzeel PL, Kuijper PH, Kapp A, Warringa RA, Betz S, Bruijnzeel-Koomen CA. The involvement of eosinophils in the patch test reaction to aeroallergens in atopic dermatitis: its relevance for the patho-genesis of atopic dermatitis. Clin Exp Allergy. 1993;23:97–109.

Bruijnzeel-Koomen CAFM, Van Wichen DF, Spry CJF, Venge P, Bruynzeel PLB. Active participation of eosinophils in patch test reactions to inhalant allergens in patients with atopic dermatitis. Br J Dermatol. 1988;118:229–38.

Büchau AS, MacLeod DT, Morizane S, Kotol PF, Hata T, Gallo RL. Bcl-3 acts as an innate immune modulator by controlling antimicrobial responses in keratinocytes. J Invest Dermatol. 2009;129:2148–55.

Buckley RH, Becker WG. Abnormalities in the regulation of human IgE synthesis. Immunol Rev. 1978;41:288–314.

Buddenkotte J, Steinhoff M. Pathophysiology and therapy of pruritus in allergic and atopic diseases. Allergy. 2010;65:805–21.

Buhl R, Hanf G, Soler M, Bensch G, et al. The anti-IgE antibody omalizumab improves asthma-related quality of life in patients with allergic asthma. Eur Resp J. 2002;20:1088–94.

Buhles N, Wehrmann J, Amon K. Dermatologische stationäre Rehabilitation bei atopischer Dermatitis Erwachsener. J Deutsch Derm Ges. 2003;3:238–41.

Bunikowski R, Mielke M, Skarabis H, et al. Prevalence and role of serum IgE antibodies to the Staphylococcus aureus-derived superantigens SEA and SEB in children with atopic dermatitis. J Allergy Clin Immunol. 1999;103:119–24.

Bunikowski R, Staab D, Kussebi F, Brautigam M, Weidinger G, Renz H, Wahn U. Low-dose cyclosporin A microemulsion in children with severe atopic dermatitis: clinical and immunological effects. Pediatr Allergy Immunol. 2001;12:216–23.

Burks AW, Laubach S, Jones SM. Oral tolerance, food allergy, and immunotherapy: implications for future treatment. J Allergy Clin Immunol. 2008;121: 1344–50.

Buske-Kirschbaum A, Geiben A, Hellhammer D. Psychobiological aspects of atopic dermatitis: an overview. Psychother Psychosom. 2001;70:6–16.

Buslau M, Thaci D. Atopic dermatitis: borage oil for systemic therapy. Z Dermatol. 1996;182:131–6.

Busse WW, Lantis SOH. Decrease H2 histamine granulocyte response in atopic eczema. J Invest Dermatol. 1979;73:184–9.

Bussmann C, Böckenhoff A, Henke H, Werfel T, Novak N. Does allergen-specific immunotherapy represent a therapeutic option for patients with atopic dermatitis? J Allergy Clin Immunol. 2006;118:1292–8.

Bussmann C, Weidinger S, Novak N. Genetics of atopic dermatitis. JDDG. 2011;9:670–6.

Butler JM, Ebert M, Chan M, Stevens SR, Szobieszczuk D, Hanifin JM. Basophil histamine release in atopic dermatitis and its relationship to disordered cyclic nucleotide metabolism. Acta Derm Venereol [Suppl] (Stockh). 1985;114:55–61.

Camargo Jr CA, Ganmaa D, Sidbury R, Erdenedelger K, Radnaakhand N, Khandsuren B. Randomized trial of vitamin D supplementation for winter-related atopic dermatitis in children. J Allergy Clin Immunol. 2014;134:831–5.

Cap F. Bemerkungen eines Physikers zur Bioresonanz. Allergologie. 1995;18:235–7.

Caputo R, Vanotti P, Bertani E. Netherton's syndrome in two adult brothers. Arch Dermatol. 1984;120:220–2.

Carlsson CP, Wallengren J. Therapeutical and experimental therapeutic studies on acupuncture and itch: review of the literature. J Eur Acad Dermatol Venereol. 2010;24:1013–6.

Caruso C, Gaeta F, Valluzzi RL, Romano A. Omalizumab efficacy in a girl with atopic eczema. Allergy. 2010;65:278–9.

Cassano N, Loconsole F, Coviello C, Vena GA. Infliximab in recalcitrant severe atopic eczema associated with contact allergy. Int J Immunopathol. 2006;19: 237–40.

Cavani A, Albanese C, Traidl C, Sebastiani S, Girolomoni G. Effector and regulatory T cells in allergic contact dermatitis. Trends Immunol. 2001;22:118–20.

Chan SC, Li SH, Hanifin JM. Increased interleukin-4 production by atopic mononuclear leukocytes correlates with increased cyclic adenosine monophosphate-phosphodiesterase activity and is reversible by phosphodiesterase inhibition. J Invest Dermatol. 1993;100:681–4.

Charman CR, Williams HC. Outcome measures of disease severity in atopic eczema. Arch Dermatol. 2000;136:763–9.

Chatzi L, Torrent M, Romieu I, Garcia-Esteban R, Ferrer C, Vioque J, Kogevinas M, Sunyer J. Mediterranean diet in pregnancy is protective for wheeze and atopy in childhood. Thorax. 2008;63:507–13.

Chen W, Mempel M, Schober W, Behrendt H, Ring J. Gender differences, sex hormones and immediate hypersensitivity. Allergy. 2008;63:1418–27.

Cheng H-M, Chiang L-C, Jan Y-M, Chen G-W. The efficacy and safety of a Chinese herbal product (Xiao-Feng-San) for the treatment of refractory atopic dermatitis: a randomized, double-blind, placebo-controlled trial. Int Arch Allergy Immunol. 2011;155:141–8.

Chida Y, Hamer M, Steptow A. A bidirectional relationship between psychosocial factors and atopic disorders: A systematic review and metaanalysis. Psychosom Med. 2008;70:102–16.

Christiansen JV, Gadborg E, Kleiter I, et al. Efficacy of bufexamac cream in skin diseases. A double-blind multicentre trial. Dermatologica. 1977;154:177–84.

Church MK. Non-H1-receptor effects of antihistamines. Clin Exp Allergy. 1999;29 Suppl 3:39–48.

Coca AF. Familial non-reaginic food allergy. Springfield: Charles C Thomas; 1943.

Coca AF, Cooke RA. On the classification of the phenomena of hypersensitiveness. J Immunol. 1923;8:163–82.

Coca AF, Grove E. Studies in hypersensitiveness. XIII. A study of the atopic reagins. J Immunol. 1925;10:445.

Coffmann RL, von der Weid T. Multiple passways for the initiation of T helper 2 (Th2) reponses. J Exp Med. 1997;185:373–5.

Colcha W, Leuschner J, Leuschner F. The adverse effects of dark sulfonated shale oil following local and systemic administration. Arzneimittelforschung. 1994;44:844–9.

Colver GB, Mortimer PS, Millard PR. The "dirty neck" – a reticulate pigmentations in atopics. Clin Exp Dermatol. 1987;12:1–4.

Conroy MC, Adkinson NF, Lichtenstein LM. Measurement of IgE in human basophils; relation to serum IgE and anti-IgE-induced histamine release. J Immunol. 1977;118:1317–24.

Cookson WO, Moffatt MF. The genetics of atopic dermatitis. Curr Opin Allergy Immunol. 2002;2:283–387.

Cookson WOCM, Young RP, Sandford A, et al. Maternal inheritance of atopic IgE responsivenesson chromosome 11q. Lancet. 1992;340:381–4.

Cookson WO, Ubhi B, Lawrence R, et al. Genetic linkage of childhood atopic dermatitis to psoriasis susceptibility loci. Nat Genet. 2001;27:372–3.

Corbo GM, Ferrante E, Macciocchi B, Foresi A, De Angelis V, Fabbri L, Ciappi G. Bronchial hyperresponsiveness in atopic dermatitis. Allergy. 1989;44:595–8.

Cork MJ. The importance of skin barrier function. J Dermatol Treat. 1997;8:S7–13.

Cork MJ, Robinson D, Vasilopoulos Y, Ferguson A, Moustafa M, Mac Gowan A, Ward SJ, Tazi-Ahnini R. Predisposition to sensitive skin and atopic eczema. Community Pract. 2005;78:440–2.

Cork MJ, Danby SG, Vasilopoulos Y, Hadgraft J, Lane ME, Moustafa M, Guy RH, MacGowan AL, Tazi-Ahnini R, Ward SJ. Epidermal barrier dysfunction in atopic dermatitis. J Invest Dermatol. 2009;129:1892–908.

Cowden JM, Zhang M, Dunford PJ, Thurmond RL. The histamine H_4 receptor mediates inflammation and pruritus in Th2-dependent dermal inflammation. J Invest Dermatol. 2010;130:1023–33.

Cox L, Platts-Mills TA, Finegold I et al. American Academy of Allergy, Asthma & Immunolo-gy/American College of Allergy, Asthma and Immunology Joint Task Force. Report on omalizumab-associated anaphylaxis. J Allergy Clin Immunol. 2007;120:1373–7.

Cramer C, Ranft U, Ring J, Möhrenschlager M, Behrendt H, Oppermann H, Wilhelm M, Krämer U. Allergic sensitization and disease in mother-child pairs from Germany: role of early childhood environment. Int Arch Allergy Immunol. 2007;143:282–9.

Crameri R, Faith A, Hemmann S, Jaussi R, Ismail C, Menz G, Blaser K. Humoral and cell-mediated autoimmunity in allergy to Aspergillus fumigatus. J Exp Med. 1996;184:265–70.

Czarnecka-Operacz M, Silny W. Specific immunotherapy in atopic dermatitis – four-year treatment in different age and airborne allergy type subgroups. Acta Dermatovenerol Croat. 2006;14(4):230–40.

Czerny A. Die exsudative Diathese. Jb Kinderheilk. 1905;61:3–199.

Dale HH, Laidlaw BP. The physiological action of β-Imidazolylethylamine. J Physiol. 1910;41:318.

Darsow U, Sbornik M, Rombold S, Katzer K, von Krempelhuber A, Chaplin P, Baedeker N, Sobek V, Vollmar J, Rösch S, von Sonnenburg F, Behrendt H, Ring J. Long-term safety of replication-defective smallpox vaccine (MVA-BN) in atopic eczema and allergic rhinitis. (in prep).

Darsow U, Ring J. Airborne and dietary allergens in atopic eczema: a comprehensive review of diagnostic tests. Clin Exp Dermatol. 2000;25:544–51.

Darsow U, Vieluf U, Ring J. The atopy patch test: an increased rate of reactivity in patients who have an air-exposed pattern of atopic eczema. Br J Dermatol. 1996;135:182–6.

Darsow U, Mautner VF, Bromm B, Scharein E, Ring J. Der Eppendorfer Juckreizfragebogen. Hautarzt. 1997a;48:730–3.

Darsow U, Scharein E, Bromm B, Ring J. Skin testing of the pruritogenic activity of histamine and cytokines (interleukin-2 and tumor necrosis factor-alpha) at the dermal-epidermal junction. Br J Dermatol. 1997b;137:415–7.

Darsow U, Vieluf D, Ring J. Evaluating the relevance of aeroallergen sensitization in atopic eczema with the atopy patch test: a randomized, double-blind multicenter study. Atopy Patch Test Study Group. J Am Acad Dermatol. 1999;40:187–93.

Darsow U, Drzezga A, Frisch M, Munz F, Weilke F, Bartenstein P, Schwaiger M, Ring J. Processing of histamine-induced itch in the human cerebral cortex: a correlation analysis with dermal reactions. J Invest Dermatol. 2000;115:1029–33.

Darsow U, Scharein E, Simon D, Walter G, Bromm B, Ring J. New aspects of itch physiopathology: component analysis of atopic using the "Eppendorf Itch Questionnaire". Int Arch Allergy Immunol. 2001;124:326–31.

Darsow U, Forer I, Ring J. Spezifische Hyposensibilisierung bei atopischem Ekzem. Allergologie. 2005;28:53–61.

Darsow U, Wollenberg A, Simon D, Taïeb A, Werfel T, Oranje A, Gelmetti C, Svensson A, Deleuran M, Calza A-M, Giusti F, Lübbe J, Seidenari S, Ring J. ETFAD/EADV eczema task force 2009 position paper on diagnosis and treatment of atopic dermatitis. J Eur Acad Dermatol Venereol. 2010;24:317–28.

Darsow U, Forer I, Ring J. Allergen-specific immunotherapy in atopic eczema. Curr Allergy Asthma Rep. 2011;11:277–83.

Darsow U, Wollenberg A, Simon D, Taïeb A, Werfel T, Oranje A, Gelmetti C, Svensson A, Deleuran M, Calza A-M, Giusti F, Lübbe J, Seidenari S, Ring J, for the European Task Force on Atopic Dermatitis/EADV Eczema Task Force. Difficult to control atopic dermatitis. WAO J. 2013;6:1–5.

David TJ. Short stature in children with atopic eczema. Acta Derm Venereol Suppl. 1989;144:41–4.

David TJ, Cambridge GC. Bacterial infection and atopic eczema. Arch Dis Child. 1986;61:20–3.

David TJ, Waddington E, Stanton RHJ. Nutritional hazards of elimination diets in children with atopic eczema. Arch Dis Child. 1984;59:323–5.

David TJ, Wells FE, Sharpe TC, Gibbs AC, Devlin J. Serum levels of trace metals in children with atopic eczema. Br J Dermatol. 1990;122:485–9.

Dawe RS. Ultraviolet A1 phototherapy. Br J Dermatol. 2003;148:626–37.

De Benedetto A, Qualia CM, Baroody FM, Beck LA. Filaggrin expression in oral, nasal and esophageal mucosa. J Invest Dermatol. 2008;128:1594–7.

De Benedetto A, Agnihothri R, McGirt LY, Bankova LG, Beck L. Atopic dermatitis: a disease caused by innate immune defects? J Invest Dermatol. 2009;129:14–30.

de Weck AL. What can we learn from the allergic zoo? Int Arch Allergy Immunol. 1995;107:13–8.

de Weck A. Memories: failures and dreams, One life, many dreams, vol. 1. Berlin: Pro Business; 2008.

De Weert J, Timmerman L, Kint A. Alopecia areata and atopy. Dermatologica. 1984;168:224–9.

Deo M, Yung A, Hill S, Rademaker M. Methotrexate for treatment of atopic dermatitis in children and adolescents. Int J Dermatol. 2014;53:1037–41.

Degos R. Dermatologie. Paris: Flammarion; 1953.

Deleuran M, Ellingsen AR, Paludan K, Schou C, Thestrup-Pedersen K. Purified Der p1 and p2 patch tests in patients with atopic dermatitis: evidence for both allergenicity and proteolytic irritancy. Acta Derm Venereol. 1998;78:241–3.

Desai NS, Poindexter GB, Monthrope YM, Bendeck SE, Swerlick RA, Chen SC. A pilot quality-of-life instrument for pruritus. J Am Acad Dermatol. 2008;59(2):234–44. doi:10.1016/j.jaad.2008.04.006. Epub 11 June 2008.

Devillers ACA, de Waard-van der Spek FB, Mulder PGH, Oranje AP. Treatment of refractory atopic dermatitis using "wet-wrap" dressings and diluted corticosteroids: results of standardized treatment in both children and adults. Dermatology. 2002;204:50–5.

Devos SA, van der Valk PG. The relevance of skin prick tests for Pityrosporum ovale in patients with head and neck dermatitis. Allergy. 2000;55:1056–8.

Diebschlag W, Diebschlag B. Hausstauballergien. Gesundheitliche und hygienische Aspekte. 2nd ed. Munich: Herbert Utz; 2000.

Diepgen TL. Atopic dermatitis – the role of social factors. J Am Acad Dermatol. 2001;45:44–8.

Diepgen TL. Early treatment of the atopic child study group. Long-term treatment with cetirizine of infants with atopic dermatitis: a multi-country, double-blind, randomized, placebo-controlled trial (the ETAC trial) over 18 months. Pediatr Allergy Immunol. 2002;13:278–86.

Diepgen TL, Coenraads PJ. The epidemiology of occupational contact dermatitis. In: Kamerva L, Elsner P, Wahlberg JE, Maibach HI, editors. Handbook of occupational dermatology. Berlin: Springer; 2000. p. 3–16.

Diepgen TL, Fartasch M, Hornstein OP. Kriterien zur Beurteilung der atopischen Hautdiathese. Dermatosen. 1991;39:79–83.

Diepgen T, Fartasch M, Ring J, Scheewe S, Staab D, Szcepanski R, Werfel T, Wahn U, Gieler U. Neurodermitisschulung. Hautarzt. 2003;54:946–51.

Diepgen TL, Andersen KE, Brandao FM, Bruze M, Bruynzeel DP, Frosch P, Goncalo M, Goossens A, Le Coz CJ, Rustemeyer T, White IR, Agner T. Hand eczema classification: a cross-sectional, multicentre study of the aetiology and morphology of hand eczema. Br J Dermatol. 2009;160:323–58.

Dieris-Hirche J, Gieler U, Kupfer JP, Milch WE. Suizidgedanken, Angst und Depression bei erwachsenen Neurodermitikern. Hautarzt. 2009;60:641–6.

Diezel W, Gruner S, Anhalt GJ. ATPase positive epidermal Langerhans cells: inhibition of ATPase by ammonium bituminosulfonate (Ichthyol) and pix lithanthracis. Hautarzt. 1992;43:22–4.

Dinkloh A, Worm M, Geier J, Schnuch A, Wollenberg A. Contact sensitization in patients with suspected cosmetic intolerance: results of the IVDK 2006–2011. J Eur Acad Dermatol Venereol. 2015;29:1071–81.

Dittmar HC, Pflieger D, Schempp CM, Schöpf E, Simon JC. Vergleichsstudie Solebäder plus UVA/B versus UVA/B Monotherapie bei Patienten mit subakuter atopischer Dermatitis. Hautarzt. 1999;50:649–53.

Dondi A, Ricci L, Neri I, Ricci G, Patrizi A. The switch from non-IgE-associated to IgE-associated atopic dermatitis occurs early in life. Allergy. 2013;68:259–60.

Dorsch W, Ring J. Komplementärverfahren oder sogenannte Alternativmethoden in der Allergologie. Allergo J. 2002;11:163–70.

Dorsch W, Sitzmann FC, editors. Naturheilkunde in der Kinderheilkunde. 2nd ed. Stuttgart: Hippokrates; 2001.

Dorsch W, Ring J, Reimann HY, Geiger R. Mediator studies in skin blister fluids from parents with dual skin reactions. J Allerg Clin Immunol. 1982;70: 236–44.

Droitcourt C, TouboulD GC, Ezzedine K, Cario-André M, de Verneuil H, Colin J, Taïeb A. A prospective study of filaggrin null mutations in keratoconus patients with or without atopic disorders. Dermatology. 2011;222:336–41.

Drzimalla K, Wagner SA, Disch R, Borelli S. Longterm results after high-altitude climatotherapy in Davos –a follow-up study. Präv Rehab. 1999;11:18–27.

Du Toit G, Roberts G, Sayre PH, Bahnson HT, Radulovic S, Santos AF, Brough HA, Phippard D, Basting M, Feeney M, Turcanu V, Sever ML, Gomez Lorenzo M, Plaut M, Lack G, LEAP Study Team. Randomized trial of peanut consumption in infants at risk for peanut allergy. N Engl J Med. 2015;372(9):803–13. doi:10.1056/NEJMoa1414850. Epub 23 Feb 2015.

Dubowitz V. Familial low birth weight dwarfism with an unusual facies and skin eruption. J Med Genet. 1965;2:12–7.

Dunstan JA, Mori TA, Barden A, Beilin LJ, Holt PG, Calder PC, Taylor AL, Prescott SL. Effects of n-3 polyunsaturated fatty acid supplementation in pregnancy on maternal and fetal erythrocyte fatty acid composition. Eur J Clin Nutr. 2004;58:429–37.

Dupré MMA, Christol B, Bonafe JL. La dermatite du toboggan (variant de "frictional lichenoid eruption in children"). Bull Soc Fr Dermatol Syphiligr. 1974;81:203–5.

Dupré AS, Christol B, Bonafe JL, Lassere J. Orf and atopic dermatitis. Br J Dermatol. 1981;105:103–4.

Dutoit G, Kats Y, Sasieni P, et al. Early consumption of peanuts in infancy is associated with a low prevalence of peanut allergy. J Allergy Clin Immunol. 2008;22:984–91.

Eberlein B, Eicke C, Reinhardt H-W, Ring J. Adjuvante Therapie mit einer N-Palmitoylethanolamin-haltigen Creme bei Kindern mit atopischem Ekzem (ATOPA-Studie). Akt Dermatol. 2009a;35:339–41.

Eberlein B, Gulyas AF, Schultz K, Lecheler J, Flögel S, Wolfmeyer C, Thiessen K, Jakob T, Schuster T, Hollweck R, Ring J, Behrendt H. Domestic allergens and endotoxin in three hospitals offering in-patient rehabilitation for allergic disease in the alpine mountain climate of Bavaria – The AURA study. Int J Hyg Environ Health. 2009b;212:21–6.

Eberlein-König B, Spiegl A, Przybilla B. Change of skin roughness due to lowering air humidity in a climate chamber. Acta Derm Venereol. 1996;76:447–9.

Eberlein-König B, Przybilla B, Kühnl P, Pechak J, Gebefügi I, Kleinschmidt J, Ring J. Influence of airborne nitrogen dioxide or formaldehyde on parameters of skin function and cellular activation in patients with atopic eczema and control subjects. J Allergy Clin Immunol. 1998;101:141–3.

Eberlein-König B, Schäfer T, Huss-Marp J, Darsow U, Möhrenschlager M, Herbert O, Abeck D, Krämer U, Behrendt H, Ring J. Skin surface pH, stratum corneum hydration, trans-epidermal water loss and skin roughness related to atopic eczema and skin dryness in a population of primary school children. Acta Derm Venereol. 2000;80(3):188–91.

Edgren G. Prognose und Erblichkeitsmomente bei Eczema infantum. Eine klinisch-statistische Untersuchung von Allergieerscheinungen. Acta Paediatr Scand. 1943;30 Suppl 2:1–204.

Ege MJ, Herzum I, Büchele G, et al., Protection Against Allergy Study Rural Environments (PASTURE) Study group. Prenatal exposure to a farm environment modifies atopic sensitization at birth. J Allergy Clin Immunol, 2008a;122:407–12.

Ege MJ, Herzum I, Büchele G, Krauss-Etschmann S, Lauener RP, Roponen M, et al. Prenatal exposure to a farm environment modifies atopic sensitization at birth. J Allergy Clin Immunol. 2008b;122:407–12.

Egelrud T. Purification and preliminary characterization of stratum corneum chymotryptic enzyme: a protein-ase which may be involved in desquamation. J Invest Dermatol. 1993;101:200–4.

Egle UT, König U, Dorsch W. Zur pathogenetischen Bedeutung früher psychosozialer Einflussfaktoren bei atopischer Dermatitis. Allergologie. 2002;25:291–9.

Ehlers A, Stangier U, Gieler U. Treatment of atopic dermatitis. A comparison of psychological and dermatological approaches to relapse prevention. J Consult Clin Psychol. 1995;63:624–35.

Ehlken B, Möhrenschlager M, Kugland B, Berger K, Quednau K, Ring J. Krankheitskostenstudie bei Patienten mit atopischem Ekzem in Deutschland. Hautarzt. 2005;56:1144–51.

Ehnert B, Lau-Schadendorf S, Weber A, Buettner P, Schou C, Wahn U. Reducing domestic dust mite allergen reduces bronchial hyperreactivity in sensitive children with asthma. J Allergy Clin Immunol. 1992;90:135–8.

Ehrlich P. Beiträge zur Kenntnis der der Anilinfärbungen und ihrer Verwendung in der mikroskopischen Technik. Arch mikr Anat. 1877;13:263, T-XXI, 5.

Eichenfield LF, Lucky AW, Boguniewicz M, Langley RG, Cherill R, Marshall K, Bush C, Graeber M. Safety and efficacy of pimecrolimus (ASM 981) cream 1 % in the treatment of mild and moderate atopic dermatitis in children and adolescents. J Am Acad Dermatol. 2002;46:495–504.

Eigenmann PA, Sicherer SH, Borkowski TA, Cohen BA, Sampson HA. Prevalence of IgE-mediated food allergy among children with atopic dermatitis. Pediatrics. 1998;101:E8.

Elias PM, Menon GK. Structural and lipid biochemical correlates of the epidermal permeability barrier. Adv Lipid Res. 1991;24:1–26.

Ellinghaus D, Baurecht H, Esparza-Gordillo J, Rodríguez E, Matanovic A, Marenholz I, Hübner N, Schaarschmidt H, Novak N, Michel S, Maintz L, Werfel T, Meyer-Hoffert U, Hotze M, Prokisch H, Heim K, Herder C, Hirota T, Tamari M, Kubo M, Takahashi A, Nakamura Y, Tsoi LC, Stuart P, Elder JT, Sun L, Zuo X, Yang S, Zhang X, Hoffmann P, Nöthen MM, Fölster-Holst R, Winkelmann J, Illig T, Boehm BO, Duerr RH, Büning C, Brand S, Glas J, McAleer MA, Fahy CM, Kabesch M, Brown S, McLean WH, Irvine AD, Schreiber S, Lee YA, Franke A, Weidinger S. High-density genotyping study identifies four new susceptibility loci for atopic dermatitis. Nat Genet. 2013;45:808–12.

Ellis CN, Drake LA, Prendergast MM, Abramovits W, Boguniewicz DR, Lebwohl M, Stevens SR, Whitaker-Worth DL, Cheng JW. Cost of atopic dermatitis and eczema in the United States. J Am Acad Dermatol. 2002;46:361–70.

Ellis C, Luger T, Abeck D, Allen R, Graham-Brown RA, De Prost Y, Eichenfield LF, Ferrandiz C, Gian-netti A, Hanifin J, Koo JY, Leung D, Lynde C, Ring J, Ruiz-Maldonado R, Saurat JH. International Consensus Conference on Atopic Dermatitis II (ICCAD II): clinical update and current treatment strat-egies. Br J Dermatol. 2003;148 Suppl 63:3–10.

Elman S, Hynan LS, Gabriel V, Mayo MJ. The 5-D itch scale: a new measure of pruritus. Br J Dermatol. 2010;162:587–93.

Elsner I, Kapp A. Regulation and modulation of eosinophil effector functions. Allergy. 1999;54:15–26.

Emerson RM, Charman CR, Williams HC. The Nottingham Eczema Severity Score: preliminary refinement of the Rajka and Langeland grading. Br J Dermatol. 2000;142:288–97.

Enders F, Przybilla B, Ring J, Burg G, Braun-Falco O. Epikutantestung mit einer Standardreihe. Hautarzt. 1988;39:779–86.

Engman MF, Weiss RS, Engman ME. Eczema and environment. Med Clin North Am. 1936;20:651–63.

Engst R, Vocks E. Hochgebirgsklimatherapie bei Dermatosen und Allergien. Wirkmechanismen, Ergebnisse und Einflüsse auf immunologische Parameter. Rehabilitation. 2000;39:215–22.

Enk AH, Katz SI. Early events in the induction phase of contact sensitivity. J Invest Dermatol. 1992; 99:9–41.

Ernst E, Barnes J. Are homeopathic remedies effective for delayed-onset muscle soreness? A systemic review of placebo-controlled trials. Perfusion. 1998;11:4–8.

Esparza-Gordillo J, Weidinger S, Fölster-Holst R, Bauerfeind A, Ruschendorf F, Patone G, Rohde K, Marenholz I, Schulz F, Kerscher T, Hubner N, Wahn U, Schreiber S, Franke A, Vogler R, Heath S, Baurecht H, Novak N, Rodriguez E, Illig T, Lee-Kirsch MA, Ciechanowicz A, Kurek M, Piskackova T, Macek M, Lee YA, Ruether A. A common variant on chromosome 11q13 is associated with atopic dermatitis. Nat Genet. 2009;41:596–601.

European Task Force on Atopic Dermatitis. Severity scoring of atopic dermatitis: the SCORAD Index. Consensus report of the European task force on atopic dermatitis. Dermatology. 1993;186:23, 31.

Ewing CI, Ashcroft C, Gibbs AC, Jones GA, Connor PJ, David TJ. Flucloxacilin in the treatment of atopic dermatitis. Br J Dermatol. 1998;138:1022–9.

Exl BM, Deland U, Secretin MC, Preysch U, Wall M, Shmerling DH. Improved general health status in an unselected infant population following an allergen-reduced dietary intervention programme: the ZUFF-STUDY-PROGRAMME. Part II: infant growth and health status to age 6 months. Zug-FrauenFeld. Eur J Nutr. 2000;39:145–56.

Eyerich K, Novak N. Immunology of atopic eczema: overcoming the Th1/Th2 paradigm. Allergy. 2013;68:974–82.

Eyerich K, Foerster S, Rombold S, Seidl HP, Behrendt H, Hofmann H, Ring J, Traidl-Hoffmann C. Patients with chronic mucocutaneous candidiasis exhibit reduced production of Th17-associated cytokines IL-17 and IL-22. J Invest Dermatol. 2008;128:3640–5.

Eyerich K, Pennino D, Scarponi C, Foerster S, Nasorri F, Behrendt H, Ring J, Traidl-Hoffmann C, Albanesi C. IL-17 in atopic eczema: linking allergen-specific adaptive and microbial-triggered innate immune response. J Allergy Clin Immunol. 2009a;123:59–66.

Eyerich S, Eyerich K, Pennino D, Carbone T, Nasorri F, Pallotta S, Cianfarani F, Odorisio T, Traidl-Hoffmann C, Behrendt H, Durham SR, Schmidt-Weber CB, Cavani A. Th22 cells represent a distinct human T cell subset involved in epidermal immunity and remodeling. J Clin Invest. 2009b;119:3573–85.

Eyerich S, Onken AT, Weidinger S, Franke A, Nasorri F, Pennino D, Grosber M, Pfab F, Schmidt-Weber CB, Mempel M, Hein R, Ring J, Cavani A, Eyerich K. Mutual antagonism of T cells causing psoriasis and atopic eczema. N Engl J Med. 2011;365(3):231–8.

Fajt ML, Wenzel SE. Biologic therapy in asthma: entering the new age of personalized medicine. J Asthma. 2014;51(7):669–76.

Falk ES. Ketotifen in the treatment of atopic dermatitis. Results of a double-blind study. Rev Eur Sci Med Farmacol. 1993;15(2):63–6.

Falth-Magnusson K, Kjellmann NI. Allergy prevention by maternal elimination diet during late pregnancy – a 5-year follow-up of a randomized study. J Allergy Clin Immunol. 1992;89:709–13.

Farahmand S, Tien L, Hui X, Maibach HI. Measuring transepidermal water loss: a comparative in vivo study of condenser-chamber, unventilated-chamber and open-chamber systems. Skin Res Technol. 2009;15: 392–8.

Farin E, Gerdes N, Jäckel WH, Follert P, Klein K, Glattacker M. "Qualitätsprofile" von Rehabilitationskliniken als Modell der Qualitätsmessung in Einrichtungen des Gesundheitswesens. Gesundh ökon Qual Manag. 2003;8:191–204.

Fartasch M, Diepgen TL, Hornstein OP. Atopic dermatitis – ichthyosis vulgaris – hyperlinear palms – an ultrastructural study. Dermatologica. 1989;178:202–5.

Felix R, Shuster S. A new method for the measurement of itch and the response to treatment. Br J Dermatol. 1975;93:303–12.

Ferguson JE, Chalmers RJ, Rowlands DJ. Reversible dilated cardiomyopathy following treatment of atopic eczema with Chinese herbal medicine. Br J Dermatol. 1997;136:592–3.

Ferié J, Dinkela A, Mbata M, Idindili B, Schmid-Grendelmeier P, Hatz C. Skin disorders among school children in rural Tanzania and an assessment of therapeutic needs. Trop Doct. 2006;36:219–21.

Finlay AY. Measurement of disease activity and outcome in atopic dermatitis. Br J Dermatol. 1996a;135:509–15.

Finlay AY. Measures of the effect of severe atopic dermatitis on quality of life. J Eur Acad Dermatol Venereol. 1996b;7:149–59.

Finlay AY. Quality of life measurement in dermatology: a practical guide. Br J Dermatol. 1997;136:305–14.

Finlay AY, Khan GK. Dermatology Life Quality Index (DLQI): a simple practical measure for routine clinical use. Clin Exp Dermatol. 1994;19:210–6.

Fisher MS, Kripke ML. Systemic alteration induced by UV light irradiation. PNAS. 1977;74:1688–92.

Flohr C, Nagel G, Weinmayer G, Kleiner A, Strachan DP, Williams HC. Lack of evidence for a protective effect of prolonged breastfeeding on childhood eczema:

lessons from the International Statistic of Asthma and Allergies in Childhood (ISAAC) phase two. Br J Dermatol. 2011;165:1280–9.
Flohr C, Irvine AD. Systemic therapies for severe atopic dermatitis in children and adults. J Allergy Clin Immunol. 2013;132:774–774.e776.
Flohr C, Mann J. New insights into the epidemiology of childhood atopic dermatitis. Allergy. 2014;69:3–16.
Fölster-Holst R, Kiene P, Brodersen JP, Christophers E. Dermatitis papulosa juvenilis. Hautarzt. 1996;47:129–31.
Fölster-Holst R, Weichenthal M, Steinsland K, Polzhofer G, Christophers E. Eczema infantum and its prognosis. Acta Derm Venereol. 2004;84:410–2.
Fölster-Holst R, Müller F, Schnopp N, Abeck D, Kreiselmaier I, Lenz T, von Rüden U, Schrezenmair J, Christophers E, Weichenthal M. Prospective, randomized controlled trial on Lactobacillus rhamnosus in infants with moderate to severe atopic dermatitis. Br J Dermatol. 2006a;155(6):1256–61.
Fölster-Holst R, Pape M, Buss YL, et al. Low prevalence of the intrinsic form of atopic dermatitis among adult patients. Allergy. 2006b;61:629–33.
Forman SB, Garrett AB. Success of omalizumab as monotherapy in adult atopic dermatitis: case report and discussion of the high-affinity immunoglobulin E receptor, FcepsilonRI. Cutis. 2007;80(1):38–40.
Frei R, Lauener RP, Cramer R, et al. Microbiota and dietary interactions: an update to the hygiene hypothesis? Allergy. 2012;67:451–61.
Freitag G, Hoppner T. Results of a postmarketing drug monitoring survey with a polidocanol-urea preparation for dry, itching skin. Curr Med Res Opin. 1997;13:529–37.
Friedländer MH. Ocular allergy. In: Middleton E, Reed CE, Ellis EF, editors. Allergy: principle and practice. 3rd ed. St Louis: Mosby; 1988.
Frosch PJ. Hautirritation und empfindliche Haut. Berlin: Rosse; 1985.
Frosch PJ, Schwanitz HJ, Macher E. A double blind trial of h1 and h2 receptor antagonists in the treatment of atopic dermatitis. Arch Dermatol Res. 1984;276(1):36–40.
Fuchs F, Hentschel G. Höhenklimatherapeutische Möglichkeiten und Erfahrungen bei Neurodermitits-Kranken auf dem Fichtelberg. Z Meteorol. 1959;13:116.
Fuhrmann T, Smith N, Tausk F. Use of complementary and alternative medicine among adults with skin disease: updated results from a national survey. J Am Acad Dermatol. 2010;63(6):1000–5.
Fujita H, Shemer A, Suarez-Farinas M, Johnson-Huang LM, Tintle S, Cardinale I, et al. Lesional dendritic cells in patients with chronic atopic dermatitis and psoriasis exhibit parallel ability to activate T-cell subsets. J Allergy Clin Immunol. 2011;128:574–82.
Furue M, Terao H, Rikihisa W, Urabe K, Kinukawa N, Nose Y, Koga T. Clinical dose and adverse effects of topical steroids in daily management of atopic dermatitis. Br J Dermatol. 2003;148(1):128–33.
Furue M, Kitahara Y, Akama H, Hojo S, Hayashi N, Nakagawa H. JAPANESE E6005 Study Investigators Safety and efficacy of topical E6005, a phosphodiesterase 4 inhibitor, in Japanese adult patients with atopic dermatitis: results of a randomized, vehicle-controlled, multicenter clinical trial. J Dermatol. 2014;41:577–85.
Galli S, editor. Anaphylaxis. Novartis Foundation symposium 157. Chichester: Wiley; 2004.
Galli SJ, Kalesnikoff J, Grimbaldeston MA, Piliponsky AM, Williams CM, Tsai M. Mast cells as "tunable" effector and immunoregulatory cells: recent advances. Annu Rev Immunol. 2005;23:749–86.
Gamble RG, Dellavalle RT. Ion-exchange water softener use and eczema. Arch Dermatol. 2011;147: 1208–10.
Garg N, Silverberg JI. Association between childhood allergic disease, psychological comorbidity, and injury requiring medical attention. Ann Allergy Asthma Immunol. 2014;112:525–32.
Garritsen FM, Brouwer MW, Limpens J, Spuls PL. Photo(chemo)therapy in the management of atopic dermatitis: an updated systemic review with implications for practice and research. Br J Dermatol. 2014;170:501–13.
Garritsen FM, ter Haar NM, Spuls PL. House dust mite reduction in the management of atopic dermatitis. A critically appraised topic. Br J Dermatol. 2013;168:688–91.
Gassner-Bachmann M, Wüthrich B. Bauernkinder leiden selten an Heuschnupfen und Asthma. Dtsch Med Wochenschr. 2000;125:924–31.
Gauger A, Mempel M, Schekatz A, Schäfer T, Ring J, Abeck D. Silver-coated textiles reduce Staphylococcus aureus colonization in patients with atopic eczema. Dermatology. 2003;207:15–21.
Gauger A, Fischer S, Mempel M, Schaefer T, Foelster-Holst R, Abeck D, Ring J. Efficacy and func-tionality of silver-coated textiles in patients with atopic eczema. J Eur Acad Dermatol Venereol. 2006;20(5):534–41. Erratum J Eur Acad Dermatol Venereol. 2006;20(6):771.
Gdalevich M, Mimouni D, David M, Mimouni M. Breast-feeding and the onset of atopic dermatitis in childhood: a systematic review and meta-analysis of prospective studies. J Am Acad Dermatol. 2001;45:520–7.
Gebert N, Hümmelink R, Könning J, et al. Efficacy of a self-management program for childhood asthma – a prospective controlled study. Patient Educ Couns. 1998;35:213–20.
Gehring W. Gezielter Einsatz von Vehikeln und Basistherapie. In: Korting HC, Sterry W, editors. Thera-peutische Verfahren in der Dermatologie. Dermatika und Kosmetika. Berlin/Wien: Blackwell Wissen-schafts-Verlag; 2001. p. 93–100.
Gehring W, Gloor M. Behandlung der Neurodermitis atopica mit einer W/O Emulsion mit und ohne Hydrocortison – Ergebnisse einer klinisch und messmethodisch kontollierten randmosierten Doppelblindstudie. Z Hautkr. 1996;71:554–60.
Gehring W, Wenz J, Gloor M. Influence of topically applied ceramide/phospholipid mixture on the barrier function of intact skin, atopic skin and experi-

mentally induced barrier damage. Int J Cosmet Sci. 1997;19:143–56.
Gelfand HH, Cinder JC, Grant SF, Soiffer M. Evaluation of histamine-gamma globulin (histaglobin) in the treatment of various allergic conditions. Ann Allergy. 1963;21:150–5.
Gelmetti C. Skin cleansing in children. J Eur Acad Dermatol Venereol. 2001;15 Suppl 1:12–5.
Gelmetti C, Wollenberg A. Atopic dermatitis – all you can do from the outside. Br J Dermatol. 2014;170: 19–24.
George AO. Atopic eczema in Nigeria. Int J Dermatol. 1989;28:237–9.
Gfesser M, Abeck D, Rügemer J, Schreiner V, Stäb F, Disch R, Ring J. The early phase of epidermal barrier regeneration is faster in patients with atopic eczema. Dermatology. 1997;195:332–6.
Giannetti A, Fantini F, Cimitan A, Pincelli C. Vasoactive intestinal polypeptide and substance P in the pathogenesis of atopic dermatitis. Acta Derm Venereol. 1992;176:90–2.
Gibbs NK, Norval M. Photoimmunosuppression: a brief overview. Photodermatol Photoimmunol Photomed. 2013;29:57–64.
Gieler U. Die Sprache der Haut. 3rd ed. Düsseldorf: Walter; 2006.
Gieler U, Ehlers A, Höhler T, Burkhard G. Die psychosoziale Situation der Patientenmit endo-genem Ekzem. Hautarzt. 1990;41:416–23.
Gieler U, Bräuer J, Freiling G. Neurodermitis-Schulung. Ein neuer, psychosomatisch orientierter Be-handlungsansatz. In: Jahrbuch der medizinischen Psychologie (Bd.9). "Hauterkrankungen aus psychologischer Sicht". Göttingen: Hogrefe Verlag; 1992.
Gieler U, Hohmann M, Niemeier V, Kupfer J, Stangler U, Ehlers A. Cost evaluation in atopic eczema. J Dermatol Treat. 1999;10 Suppl 1:15–20.
Gieler U, Ring J, Wahn U. Neurodermitisschulung. Dt Ärztebl. 2001;98:3202–9.
Girolomoni G, Sebastiani S, Albanesi C, Cavani A. T-cell subpopulations in the development of atopic and contact allergy. Curr Opin Immunol. 2001;13:733–7.
Gläser R, Meyer-Hoffert U, Harder J, Cordes J, Wittersheim M, Kobliakova J, Fölster-Holst R, Proksch E, Schröder JM, Schwarz T. The Antimicrobial Protein Psoriasin (S100A7) is Upregulated in Atopic Dermatitis and after Experimental Skin Barrier Disruption. J Invest Dermatol. 2009a;129:641–9.
Gläser R, Navid F, Schuller W, Jantschitsch C, Harder J, Schröder J, Schwarz A, Schwarz T. UV-B radiation induces the expression of antimicrobial peptides in human keratinocytes in vitro and in vivo. J Allergy Clin Immunol. 2009b;123:1117–23.
Gleich GJ. The late phase of the immunoglobulin E-mediated reaction: a link between anaphylaxis and common allergic disease? J Allergy Clin. 1982;70:160–9.
Gloor M. Sebaceous gland activity in atopic eczema. In: Ruzicka T, Ring J, Przybilla B, editors. Handbook of atopic eczema. Berlin/Heidelberg/New York: Springer; 1991. p. 287–95.
Gloor M, Gehring W. Effects of emulsions on the stratum corneum barrier and hydration (in German). Hautarzt. 2003;54:324–30.
Gloor M, Schermer W, Gehring G. Ist eine Kombinationsbehandlung von Harnstoff und Glyzerin in Externagrundlagen sinnvoll? Z Hautkr. 1997;72:509–14.
Goldblum RW, Piper WN. Artificial lichenification produced by a scratching machine. J Invest Dermatol. 1954;22:405.
Gondo A, Saeki N, Tokuda Y. Challenge reactions in atopic dermatitis after percutaneous entry of mite antigen. Br J Dermatol. 1986;115:485–93.
Granstein RB, Askari M. Cutaneous cells in activation of immunology actions: further characterization. J Invest Dermatol. 1986;97:141–9.
Grewe M. Hyposensibilisierung bei atopischem Ekzem. Allergo J. 2000;9:351–357.
Grewe M, Vogelsang K, Ruzicka T, Stege H, Krutmann J. Neurotrophin-4 production by human epidermal keratinocytes: increased expression in atopic dermatitis. J Invest Dermatol. 2000;114:1108–12.
Grootendorst DC, Dahlen SE, Bos J, et al. Benefits of high altitude allergen avoidance in atopic adolescents with moderate to severe asthma. Clin Exp Allergy. 2001;89:836–43.
Grüber C, Illi S, Lau S, Nickel R, Forster J, Kamin W, Bauer CP, Wahn V, Wahn U, MAS-90 Study Group. Transient suppression of atopy in early childhood is associated with high vaccination coverage. Pediatrics. 2003;111:282–8.
Grüber C. Probiotics and prebiotics in allergy prevention and treatment: future prospects. Expert Rev Clin Immunol. 2012;8(1):17–9. doi:10.1586/eci.11.74.
Grundmann-Kollmann M, Korting HC, Behrens S, et al. Successful treatment of severe refractory atopic dermatitis with myccophenolate mofetil. Br J Dermatol. 1999;141:175–6.
Grundmann-Kollmann M, Kaufmann R, Zollner TM. Treatment of atopic dermatitis with mycophenolate mofetil. Br J Dermatol. 2001;145:351–2.
Guillett G, Guillett MH. Natural history of sensitizations in atopic dermatitis. A 3-year. Arch Dermatol. 1992;128:187–92.
Gupta AK, Chow M. Pimercolismus: a review. J Eur Acad Dermatol Venereol. 2003;17:493–503.
Guttman-Yassky E, Suarez-Farinas M, Chiricozzi A, et al. Broad defect in epidermal cornification in atopic dermatitis identified through genomic analysis. J Allergy Clin Immunol. 2009;124:1235–44.
Gutzmer R, Langer K, Lisewski M, Mommert S, Rieckborn D, Kapp A, Werfel T. Expression of a function of histamine receptors 1 and 2 on human monocyte-derived dendritic cells. J Allergy Clin Immunol. 2002;109:524.
Gutzmer R, Mommert S, Gschwandtner M, Zwingmann K, Stark H, Werfel T. The histamine H4 recep-tor is functionally expressed on T(H)2 cells. J Allergy Clin Immunol. 2009;123:619–25.
Haapakoski R, Karisola P, Fyhrquist N, et al. Toll-like receptor activation during cutaneous allergen

sensitization blocks development of asthma through IFN-gamma-dependent mechanisms. J Invest Dermatol. 2013;133:964–72.
Hachem JP, Crumrine D, Fluhr J, Brown BE, Feingold KR, Elias PM. pH directly regulates epidermal permeability barrier homeostasis, and stratum corneum integrity/cohesion. J Invest Dermatol. 2003;121:345–53.
Haeck IM, Knol MJ, ten Berge O, van Velsen SGA, de Bruin-Weller MS, Bruijnzeel-Koomen CAFM. Enteric-coated mycophenolate sodium versus cyclosporin A as long-term treatment in adult patients with severe atopic dermatitis: a randomized controlled trial. J Am Acad Dermatol. 2011a;64:1074–84.
Haeck IM, Rouwen TJ, Timmer-de Mik L, de Bruin-Weller MS, Bruijnzeel-Koomen CA. Topical corticosteroids in atopic dermatitis and the risk of glaucoma and cataracts. J Am Acad Dermatol. 2011b;64:275–81.
Hafenreffer S. Nosodochium, in quo cutis, eique adaerentium partium, affectus omnes, singulari methodo, et cognoscendi e curandi fidelisime traduntur. Ulm: Kuhnen; 1660. p. 98–102.
Hahnemann S. Die chronischen Krankheiten, ihre eigentümliche Natur und homöopathische Heilung. Leipzig: Hauk; 1835.
Halhuber J. Der Kreislaufgesunde und –kranke im Hochgebirgsklima. Münch Med Wschr. 1959;26:1118–23.
Halken S, Hansen KS, Jacobson HP, et al. Comparison of a partially hydrolyzed infant formula with two extensively hydrolyzed formulas for allergy prevention: a prospective, randomized study. Pediatr Allergy Immunol. 2000;11:149–61.
Hamid Q, Boguniewicz M, Leung DY. Differential in situ cytokine gene expression in acute versus chronic atopic dermatitis. J Clin Invest. 1994;94:870–6.
Hamilton JD, Suarez-Farinas M, Dhingra N, Cardinale I, Li X, Kostic A, et al. Dupilumab improves the molecular signature in skin of patients with moderate-to-severe atopic dermatitis. J Allergy Clin Immunol. 2014;134:1293–300.
Han TY, Kong TS, Kim MH, Chae JD, Lee JH, Son SJ. Vitamin D status and its association with the SCORAD score and serum LL-37 level in Korean adults and children with atopic dermatitis. Ann Dermatol. 2015;27:10–14.
Hanifin JM, Lobitz Jr WC. Newer concepts of atopic dermatitis. Arch Dermatol. 1977;113:663–70.
Hanifin IM, Rajka G. Diagnostic features of atopic dermatitis. Acta Derm Venereol. 1980;92(Suppl):44–7.
Hanifin JM, Schneider LC, Leung DY, Ellis CN, Jaffe HS, Izu AE, Bucalo LR, Hirabayashi SE, Tofte SJ, Cantu-Gonzales G, et al. Recombinant interferon gamma therapy for atopic dermatitis. J Am Acad Dermatol. 1993;28:189–97.
Hanifin J, Gupta AK, Rajagopalan R. Intermittent dosing of fluticasone propionate cream for reducing the risk of relapse in atopic dermatitis patients. Br J Dermatol. 2002;147:528–37.
Hannuksela M, Karvonen J, Husa M, Jokela R, Katajamäki L, Leppisaari M. Ultraviolet light therapy in atopic dermatitis. Acta Derm Venereol. 1985;114:137–9.
Hannuksela M, Kalimo K, Lammintausta K, et al. Dose ranging study: cetirizine in the treatment of atopic dermatitis in adults. Ann Allergy. 1993;70:127–33.
Hannuksela-Svahn A, Pukkala E, Läärä E, Poikolainen K, Karvonen J. Psoriasis, its treatment, and cancer in a cohort of Finnish patients. J Invest Dermatol. 2000;114(3):587–90.
Hansen ER, Buus S, Deleuran M, Andersen KE. Treatment of atopic dermatitis with mycophenolate mofetil. Br J Dermatol. 2000;143(6):1324–6.
Happle R. The essence of alternative medicine. A dermatologist's view from Germany. Arch Dermatol. 1998;134:1455–60.
Hara J, Higuchi K, Okamoto R, Kawashima M, Imokawa G. High-expression of sphingomyelin deacylase is an important determinant of ceramide deficiency leading to barrier disruption in atopic dermatitis. J Invest Dermatol. 2000;115:406–13.
Harari M, Shani J, Seidl V, Hristakieva E. Climatotherapy of atopic dermatitis at the Dead Sea: demo-graphic evaluation and cost-effectiveness. Int J Dermatol. 2000;39(1):59–69.
Harder J, Schröder J, Gläser G. The skin surface as antimicrobial barrier: present concepts and future outlooks. Exp Dermatol. 2013;22:1–5.
Harding NJ, Birch JM, Hepworth SJ, McKinney PA. Atopic dysfunction and risk of central nervous system tumors in children. Eur J Cancer. 2008;44:92–9.
Hardyman MA, Wilkinson E, Martin E, Jayasekera NP, Blume C, Swindle EJ, Gozzard N, Holgate ST, Howarth PA, Davies DE, Collins JE. TNF-α-mediated bronchial barrier disruption and regulation by src family kinase activation. J Allergy Clin Immunol. 2013;132:665–75.
Harper JI, Ahmed I, Barclay G, et al. Cyclosporin for severe childhood atopic dermatitis: short course versus continuous therapy. Br J Dermatol. 2000;142:52–8.
Harper J, Oranje A, Prose N, editors. Textbook of pediatric dermatology. Oxford: Blackwell; 2002.
Hata TR, Audish D, Kotol P, Coda A, Kabigting F, Miller J, et al. A randomized controlled double-blind investigation of the effects of vitamin D dietary supplementation in subjects with atopic dermatitis. J Eur Acad Dermatol Venereol. 2014;28:781–9.
Hattevig G, Sigurs N, Kjellman B. Effects of maternal dietary avoidance during lactation on allergy in children in 10 years of age. Acta Pediatr. 1999;88:7–12.
Hatz HJ. Glucocorticoide. Immunologische Grundlagen, Pharmakologie und Therapierichtlinien. 1st ed. Stuttgart: Wissenschaftliche Verlagsgesellschaft mbH; 1998.
Hausen BM, Vieluf IK. Allergiepflanzen – Pflanzenallergene. Ecomed: Landsberg; 1997.
Hauser C, Saurat JH. Bedeutung der Besiedelung der Haut mit Staphylococcus aureus. Hautarzt. 1985;36:605–7.
Hauss H, Proppe A, Matthies C. Vergleichende Untersuchungen zu Behandlung von trockener, juckender Haut mit einer Zubreitung aus Harnstoff und Polidocanol sowie mit einer Linolsäure-haltigen

Fettcreme. Ergebnisse aus der Praxis. Dermatosen Beruf Umwelt. 1993;41(5):184–8.
Haxthausen H. Interpretation and value of skin tests in atopic dermatitis. Acta Derm Venereol (Stockh). 1957;3:6.
Hayashida S, Furusho N, Uchi H, Miyazaki S, Eiraku K, Gondo C, Tsuji G, Hachisuka J, Fukagawa S, Kido M, Nakahara T, Moroi Y, Hayashi J, Hagihara A, Furue M. Are lifetime prevalence of impetigo, molluscum and herpes infection really increased in children having atopic dermatitis? J Dermatol Sci. 2010;60:173–8.
Heil PM, Maurer D, Klein B, Hultsch T, Stingl G. Omalizumab therapy in atopic dermatitis: depletion of IgE does not improve the clinical course – a randomized, placebo-controlled and double blind pilot study. J Dtsch Dermatol Ges. 2010;8(12):990–8. doi:10.1111/j.1610-0387.2010.07497.x. [Article in English, German].
Hemels HGWM. The effect of propanolol on acetylcholine-induced sweat gland response in atopic and non-atopic subjects. Br J Dermatol. 1970;83:312.
Henseler T, Christophers E. Disease concomitance in psoriasis. J Am Acad Dermatol. 1995;32:982–6.
Heratizadeh A, Breuer K, Kapp A, Werfel T. Symptomatische Therapie der atopischen Dermatitis. Hautarzt. 2003;54(10):937–45.
Herbert O. Traditionalle Lebensweise als Schutz vor Allergien? Atopie und atopische Erkrankungen in fünf Dörfern auf Karkar Island Papue Neuguinea. Berlin: VWB; 2009.
Herbert OC, Barnetson R, Weninger W, Krämer U, Behrendt H, Ring J. Western lifestyle and increased prevalence of atopic diseases: an example from a small Papua New Guinean island. WAO J. 2009;2:130–7.
Herz U, Lacy P, Renz H, Erb K. The influence of infections on the development and severity of allergic disorders. Curr Opin Immunol. 2000;12:632–40.
Herzberg J. Wenig bekannte Formen der Neurodermitis. Hautarzt. 1973;24:47–51.
Hide DW, Matthews S, Matthews L, et al. Effect of allergen avoidance in infancy on allergic manifestations at age two years. J Allergy Clin Immunol. 1994;93:842–6.
Hilliquin P, Allanore Y, Coste J, Renoux M, Kahan A, Menkès CJ. Reduced incidence and prevalence of atopy in rheumatoid arthritis. Results of a case-control study. Rheumatology (Oxford). 2000;39(9):1020–6.
Hindley D, Galloway G, Murray J, Gardener L. A randomised study of "wet wraps" versus conventional treatment for atopic eczema. Arch Dis Child. 2006;91(2):164–8.
Hirota T, Takahashi A, Kubo M, Tsunoda T, Tomita K, Sakashita M, Yamada T, Fujieda S, Tanaka S, Doi S, Miyatake A, Enomoto T, Nishiyama C, Nakano N, Maeda K, Okumura K, Ogawa H, Ikeda S, Noguchi E, Sakamoto T, Hizawa N, Ebe K, Saeki H, Sasaki T, Ebihara T, Amagai M, Takeuchi S, Furue M, Nakamura Y, Tamari M. Genome-wide association study identifies eight new susceptibility loci for atopic dermatitis in the Japanese population. Nat Genet. 2012;44(11):1222–6. doi:10.1038/ng.2438. Epub Oct 2012.
Hjorth N, Clemmenson OJ. Treatment of dermatitis of the head and neck with ketoconazole in patients with type I hypersensitivity for Pityrosporum orbiculare. Semin Dermatol. 1983;2:26–9.
Hjorth N, Schmidt H, Thomsen K. Fusidic acid plus betamethasone in infected or potentially infected eczema. Pharmatherapeutica. 1985;4(2):126–31.
Ho RCM, Giam YC, Enge TP, Mack A, Goa D, Chang NWB, Cheak H, van Bever HP. The influence of childhood atopic dermatitis on health of mothers, and its impact on Asian families. Pediatr Allergy Immunol. 2010;21:501–7.
Hoare C, Li Wan Po A, Williams H. Systematic review of treatments for atopic eczema. Health Technol Assess. 2000;4:1–191.
Hoeger PH, Harper JL. Neonatal erythroderma: differential diagnosis and management of the "red baby". Arch Dis Child. 1998;79:186–91.
Holgate S, Casale T, Wenzel S, Bousquet J, Deniz Y, Reisner C. The anti-inflammatory effects of omalizumab confirm the central role of IgE in allergic inflammation. J Allergy Clin Immunol. 2005;115:459–65.
Hölscher K. Psychosomatische Aspekte in "Neurodermitis". Ring J, editor. Ecomed, Landsberg. 1998;29–44.
Holt PG, Clough JB, Holt BJ, Baron-Hay MJ, Rose AH, Robinson BW, Thomas WR. Genetic 'risk' for atopy is associated with delayed postnatal maturation of T-cell competence. Clin Exp Allergy. 1992;22:1093–9.
Hölzle E, Plewig G. Effects of dermatitis, stripping, and steroids on the morphology of corneocytes. A new bioassay. J Invest Dermatol. 1977;68:350–6.
Homey B, Zlotnik A. Chemokines in allergy. Curr Opin Immunol. 1999;11:626–34.
Homey B, Steinhoff M, Ruzicka T, Leung DY. Cytokines and chemokines orchestrate atopic skin inflammation. J Allergy Clin Immunol. 2006;118:178–89.
Hönigsmann H. Phototherapy. J Invest Dermatol. 2013;133(E1):E18–20. doi:10.1038/skinbio.2013.180.
Hotze M, Baurecht H, Rodríguez E, Chapman-Rothe N, Ollert M, Fölster-Holst R, Adamski J, Illig T, Ring J, Weidinger S. Increased efficacy of omalizumab in atopic dermatitis patients with wild-type filaggrin status and higher serum levels of phosphatidylcholines. Allergy. 2014;69:132–5.
Høst A, Andrae S, Charkin S, Diaz-Vazquez C, Dreborg S, Eigenmann PA, et al. Allergy testing in children: why, who, when and how? Allergy. 2003;58:559–69.
Høst A, Halken S, Muraro A, et al. Dietary prevention of allergic diseases in infants and small children. Pediatr Allergy Immunol. 2008;19:1–4.
Howell MD, Kim BE, Gao P, Grant AV, Boguniewicz M, De Benedetto A, et al. Cytokine modulation of atopic dermatitis filaggrin skin expression. J Allergy Clin Immunol. 2007;120:150–5.

Hradetzky S, Werfel T, Rösner LM. Autoallergy in atopic dermatitis. Allergo J Int. 2015;24:16–22.

Huang JT, Abrams M, Tlougan B, Rademaker A, Paller AS. Treatment of Staphylococcus aureus colonization in atopic dermatitis decreases disease severity. Pediatrics. 2009;123:808–14.

Hubiche T, Ged C, Benard A, Léauté-Labrèze C, McElreavey K, de Verneuil H, Taïeb A, Boralevi S. Analysis of SPINK 5, KLK 7 and FLG genotypes in a French atopic dermatitis cohort. Acta Derm Venereol. 2007;87:499–505.

Humpeler E, Skrabal F, Bartsch G. Influence of exposure to moderate altitude on the plasma concentration of cortisol, aldosterone, renin, testosterone, and gonadotropins. Eur J Appl Physiol. 1980;45:167–76.

Hünecke P. Entstellungsgefühle und strukturiertes Video-Feedback – Orientierende Befunde und Überlegungen für einen neuen psychotherapeutischen Ansatz. In: Gieler U, Stangier U, Brähler E, editors. Hauterkrankungen in psychologischer Sicht. Jahrbuch der medizinischen Psychologie (Bd. 9). Göttingen: Hofgrefe; 1993.

Hundley JL, Yosipovitch G. Mirtazapine for reducing nocturnal itch in patients with chronic pruritus. JAAD. 2004;50:889–91.

Hurrelmann K, Hoepner-Stamos F, Palentien C, Setterbulte W, Klaubert K. Gesundheitsförderung in Grundschulen – Analyse der Ausgangsbedingungen und Implementation von Maßnahmen. Bielefeld: Universität Bielefeld, Nordrhein-Westfälischer Forschungsverbund Public Health; 1998.

Hurrelmann K, Klocke A, Melzer W, Ravens-Sieberer U. Jugendgesundheitssurvey. Munich: Juventa; 2003.

Huss-Marp J, Eberlein-König B, Breuer K, Mair S, Ansel A, Darsow U, Krämer U, Mayer E, Gertis K, Ring J, Behrendt H. Influence of short term exposure to airborne Derp 1 and volatile organic compounds on skin barrier function and dermal blood flow in patients with atopic eczema and healthy individuals. Clin Exp Allergy. 2007;36:381–9.

Huss-Marp J, Darsow U, Brockow K, Pfab F, Weichenmeier I, Schober W, Petersson CJ, Borres MP, Ring J, Behrendt H. Can immunoglobulin E-measurement replace challenge tests in allergic rhinoconjunctivits to grass pollen? Clin Exp Allergy. 2011;41(8):1116–24.

Iamandescu IB. Psychoneuroallergology. 2nd ed. Bucarest: Amaltea; 2007.

Ibler K, Dam TN, Gniadecki R, Kragballe K, Jemec GB, Agner T. Efalizumab for severe refractory atopic eczema: retrospective study on 11 cases. J Eur Acad Dermatol Venereol. 2010;24:837–9.

Iikura Y, Naspitz CK, Mikawa H, Talaricoficho S, Baba M, Sole D, Nishima S. Prevention of asthma by ketotifen in infants with atopic dermatitis. Ann Allergy. 1992;68:233–6.

Illi S, Depner M, Genuneit J, Horak E, Loss G, Strunz-Lehner C, Büchele G, Boznanski A, Danielewicz H, Cullinan P, Heederik D, Braun-Fahrländer C, von Mutius E. The GABRIEL advanced studies. J Allergy Clin Immunol. 2012;129:1470–7.

Ikezawa Y, Nakazawa M, Tamura C, et al. Cyclophosphamide decreases the number, percentage and function of CD25+ CD4+ regulatory T cells. J Dermatol Sci. 2005;39:105–12.

Imokawa G. A possible mechanism underlying the ceramide deficiency in atopic dermatitis: expression of a deacylase enzyme that cleaves the N-acyl linkage of sphingomyelin and glucosylceramide. J Dermatol Sci. 2009;55:1–9.

Imokawa G, Abe A, Jin K, Higaki Y, Kawashima M, Hidano A. Decreased level of ceramides in stratum corneum of atopic dermatitis: an etiologic factor in atopic dry skin? J Invest Dermatol. 1991;96:523–7.

IPCC (Intergovernmental Panel on Climate Change). Chapter 8. Human health; 2007.

ISAAC. Worldwide variations in the prevalence of asthma symptoms: the international study of asthma and allergies in childhood (ISAAC) Steering Committee. Lancet. 1998;351:1225–32.

Ishizaka K, Ishizaka T. Identification of γE antibodies as carrier of reaginic activity. J Immunol. 1967;99:1187–98.

Isolauri E, Arvola T, Sütas Y, Moilanen E, Salminen S. Probiotics in the management of atopic eczema. Clin Exp Allergy. 2000;30:1604–10.

Jablonski NG. The evolution of human skin and skin color. Ann Rev Anthropol. 2004;33:585–623.

Jacobi A, Antoni C, Manger B, Schuler G, Hertl M. Infliximab in the treatment of moderate to severe atopic dermatitis. J Am Acad Dermatol. 2005;52:522–6.

Jacobsen E. Progressive relaxation. Chicago: University Press; 1938.

Jacquet L. La pratique dermatologique. In: Besnier E, Brocq L, Jacquet L, editors. La pratique dermatologique. 1904;5:341.

Jäger L, Wüthrich B. Nahrungsmittelallergien und -intoleranzen. Dustri, München 2001.

Jaeger T, Rothmaier M, Zander H, Ring J, Gutermuth J, Anliker MD. Acid-coated textiles (pH 5.5–6.5) – a new therapeutic strategy for stopic eczema? Acta Derm Venereol. 2015;95(6):659–63. doi:10.2340/00015555-1916.

Jakob T, Hermann K, Ring J. Eosinophil cationic protein in atopic eczema. Arch Dermatol Res. 1991;283:5–6.

Jakob T, Ring J, Udey MC. Multistep navigation of Langerhans/dendritic cells in and out of the skin. J Allergy Clin Immunol. 2001;108:688–96.

James JM, Burks AW, Roberson PK, Sampson HA. Safe administration of the measles vaccine to children allergic to eggs. N Engl J Med. 1995;332:1262–6.

Janeway CA, Medzhitov R. Innate immune recognition. Annu Rev Immunol. 2002;20:197–216.

Janmohamed SR, Oranje AP, Devillers AC, Rizopoulos D, van Praag MC, Van Gysel D, et al. The proactive wet-wrap method with diluted corticosteroids versus emollients in children with atopic dermatitis: a prospective, randomized, double-blind, placebo-controlled trial. J Am Acad Dermatol. 2014;70:1076–82.

Jekeler J, Larkö O. Phototherapy for atopic dermatitis with ultraviolet A (UVA), low dose UVB and combined UVA and UVB: two paired comparison studies. Photodermatol Photoimmunol Photomed. 1991;8:151–6.

Johansson SGO. Raised levels of a new immunoglobulin (IgND) in asthma. Lancet. 1967;2:951–5.

Johansson SGO, Hourihane JO, Bousquet J, Bruijnzeel-Koomen C, Dreborg S, Haahtela T, Kowalski ML, Mygind N, Ring J, van Cauwenberge P, van Hage-Hamsten M, Wuthrich B, EAACI (the European Academy of Allergology and Clinical Immunology) Nomenclature Task Force. A revised nomenclature for allergy. An EAACI position statement from the EAACI nomenclature task force. Allergy. 2001;56: 813–24.

Johansson C, Sandstrom MH, Bartosik J, Sarnhult T, Christiansen J, Zargari A, Back O, Wahlgren CF, Faergemann J, Scheynius A, Tenvall LM. Atopy patch test reactions to Malassezia allergens differentiate subgroups of atopic dermatitis patients. Br J Dermatol. 2003;148:479–88.

Johansson SGO, Bieber T, Dahl R, Friedmann PS, Lanier BQ, Lockey RF, Motala C, Ortega Martell JA, Platts-Mills TAE, Ring J, Thien F, Cauwenberge PV, Williams HC. Revised nomenclature for allergy for global use. Allergy Clin Immunol Int J World Allergy Org. 2004;17:4–8, (Report of the Nomenclature Review Committee of the World Allergy Organization, October 2003).

Jones HE, Rinaldi MG, Chai H, Kahn G. Apparent cross-reactivity of airborne molds and the dermatophytic fungi. J Allergy Immunol. 1973a;52:346–57.

Jones HE, Rinhardt JH, Rinaldi MG. A clinical, mycological, and immunological survey for dermatophytosis. Arch Dermatol. 1973b;108:61–5.

Juhlin L, et al. Immunoglobulin E in dermatoses: levels in atopic dermatitis and urticaria. Arch Dermatol. 1969;92:17ff.

Just HL, Deleuran M, Vestergaard C, Deleuran B, Thestrup-Pedersen K. T-cell receptor excision circles (TREC) in CD4+ and CD8+ T-cell subpopulations in atopic dermatitis and psoriasis show major differences in the emission of recent thymic emigrants. Acta Derm Venereol. 2008;88:566–72.

Jutel M, Watanabe T, Klunker S, et al. Histamine regulates T cell and antibody responses by differential expression of H1 and H2 receptors. Nature. 2001;413:420–5.

Kabashima K. New concept of the pathogenesis of atopic dermatitis: interplay among the barrier, allergy, and pruritus as a trinity. J Dermatol Sci. 2013;70(1):3–11. doi:10.1016/j.jdermsci.2013.02.001. Epub 2013 Feb 15.

Kabesch M, Peters W, Carr D, et al. Association between polymorphisms in caspase recruitment domain containing protein 15 and allergy in two German populations. J Allergy Clin Immunol. 2003;111:813–7.

Kabesch M, Schedel M, Carr D, et al. IL-4/IL-13 pathway genetics strongly influence serum IgE levels and childhood asthma. J Allergy Clin Immunol. 2006;117:269–74.

Kalliomäki M, Salminen S, Arvilommi H, Kero P, Koskinen P, Isolauri E. Probiotics in primary prevention of atopic disease: a randomized placebo-controlled trial. Lancet. 2001;357:1076–9.

Kantor I, Milbauer J, Posner M, Weinstock IM, Simon A, Thormahlen S. Efficacy and safety of emollients as adjunctive agents in topical corticosteroid therapy for atopic dermatitis. Today Ther Trends. 1993;11:157–63.

Kaposi M. Erkrankungen der Haut. 2nd ed. Wien; 1891

Kapp A, Papp K, Bingham A, Fölster-Holst R, Ortonne JP, Potter PC, Gulliver W, Paul C, Molloy S, Barbier N, Thurston M, de Prost Y, for the Flare Reduction in Ekzema with Elidel (Infants) Multicenter Investigator Study Group. Long-term management of atopic dermatitis in infants with topical pimecrolimus, a nonsteroid anti-inflammatory drug. J Allergy Clin Immunol. 2002;110:277–84.

Katagiri K, Arakawa S, Hatano Y, Fujiwara S. Tolerogenic antigen-presenting cells successfully inhibit atopic dermatitis-like skin lesion induced by repeated epicutaneous exposure to ovalbumin. Arch Dermatol Res. 2008;300:583–93.

Katsarou A, Armenaka MC. Atopic dermatitis in older patients: particular points. J Eur Acad Dermatol Venereol. 2011;25:12–8.

Kawashima M, Tango T, Noguchi T, Inagi M, Nakagawa H, Harada S. Addition of fexofenadine to a topical corticosteroid reduces the pruritus associated with atopic dermatitis in a 1-week randomized, multicentre, double-blind, placebo-controlled, parallel-group study. Br J Dermatol. 2003;148:1212–21.

Kemeny L, Szabo K. Toll-like receptors link atopic march to the hygiene hypothesis. J Invest Dermatol. 2013;133:874–8.

Kemp AS. Atopic eczema: its social and financial costs. J Paediatr Child Health. 1999;35:229–31.

Kerschenlohr K, Decard S, Darsow U, Ollert M, Wollenberg A. Clinical and immunologic reactivity to aeroallergens in "intrinsic" atopic dermatitis patients. J Allergy Clin Immunol. 2003a;111:195–7.

Kerschenlohr K, Decard S, Przybilla B, Wollenberg A. Atopy patch test reactions show a rapid influx of inflammatory dandritic and patients with intrinsic atopic dermatitis. J Allergy Clin Immunol. 2003b;111:869.

Kilpelainen M, Koskenvuo M, Helenius H, Terho EO. Stressful life events promote the manifestation of asthma and atopic disease. Clin Exp Allergy. 2002;32:256–63.

Kim E, Lee JE, Namkung JH, Kim PS, Kim S, Shin ES, Cho EY, Yang JM. Single nucleotide polymorphisms and the haplotype in the DEFB1 gene are associated with atopic dermatitis in a Korean population. J Dermatol Sci. 2009;54:25–30.

Kim KW, Myers RA, Lee JH, Igartua C, Lee KE, Kim YH, Kim EJ, Yoon D, Lee JS, Hirota T, Tamari M, Takahashi A, Kubo M, Choi JM, Kim KE, Nicolae DL, Ober C, Sohn MH. Genome-wide association study of recalcitrant atopic dermatitis in Korean children. J Allergy Clin Immunol. 2015;136(3):678–684. e4. doi:10.1016/j.jaci.2015.03.030. Epub 2015 Apr 30.

Kimura T, Miyazawa H. The 'butterfly' sign in patients with atopic dermatitis: evidence for the role of scratching in the development of skin manifestations. J Acad Dermatol. 1989;21:579–80.

Kini SP, De Long LK, Veledar E, McKenzie-Brown AM, Schaufele M, Chen SC. The impact of pruritus on quality of life: the skin equivalent of pain. Arch Dermatol. 2011;147:312–9.

Kissling S, Wüthrich B. Verlauf der atopischen Dermatitis nach dem Kleinkindesalter. Hautarzt. 1993;44:569–73.

Kitamura K, Takahashi Y, Sasagawa S. (in Japanese). Jpn J Dermatol. 1950;60:59.

Kjellmann NIM. Atopic disease in seven-year-old children. Incidence in relation to family history. Acta Pediatr Scand. 1977;66:465–71.

Kleijnen J, Kniepschild P, ter Riet G. Clinical trials in homoepathy. Br Med J. 1991;302:316–23.

Klein PA, Clark RA. An evidence-based review of the efficacy of antihistamines in relieving pruritus in atopic dermatitis. Arch Dermatol. 1999;135:1522–5.

Kleine-Tebbe J, Lepp U, Niggemann B, et al. In-vitro-Diagnostik von Nahrungsmittelallergien. Leitlinie von DGAKI, ÄDA, GPA, SGAI, ÖGAI. Allergo J. 2009;18:132–46, (AWMF-Leitlinienregister Nr. 061/008, www.awmf-online.de).

Kneipp S. Meine Wasser-Kur. 50th ed. Kempten: Kösel'sche Buchhandlung; 1984.

Knobler RM. Photophoresis – extracorporal irradiation of 8-MOP containing blood – a new therapeutic modality. Blood. 1987;54:247–50.

Kobayashi H, Mizuno N, Teramae H, Kutsuna H, Ueoku S, Onoyama J, Yamanaka K, Fujita N, Ishii M. The effects of Hochu-ekki-to in patients with atopic dermatitis resistant to conventional treatment. Int J Tissue React. 2004;26:113–7.

Koblenzer CS. Itching and the atopic skin. J Allergy Clin Immunol. 1999;104:109–13.

Kodama A, Horikawa T, Suzuki T, Ajiki W, Takashima T, Harada S, Ichihasha M. Effects of stress on atopic dermatitis: investigations in patients after the great Hanshin earthquake. J Allergy Clin Immunol. 1999;104:173–6.

Kofler H, Ulmer H, Mechter E, Falk M, Fritsch PO. Bioresonanz bei Pollinose: Eine vergleichende Un-tersuchung zur diagnostischen und therapeutischen Wertigkeit. Allergologie. 1996;19:114–22.

Kondo H, Ichikawa Y, Imokawa G. Percutaneous sensitization with allergens through barrier-disrupted skin elicits a Th2-dominant cytokine response. Eur J Immunol. 1998;28:769–79.

Kong HH, Oh J, Deming C, Conlan S, Grice EA, Beatson MA, et al. Temporal shifts in the skin microbiome associated with disease flares and treatment in children with atopic dermatitis. Genome Res. 2012;22:850–9.

Korting GW. Zur Pathogenese des endogenen Ekzems. Stuttgart: Thieme; 1954.

Korting HC. Äußerliche Dermatotherapie. In: Braun-Falco O, Plewig G, Wolff HH, editors. Dermatologie und Venerologie. 4th ed. Berlin: Springer; 1995. p. 1488–529.

Kowalzick L, Kleinheinz A, Weichenthal M, Ring J. Low-dose versus medium-dose UVA1 treatment in severe atopic eczema. Acta Derm Venereol. 1995;75:43–5.

Kramer MS, Kakuma R. Maternal dietary antigen avoidance during pregnancy and/or lactation for preventing or treating atopic disease in the child. Cochrane Database Syst Rev 2003;(4):CD000133.

Krämer U, Link E, Behrendt H, Ring J. Trends und Risikofaktoren von Asthma und allergischen Er-krankungen bei Kindern und Jugendlichen in Deutschland. Miriam-Studie Augsburg. 1996; 2001(01 EE 9501/2):1–27.

Krämer U, Altmann L, Behrendt H, Dolgner R, Islam MS, Kaysers HG, Ring J, Stiller-Winkler R, Turfeld M, Weishoff-Houben M, Willer H, Winneke G. Comparison of the influence of socioeconomic factors on air pollution health effects in West and East Germany. In: Jantunen H, editor. Socioeconomic and cultural factors in air pollution epidemiology, Air pollution epidemiology report series, vol. 8. Bruxelles: EU; 1997. p. 41–9.

Krämer U, Behrendt H, Dolgner R, Ranft U, Ring J, Willer H, Schlipköter HW. Airway disease and allergies in East and West German children during the first 5 years after reunification: time trends and the impact of sulphur dioxide and total suspended particles. Int J Epidemiol. 1999a;28:865–73.

Krämer U, Heinrich J, Wjst M, Wichmann HE. Age of entry to day nursery and allergy in later child-hood. Lancet. 1999b;353:450–4.

Krämer U, Oppermann H, Ranft U, Schäfer T, Ring J, Behrendt H. Veränderungen in den Prävalenzen von allergischen Erkrankungen bei sechsjährigen Kindern aus Ost- und Westdeutschland seit 1991. Allergo J. 1999c;8:305–9.

Kramer MS, Chalmers B, Hodnett ED, et al. Promotion of breastfeeding intervention trial (PROBIT): a randomized trial in the Republic of Belarus. JAMA. 2001;285:413–20.

Krämer U, Link E, Oppermann H, et al. Die Schulanfängerstudie in West- und Ostdeutschland (SA-WO). Trends von Allergien und Sensibilisierungen 1991–2000. Gesundheitswesen. 2002;64:657–63.

Krämer U, Lemmen CH, Behrendt H, Link E, Schäfer T, Gostomzyk J, Scherer G, Ring J. The effect of environmental tobacco smoke on eczema and allergic sensitization in children. Br J Dermatol. 2004;150:111–8.

Krämer U, Weidinger S, Darsow U, Möhrenschlager M, Ring J, Behrendt H. Seasonality in symptom severity influenced by temperature or grass pollen: results of a panel study in children with eczema. J Invest Dermatol. 2005;124:514–23.

Krämer U, Schmitz R, Ring J, Behrendt H. What can reunification of East and West Germany tell us about the cause of the allergy epidemic? Clin Exp Allergy. 2015;45(1):94–107. doi:10.1111/cea.12458.

Kreft B, Wohlrab J, Fischer M, Uhlig H, Skolziger R, Marsch WC. Analyse des Serumzinkspiegels bei

Patienten mit atopischer Dermatitis, Psoriasis vulgaris und Hautgesunden. Hautarzt. 2000;51:931–4.

Krönauer C, Eberlein-König B, Ring J, Behrendt H. Influence of UVB, UVA and UVA1 irradiation on histamine release from human basophils and mast cells in vitro in the presence and absence of antioxidants. Photochem Photobiol. 2003;77(5):531–4.

Krueger JG, Ferris LK, Menter A, Wagner F, White A, Visvanathan S, Lalovic B, Aslanyan S, Wang EE, Hall D, Solinger A, Padula S, Scholl P. Anti-IL-23A mAb BI 655066 for treatment of moderate-to-severe psoriasis: safety, efficacy, pharmacokinetics, and biomarker results of a single-rising-dose, randomized, double-blind, placebo-controlled trial. J Allergy Clin Immunol. 2015;136(1):116–124.e7. doi:10.1016/j.jaci.2015.01.018. Epub 2015 Mar 11.

Krutmann J, Hönigsmann H. Handbuch der dermatologischen Phototherapie und Photodiagnostik. Berlin/Heidelberg: Springer; 1997.

Krutmann J, Czech W, Diepgen T, Niedner R, Kapp A, Schopf E. Highdose UVA-1 therapy in the treatment of patients with atopic dermatitis. J Am Acad Dermatol. 1992;26:225–30.

Krutmann J, Diepgen TL, Luger TA, Grabbe S, Meffert H, Sönnichsen N, Czech W, Kapp A, Stege H, Grewe M, Schöpf E. High-dose UVA 1 therapy for atopic dermatitis: results of a multicenter trial. J Am Acad Dermatol. 1998;38:589–93.

Krutmann J, Morita A, Chung JH. Sun exposure: What molecular photodermatology tells us about its good and bad sides. J Invest Dermatol. 2012;132:976–84.

Kuehr J. Asthma und Allergien bei Kindern. Studien in Süddeutschland. Allergologie. 1999;22:48–53.

Kukutsch NA. Darstellung und Diskussion alternativer/komplementärer diagnostischer und/oder therapeutischer Konzepte im Hinblick auf atopische Erkrankungen. Dissertation, Universität Hamburg, 1997

Kunz B, Ring J. Clinical features and diagnostic criteria of atopic dermatitis. In: Harper J, Oranje A, Prose N, editors. Textbook of pediatric dermatology. Oxford: Blackwell Science; 2000. p. 199–215.

Kunz B, Ring J, Überla K. Frequency of contact dermatitis and contact sensitization in preschool children. Arch Derm Res. 1990;281:544.

Kunz B, Oranje AP, Labreze L, Stalder JF, Ring J, Taïeb A. Clinical validation and guidelines for the SCORAD index: consensus report of the European Task Force on Atopic Dermatitis. Dermatology. 1997;195:10–9.

Kunz B, Lüdtke R, Leeber N, Ring J. Test-retest-reliability and validity of the kinesiology muscle test. Complement Ther Med. 2001;9:141–5.

Kwiek B, Novak N. Immunosupressants as treatment for atopic dermatitis. In: Pawankar R et al., editors. Allergy frontiers: therapy and prevention. Berlin/New York: Springer; 2010. p. 291–310.

La Rosa M, Ranno C, Musarra I, Guglielmo F, Corrias A, Bellanti JA. Double-blind study of cetirizine in atopic eczema in children. Ann Allergy. 1994;73(2):117–22.

Lack G, Fox D, Northstone K, Golding J, Avon Longitudinal Study of Parents and Children Study Team. Factors associated with development with peanut allergy in childhood. N Engl J Med. 2003;348:977–85.

Lacour M, Hauser C. The role of microorganisms in atopic dermatitis. Clin Rev Allergy. 1993;11:491–522.

Langan SM, Silcocks P, Williams HC. What causes flares of eczema in children? Br J Dermatol. 2009;161:640–6.

Langeland T, Fagertum HE, Larsen S. Therapeutic effect of loratadine on pruritus in patients with atopic dermatitis. A multi-crossover-designed study. Allergy. 1994;49(1):22–6.

Langer H, Hauswald B. Langzeitstudie über die Therapie der Rhinopathia pollinosa mittels Akupunktur bzw. Laserakupunktur Erfahrungsheilkunde. 1992;4:262–7.

Langerhans P Über die Nerven der menschlichen Haut. Arch Pathol Anatom. 1868;44:325-37

Langeveld-Wildschut EG, Riedl H, Thepen T, Bihari IC, Bruijnzeel PL, Bruijnzeel-Koomen CA. Modulation of the atopy patch test reaction by topical corticosteroids and tar. J Allergy Clin Immunol. 2000;106:737–43.

Lanzavecchia A, Sallusto F. The instructive role of dentritic cells on T cells responses: lineages, plastic and kinetics. Curr Opin Immunol. 2001;13:291.

Lara-Corrales I, Gomez G, De Los RC, Pope E. Vitamin D in patients dermatitis: a randomized, double-blinded, placebo-controlled study preliminary analysis. Pediatr Dermatol. 2013;30:638.

Larkö O, Swanbeck G. Is UVB treatment of psoriasis safe? A study of extensively UVB-treated psoriasis patients compared with a matched control group. Acta Derm Venereol. 1982;62(6):507–12.

Lau S, Falkenhorst G, Weber A, et al. High mite-allergen exposure increases the risk of sensitization in atopic children and young adults. J Allergy Clin Immunol. 1989;84:718–25.

Lauffer F, Ring J. Target oriented therapy – emerging specific drugs for atopic dermatitis. Emerging Drugs, 2016.

Lee YA, Wahn U, Kehrt R, et al. A major susceptibility locus for atopic dermatitis maps to chromosome 3q21. Nat Genet. 2000;26:470473.

Lee YL, Su HJ, Scheu HM, Yu HS, Guo YL. Traffic-related air pollution, climate, and prevalence of eczema in Taiwanese school children. J Invest Dermatol. 2008;128:2412–20.

Leonardi A, Bogacka E, Fauquert JL, Kowalski ML, Groblewska A, Jedrzejczak-Czechowicz M, Doan S, Marmouz F, Demoly P, Delgado L. Ocular allergy: recognizing and diagnosing hypersensitivity disorders of the ocular surface. Allergy. 2012;67:1327–37.

Leung DY. Role of Staphylococcus aureus in atopic dermatitis. In: Bieber T, Leung DYM, editors. Atopic dermatitis. New York: Marcel Dekker; 2002. p. 401–18.

Leung DY. Infection in atopic dermatitis. Curr Opin Pediatr. 2003;15:399–404.

Leung AK, Barber KA. Managing childhood atopic dermatitis. Adv Ther. 2003;20:129–37.

Leung DY, Bieber T. Atopic dermatitis. Lancet. 2003;361:151.

Leung DY, Hirsch RL, Schneider L, et al. Thymopentin therapy reduces the clinical severity of atopic dermatitis. J Allergy Clin Immunol. 1990;85:927–33.

Leung DY, Harbeck R, Bina P, Reiser RF, Yang E, Norris DA, Hanifin JM, Sampson HA. Presence of IgE antibodies to staphylococcal exotoxins on the skin of patients with atopic dermatitis. J Clin Invest. 1993;92:1374–80.

Leung DY, Sampson HA, Yunginger JW, Burks Jr AW, Schneider LC, Wortel CH, Davis FM, Hyun JD, Shanahan Jr WR. Effect of anti-IgE therapy in patients with peanut allergy. N Engl J Med. 2003;348:986.

Leutgeb C, Bandmann HJ, Breit R. Handlinienmuster, Ichthyosis vulgaris und Dermatitis atopica. Arch Dermatol Forsch. 1972;244:344–56.

Lever R, Hadley K, Downey D, Mackie R. Staphylococcal colonization in atopic dermatitis and the effect of topical mupirocin therapy. Br J Dermatol. 1988;119:189–98.

Lewis-Jones S. Quality of life and childhood atopic dermatitis: the misery of living with childhood eczema. Int J Clin Pract. 2006;60:1251–8.

Lewis-Jones MS, Finlay AY, Dykes PJ. The infants' dermatitis quality of life index. Br J Dermatol. 2001;144:104–10.

Leyden JJ, et al. Staphylococcus aureus in the lesions of atopic dermatitis. Br J Dermatol. 1975;90:525 ff.

Lichtenstein LM. The mechanism of basophil histamine release induced by antigen and by the calcium ionophore A 23187. J Immunol. 1975;114:1692–9.

Lim A, Luderschmidt S, Weidinger A, Schnopp C, Ring J, Hein R, Ollert M, Mempel M. The IgE repertoire in PB-MCs of atopic patients is characterized by individual rearrangements without variable region of the heavy immunoglobulin chain bias. J Allergy Clin Immunol. 2007;120:696–706.

Lipozencic J, Wolf R. Atopic dermatitis: an update and review of the literature. Dermatol Clin. 2007;25:605–12.

Lob-Corzilius T, Petermann F. Asthmaschulung – Wirksamkeit bei Kindern und Jugendlichen. Beltz: Weinheim; 1997.

Lobitz WC, Campbell CJ. Physiologic studies in atopic dermatitis (disseminated neurodermitits) I. The local cutaneous response to intradermally injected acetylcholine and epinephrine. Arch Dermatol Syphil. 1953;67:575.

Loden M, Anderson AC, Lindberg M. Improvement in skin barrier function in patients with atopic dermatitis after treatment with a moisturizing cream (Canoderm). Br J Dermatol. 1999a;140:264–7.

Loden M, Andersson AC, Lindberg M. The effect of two urea-containing creams on dry, eczematous skin in atopic patients. II Adverse effects. J Dermatolog Treat. 1999b;10(3):171–5.

Lonne-Rahm SB, Rickberg H, El-Nour H, Mårin P, Azmitia EC, Nordlind K. Neuroimmune mechanisms in patients with atopic dermatitis during chronic stress. J Eur Acad Dermatol Venereol. 2008;22:11–8.

Lord GM. Nephropathy caused by Chinese herbs in the UK. Lancet. 1999;354:481–2.

Lü ZR, Park TH, Lee ES, Kim KJ, Park D, Park YD, Yang JM. Dysregulated genes of extrinsic type of atopic dermatitis: 34 K microarray and interactomic analyses. J Dermatol Sci. 2009;53:146–50.

Lubbe J. Klinische Erfahrungen mit topischen Calcineurininhibitoren in der Praxis. Hautarzt. 2003;54(5):432–9.

Luger TA. Balancing efficacy and safety in the management of atopic dermatitis: the role of methylprednisolone aceponate. J Eur Acad Dermatol Venereol. 2010;25:251–8.

Luger TA, Van Leent EJ, Graeber M, Hedgecock S, Thurston M, Kandra A, Berth Jones J, Bjerke J, Christophers E, Knop J, Knulst AC, Morren M, Morris A, Reitamo S, Roed-Petersen J, Schöpf E, Thestrup-Pedersen K, Van der Valk PGM, Bos J. SDZ ASM981: an emerging new standard for the treatment of atopic dermatitis. Br J Dermatol. 2001;144:788–94.

Luger T, Loske K, Elsner P, et al. Topical skin therapy with glucocorticosteroids – therapeutic index. J Dtsch Dermatol Ges. 2004;7:629–34.

Luger TA, Bieber T, Meurer M, et al. Therapie des atopischen Ekzems mit Calcineurin-Inhibitoren. Leitlinie der Deutschen Dermatologischen Gesellschaft. J Dtsch Dermatol Ges. 2005;3:385–91.

Luger T, Boguniewicz M, Carr W, Cork M, Deleuran M, Eichenfield L, Eigenmann P, Fölster-Holst R, Gelmetti C, Gollnick H, Hamelmann E, Hebert AA, Muraro A, Oranje AP, Paller AS, Paul C, Puig L, Ring J, Siegfried E, Spergel JM, Stingl G, Taieb A, Torrelo A, Werfel T, Wahn U. Pimecrolimus in atopic dermatitis: consensus on safety and the need to allow use in infants. Pediatr Allergy Immunol. 2015;26:306–15.

Lyakhovitsky A, Barzilai A, Heyman R, Baum S, Amichai B, Solomon M, Shpiro D, Trau H. Low-dose methotrexate treatment for moderate-to-severe atopic dermatitis in adults. J Eur Acad Dermatol Venereol. 2010;24:43–9.

Mackie RM, Husain SL. Juvenile plantar dermatosis: a new entity? Clin Exp Dermatol. 1976;1:253–60.

Maeda K, Yamamoto K, Tanaka Y, Anan S, Yoshida H. House dust mite (HDM) antigen in naturally occurring lesions of atopic dermatitis (AD): the relationship between HDM antigen in the skin and HDM antigen-specific IgE antibody. J Dermatol Sci. 1992;3:73–7.

Mailhol C, Lauwers-Cances V, Rancé F, Paul C, Giordano-Labadie F. Prevalence and risk factors for allergic contact dermatitis to topical treatment in atopic dermatitis: a study in 641 children. Allergy. 2009;64:801–6.

Manenti L, Vaglio A. Gabapentin for uraemic pruritus. Nephrol Dial Transpl. 2005;20:1278–9.

Mao XQ, Shirakawa T, Yoshikawa T, Yoshikawa K, Kawai M, Sasaki S, Enomoto T, Hashimoto T, Furuyama J, Hopkin JM, Morimoto K. Association between genetic variants of mast-cell chymase and eczema. Lancet. 1996;348:581–3.

Marchionini A, Borelli S. Klimabehandlung der Neurodermitis disseminata. Dtsch Med Wschr. 1956;81:811–6.

Marchionini A, Hausknecht W. Säuremantel der Haut und Bakterienabwehr. Klein Wochenschr. 1938;17:633–66.

Marghescu S. Patch test reactions in atopic patients. Acta Derm Venereol. 1985;114:113–7.

Marsella R, Girolomoni G. Canine models of atopic dermatitis: a useful tool with untapped potential. J Invest Dermatol. 2009;129:2351–7.

Marsh DG, Meyers DA, Bias WB. The epidemiology and genetics of atopic allergy. N Engl J Med. 1981;305:1551–9.

Marsh DG, Neely JD, Breazeale DR, et al. Linkage analysis of IL4 and other chromosome 5q31.1 markers and total serum immunoglobulin E concentrations. Science. 1994;264:1152–6.
Marty P. La relation objectale allergique. Rev Franc Psychoanal. 1958;22:5–35.
Massoumi R. The central role of Bcl-3 in atopic dermatitis. J Invest Dermatol. 2009;129:2088–90.
Matzinger P. Memories are made of this? Nature. 1994;369:605–6.
Maurer D, Fiebiger E, Reininger B, Wolff-Winiski B, Jouvin MH, Kilgus O, Kinet JP, Stingl G. Expression of functional high affinity immunoglobulin E receptors (Fc epsilon RI) on monocytes of atopic individuals. J Exp Med. 1994;179:745.
Maurer M, Church M, Gonçalo M, Sussman G, Sánchez-Borges M. Management and treatment of chronic urticaria (CU). J Eur Acad Dermatol Venereol. 2015; (29 Suppl 3):16–32.
Maurer M, Rosén K, Hsin-Ju HJ, Saini S, Grattan C, Gimenéz-Arnau A, Agarwal S, Doyle R, Canvin J, Kaplan A, Casale T. Omalizumab for the treatment of chronic idiopathic or spontaneous urticaria. N Engl J Med. 2013;368:2340–3.
Mayaux MJ, Guihard-Moscato ML, Schwartz D, Benveniste J, Coquin Y, Crapanne JB, Poiterin B, Rodary M, Chevrel JP, Mollet M. Controlled clinical trial of homoeopathy in postoperative ileus. Lancet. 1988;8584:528–9.
Mayr A, Stickl H, Muller HK, Danner K, Singer H. [The smallpox vaccination strain MVA: marker, ge-netic structure, experience gained with the parenteral vaccination and behavior in organisms with a debilitated defence mechanism (author's transl)]. Zentralbl Bakteriol B. 1978;167:375–90.
Mayser P, Kupfer J, Nemetz D, Schäfer U, Nilles M, Hort W, Gieler U. Treatment of head and neck dermatitis with ciclopiroxolamine cream – results of a double-blind, placebo-controlled study. Skin Pharmacol Physiol. 2006;19(3):153–9.
McNally NJ, Williams HC, Phillips DR, et al. Atopic eczema and domestic water hardness. Lancet. 1998;352:527–31.
Mee AS, Brown D, Jewell DP. Atopy in inflammatory bowel disease. Scand J Gastroenterol. 1979;14(6): 743–6.
Meerwaldt R, Odink RJ, Landaeta R, Aarts F, Brunekr FB, Gerritsen J, van Aalderen WM, Hoekstra MO. A lower prevalence of atopy symptoms in children with tpy 1 diabetes mellitus. Clin Exp Allergy. 2002; 32:254–5.
Meggitt SJ, Gray JC, Reynolds NJ. Azathioprine dosed by thiopurine methyltransferase activity for moderate-to-severe atopic eczema: a double-blind, randomised controlled trial. Lancet. 2006;367(9513):839–46.
Meingassner JG, Grassberger M, Fahrngruber H, Moore HD, Schuurman H, Stutz A. A novel anti-inflammatory drug, SDZ ASM 981, for the topical and oral treatment of skin diseases: in vivo pharmacology. Br J Dermatol. 1997;137:568–76.
Melin L, Frederiksen T, Noren P, Swebilius BG. Behavioural treatment of scratching in patients with atopic dermatitis. Br J Dermatol. 1986;115(4): 467–74.
Mempel M, Hojka M, Schnopp C, Ring J, Abeck D. Colonization features of Staphylococcus aureus in children with atopic eczema. Ann Dermatol Venereol. 1998;125 Suppl 1:S63.
Menz G, Kronenberger H, Lecheler J, Schulz K. Rehabilitation bei Asthma bronchiale. Pneumologie. 2007;61:710–20.
Mercuriali H. De morbis cutaneis et omnibus corporis humani excrementis tractatus. Venetiis: Aput Iuntas; 1601.
Merk HF, Bickers DR. Dermatopharmatologie und Dermatopharmazie. Berlin: Blackwell; 1992.
Metzger H, Rivnay B, Henkart M, Kanner B, Kinet JP, Perez-Montfort R. Analysis of the structure and function of the receptor for immunoglobulin E. Mol Immunol. 1984;21:1167–75.
Meurer M, Fölster-Holst R, Wozel G, Weidinger G, Junger M, Bräutigam M. CASM-DE-01 study group: Efficacy and safety of pimecrolimus cream in the long-term management of atopic dermatitis in adults: a six-month study. Dermatology. 2002;205:271–7.
Meurer M, Fartasch M, Albrecht G, et al. Long-term efficacy and safety of pimecrolimus cream 1 % in adults with moderate atopic dermatitis. Dermatology. 2004;208:365–72.
Meyerson LW. A peculiar papulosquamos eruption involving pigmented nevi. Arch Dermatol. 1971;103: 510–2.
Mier PD. Earliest description of the atopic syndrome? Br J Dermatol. 1975;92:359.
Mihm MC, Soter NA, Dvorak HF, Austen KF. The structure of normal skin and the morphology of atopic eczema. J Invest Dermatol. 1976;67:305–12.
Mildner M, Jin J, Eckhart L, Kezic S, Gruber F, Barresi C, Stremnitzer C, Buchberger M, Mlitz V, Ballaun C, Sterniczky B, Födinger D, Tschachler E. Knockdown of filaggrin impairs diffusion barrier function and increases UV sensitivity in a human skin model. J Invest Dermatol. 2010;130:2286–94.
Milgrom H, Berger W, Nayak A, Gupta N, Pollard S. Treatment of childhood asthma with anti-immunoglobulin E antibody (omalizumab). Pediatrics. 2001;108:36–45.
Milingou M, Antille C, Sorg O, Saurat JH, Lubbe J. Alcohol intolerance and facial flushing in patients treated with topical tacrolimus. Arch Dermatol. 2004;140(12):1542–4.
Mitchell EB, Crow J, Chapman MD, Jouhal SS, Pope FM, Platts-Mills TAE. Basophils in allergen-induced patch test sites in atopic dermatitis. Lancet. 1982;1: 127–30.
Mitschenko AV, Lwow AN, Kupfer J, Niemeier V, Gieler U. Neurodermitis und Stress. Hautarzt. 2008;59:314–8.
Mitsuyama K, Niwa M, Masuda J, Yamasaki H, Kuwaki K, Takedatsu H, Kobayashi T, Kinjo F, Kishimoto K, Matsui T, Hirai F, Makiyama K, Ohba K, Abe H, Tsubouchi H, Fujita H, Maekawa R, Yoshida H, Sata M, Kyushu ACP Study Group. Possible diagnostic role of antibodies to Crohn's disease peptide (ACP):

results of a multicenter study in a Japanese cohort. J Gastroenterol. 2014;49(4):683–91. doi:10.1007/s00535-013-0916-9.

Mittermann I, Reininger R, Zimmermann M, Gangl K, Reisinger J, Aichberger KJ, Greisenegger EK, Niederberger V, Seipelt J, Bohle B, Kopp T, Akdis CA, Spitzauer S, Valent P, Valenta R. The IgE-reactive autoantigen Hom s 2 induces damage of respiratory epithelial cells and keratinocytes via induction of IFN-γ. J Invest Dermatol. 2008;128:1451–9.

Miyagaki T, Sugaya M. Erythrodermic cutaneous T cell lymphoma: how to differentiate this rare disease from atopic dermatitis. J Dermatol Sci. 2011;64:1–6.

Miyake Y, Yokoyama T, Yura A, Iki M, Shimizu T. Ecological association of water hardness with prevalence of childhood atopic dermatitis in a Japanese urban area. Environ Res. 2004;94:33–7.

Moffatt M, Cookson W. The genetics of asthma. Maternal effects in atopic disease. Clin Exp Allergy. 1998;28 Suppl 1:56–61.

Moffatt MF, Hill MR, Cornelis J, Schou C, et al. Genetic linkage of T-cell α/δ complex specific IgE responses. Lancet. 1994;343:1597–600.

Moffatt MF, Kabesch M, Lian L, et al. Genetic variants regulating ORMDL3 expression contribute to the risk of childhood asthma. Nature. 2007;448:470–3.

Möhrenschlager M, Ring J. Allergy to peanut oil – clinically relevant? J Eur Acad Dermatol Venereol. 2007;21:452–5.

Möhrenschlager M, Schäfer T, Williams HC, von der Werth J, Krämer U, Behrendt H, Ring J. Überset-zung und Validierung der britischen Diagnosekriterien des atopischen Ekzems bei 8- und 9-jährigen Schulkindern in Augsburg. Allergol J. 1998;7:373–7.

Möhrenschlager M, Beham A, Abeck D, Ring J. Atopic eczema in monozygotic twins with Dubowitz syndrome. Br J Dermatol. 1998;138:1091–2.

Möhrenschlager M, Weidinger S, Huss-Marp J, Krämer U, Behrendt H, Ring J. Do gender-specific differences in eyelash length in 5- to 6-year old preschoolchildren with and without atopic eczema exist? Results from the MIRIAM study conducted in Augsburg, Germany. Pediatr Dermatol. 2005;22:576–7.

Möhrenschlager M, Darsow U, Schnopp C, Ring J. Atopic Eczema: what's new? J Eur Acad Dermatol Venereol. 2006a;20:503–13.

Möhrenschlager M, Schäfer T, Huss-Marp J, Eberlein-König B, Weidinger S, Ring J, Behrendt H, Krämer U. The course of eczema in children aged 5–7 years and its relation to atopy: differences be-tween boys and girls. Br J Dermatol. 2006b;3:505–13.

Möller H. Atopic winter feet in children. Acta Derm Verneol. 1972;52:401–5.

Molin S, Vollmer S, Weiss EH, Ruzicka T, Prinz JC. Filaggrin mutations may confer susceptibility to chronic hand eczema characterized by combined allergic and irritant contact dermatitis. Br J Dermatol. 2009;161(4):801–7. doi:10.1111/j.1365-2133.2009.09245.x. Epub 2009 Apr 22.

Morgan DB. A suggestive sign of allergy. Arch Dermatol. 1948;57:1050.

Morgenstern V, Zutavern A, Cyrys J, Brockow K, Koletzko S, Krämer U, Behrendt H, Herbarth O, von Berg A, Bauer CP, Wichmann HE, Heinricht J, GINI Study Group; LISA Study Group. Atopic diseases, allergic sensitization and exposure to traffic-related air pollution in children. Am J Respir Crit Care Med. 2008;177:1331–7.

Mossmann TR, Saat S. The expanding universe of T-cell subsets: Th1, Th2 and more. Immunol Today. 1996;17:138–46.

Mostafa-Kara N, Pauwels A, Pinus E, Biuor M, Levy VG. Fatal hepatitis after herbal tea. Lancet. 1992;340:674.

Moustafa F, Feldman SR. A review of phosphodiesterase-inhibition and the potential role for phosphodiesterase 4-inhibitors in clinical dermatology. Dermatol Online J. 2014;16:22608.

Mrabet-Dahbi S, Maurer M. Does allergy impair innate immunity? Leads and lessons from atopic dermatitis. Allergy. 2010;65:1351–6.

Muche-Borowski C, Kopp M, Reese I, Sitter H, Werfel T, Schäfer T, German Society for Allergology and Clinical Immunology (DGAKI); Society of German Allergologists (ADA); German Society for Pediatric and Adolescent Medicine (DGKJ); German Society of Dermatology (DDG); German Society of Pediatric Allergology (GPA). Allergy prevention. J Dtsch Dermatol Ges. 2010;8:718–24.

Münch D. Music therapy in atopic eczema. In: Ring J, Przybilla B, Ruzicka T, editors. Handbook of atopic eczema. 2nd ed. Berlin/New York/Tokio: Springer; 2006. p. 565–9.

Munkvad M. A comparative trial of Clinitar versus hydrocortisone cream in the treatment of atopic eczema. Br J Dermatol. 1989;121:763–6.

Münzel K. Psychosoziale Belastung als Einflußfaktor bei der atopischen Dermatitis. In: Petermann F, Warschburger P, editors. Neurodermitis. Göttingen: Hogrefe; 1999.

Münzel K, Schandry R. Atopisches Ekzem. Pathophysiologische Reaktivität unter standardisierter Belastung. Hautarzt. 1990;41:606–11.

Murota H, Kitaba S, Tani M, Wataya-Kaneda M, Azukizawa H, Tanemura A, Umegaki N, Terao M, Kotobuki Y, Katayama I. Impact of sedative and non-sedative antihistamines on the impaired productivity and quality of life in patients with pruritic skin diseases. Allergol Int. 2010;59:345–54.

Murphy LA, Atherton DJ. A retrospective evaluation of azathioprine in severe childhood atopic eczema, using thiopurine methyl transferase levels to exclude patients at high risk of myelosuppression. Br J Dermatol. 2002;147:324–30.

Murray CS, Rees J. Are subjective accounts of itch to be relied on? The lack of relation between visual analogue itch scores and actigraphic measures of itch. Acta Derm Venereol. 2011;91:18–23.

Müseler A, Rakoski J, v. Zumbusch R, Henning M, Borelli S. Vergleichende hautphysiologische Untersuchung zur Wirksamkeit von Zinkschüttelmixtur bei akuter Neurodermitis. Z Hautkr. 1995;70:803–7.

Mustakallio KK, Kiistala U, Piha HJ, Nieminen E. Epidermal lipids in Besnier's prurigo (atopic eczema). Ann Med Exp Biol Fenn. 1967;45:323–5.

Nagelkerken L, Verzaal P, Lagerweij T, Persoon-Deen C, Berbee JFP, Prens EP, Havekes LM, Oranje AP. Development of atopic dermatitis in mice transgenic for human apolipoprotein C1. J Invest Dermatol. 2007;128:1165–72.

Nahm D-H, Lee ES, Park H-J, Kim H-A. Treatment of atopic dermatitis with a combination of allergen-specific immunotherapy and a histamine-immunoglobulin complex. Int Arch Allergy. 2008;146:235–40.

Nakano T, Shimojo N, Okamoto Y, Ebisawa M, Kurihara K, Hoshioka A, Yamaguchi K, Ito K, Fujisawa T, Kameda M, Suehiro Y, Ogura H, Shibata R, Suzuki S, Takahashi Y, Ikeda M, Kohno Y. The use of complementary and alternative medicine by pediatric food-allergic patients in Japan. Int Arch Allergy Immunol. 2012;159:410–5.

Naldi L, Mercury SR. Chronic pruritus management: a plea for improvement – can itch clinics be an option? Dermatology. 2010;221:216–8.

Napadow V, Li A, Loggia M, Kim J, Mawla I, Desbordes G, Schalock PC, Lerner EA, Tran TN, Ring J, Rosen BR, Kaptchuk TJ, Pfab F. The imagined itch: brain circuitry supporting nocebo-induced itch in atopic dermatitis patients. Allergy. 2015;17:10.1111–12727, in press.

Natter S, Seiberler S, Hufnagl P, Binder BR, Hirschl AM, Ring J, Abeck D, Schmidt T, Valent P, Valen-ta R. Isolation of cDNA clones coding for IgE autoantigens with serum IgE from atopic dermatitis patients. FASEB J. 1998;12:1559–69.

Neis MM, Peters B, Dreuw A, Wenzel J, Bieber T, Mauch C, et al. Enhanced expression levels of IL-31 correlate with IL-4 and IL-13 in atopic and allergic contact dermatitis. J Allergy Clin Immunol. 2006;118:930–7.

Nemoto-Hasebe I, Akiyama M, Nomura T, Sandilands A, McLean WI, Shimizu H. Clinical Severity Correlates with Impaired Barrier in Filaggrin-Related Eczema. J Invest Dermatol. 2009;129:682–9.

Nenoff P, Reinl P, Haustein UF. Der Hefepilz Malassezia. Erreger, Pathogenese und Therapie. Hautarzt. 2001;52:73–86.

Neuber K, Gerhard C, Held KR, Ring J. Dramatic improvement of nummular eczema after parenteral testosterone substitution in a patient with mixed gonadal dysgenesia. Allergo J. 1993;5:77–8.

Neuber K, Steinrücke K, Ring J. Staphylococcal Enterotoxin B Affects in vitro IgE Synthesis, Interfer-on-γ, Interleukin-5 production in Atopic Eczema. Int Arch Allergy Immunol. 1995;107:179–82.

Neuber K, Schwartz I, Itschert G, Dieck AT. Treatment of atopic eczema with oral mycophenolate mofetil. Br J Dermatol. 2000;143:385–91.

Neumann C. Contact allergy and atopic eczema. In: Ruzicka T, Ring J, Przybilla B, editors. Handbook of atopic eczema. Berlin/New York: Springer; 1991.

Niebel G. Verhaltensmedizinisches Gruppentraining für Patienten mit atopischer Dermatitis in Ergän-zung zur dermatologischen Behandlung; Pilotstudie zur Erprobung von Selbsthilfestrategien. Verhaltenmodifikation und Verhaltensmedizin. 1990; 11:24–44.

Niebel G. Verhaltensmedizin der chronischen Hautkrankheiten. Huber Verlag: Bern; 1995.

Niggemann B, Reibel S, Wahn U. The atopy patch test (APT) – a useful tool for the diagnosis of food allergy in children with atopic dermatitis. Allergy. 2000;55:281–5.

Niggemann B, Reibel S, Roehr CC, Felger D, Ziegert M, Sommerfeld C, Wahn U. Predictors of posi-tive food challenge outcome in non-IgE-mediated reactions to food in children with atopic dermatitis. J Allergy Clin Immunol. 2001;108:1053–8.

Nishioka K, Yasueda H, Saito H. Preventive effect of bedding encasement with microfine fibers onmite sensitization. J Allergy Clin Immunol. 1998;101: 28–32.

Noda S, Krueger JG, Guttmann-Yassky E. The translational revolution and use of biologics in patients with inflammatory skin diseases. J Allergy Clin Immunol. 2015;135:324–36.

Novak N. New insights into the mechanism and management of allergic diseases: atopic dermatitis. Allergy. 2009;64:265–75.

Novak N, Bieber T. Allergic and nonallergic forms of atopic diseases. J Allergy Clin Immunol. 2003;112:252–62.

Novak N, Allam JP, Bieber T. Allergic hyperreactivity to microbial components: a trigger factor of "intrinsic" atopic dermatitis? J Allergy Clin Immunol. 2003;112:215–6.

Novak N, Yu CF, Bussmann C, Maintz L, Peng WM, Hart J, et al. Putative association of a TLR9 promoter polymorphism with atopic eczema. Allergy. 2007;62:766–72.

Novak N, Bieber T, Hoffmann M, Fölster-Holst R, Homey B, Werfel T, Sager A, Zuberbier T. Efficacy and safety of subcutaneous allergen-specific immunotherapy with depigmented polymerized mite extract in atopic dermatitis. J Allergy Clin Immunol. 2012;130: 925–31.

Novembre E, Cianferoni A, Lombardi E, Bernardini R, Pucci N, Vierucci A. Natural history of "intrinsic" atopic dermatitis. Allergy. 2001;56:453–4.

Nowak D, Heinrich J, Jörres R. Prevalence of respiratory symptoms, bronchial hyperresponsiveness and atopy among adults: West and East Germany. Eur Respir J. 1996;9:2541–52.

Nürnberg W. Stationäre Rehabilitation von Hauterkrankungen am Beispiel des atopischen Ekzems. Hautarzt. 2005;56:644–8.

O'Driscoll J, Burden AD, Kingston TP. Potent topical steroid obtained from a Chinese herbalist. Br J Dermatol. 1992;127:543–4.

Ochs HD, Oukka M, Torgerson TR. TH17 cells and regulatory T cells in primary immunodeficiency diseases. J Allergy Clin Immunol. 2009;123:977–83.

Oepen J. Unkonventionelle diagnostische und therapeutische Methoden in der Umweltmedizin. Gesundheitswesen. 1998;60:420–30.

Oh SH, Bae BG, Park CO, Noh JY, Park IH, wu WH, Lee KH. Association of stress with symptoms of atopic dermatitis. Acta Derm Venereol. 2010;90: 582–8.

Ohman S, Johansson SGO. Immunoglobulins in atopic dermatitis with special reference to IgE. Acta Derm Venerol (Stockh). 1974;54:193–202.

Ohtsuka T, Matsumaru S, Uchida K, et al. Time course of plasma histamine and tryptase following food challenges in children with suspected food allergy. Ann Allergy. 1993;71:139–46.

Oji V, Eckl K-M, Aufenvenne K, Nätebus M, Tarinski T, Ackermann K, Seller N, Metze D, Nürnberg G, Fölster-Holst R, Schäfer-Korting M, Hausser I, Traupe H, Hennies HC. Loss of corneodesmosin leads to severe skin barrier defect, pruritus, and atopy: unraveling the peeling skin disease. Am J Hum Genet. 2010;87:1–8.

Olaiwan A, Chandesris MO, Fraitag S, Lortholary O, Hermine O, Fischer A, de Prost Y, Picard C, Bodemer C. Cutaneous findings in sporadic and familial autosomal dominant hyper-IgE syndrome: a retrospective, single-center study of 21 patients diagnosed using molecular analysis. J Am Acad Dermatol. 2011;65:1167–72.

Oldhoff JM, Darsow U, Werfel T, Katzer K, Wulf A, Laifaoui J, Hijnen DJ, Plotz S, Knol EF, Kapp A, Bruijnzeel-Koomen CA, Ring J, de Bruin-Weller MS. Anti-IL-5 recombinant humanized monoclonal antibody (mepolizumab) for the treatment of atopic dermatitis. Allergy. 2005;60:693–6.

Olesen AB. Diseases rarely associated with atopic eczema. In: Ring J, Przybilla B, Ruzicka T, editors. Handbook of atopic eczema. 2nd ed. Berlin/New York/Tokio: Springer; 2006. p. 144–9.

Olesen AB, Ellingsen AR, Larsen ES, Larsen PO, Veien NK, Thestrup-Pedersen K. Atopic dermatitis may be lined to whether a child is first or second born and/or the age of the mother. Acta Derm Venerol (Stockh). 1996;76:457–60.

Olesen AB, Ellingsen AR, Olesen H, Juul S, Thestrup PK. Atopic dermatitis and birth factors: historical follow-up by record linkage. BMJ. 1997;314:1003–8.

Olesen AB, Juul S, Birkebaek N, Thestrup-Pedersen K. Association between atopic dermatitis atopic dermatitis and insulin-dependent diabetes mellitus: a case-control study. Lancet. 2001;357:1749–52.

Olesen AB, Juul S, Thestrup-Pedersen K. Atopic dermatitis is increased following vaccination for measles, mumps and rubella or measles infection. Acta Derm Venereol. 2003;83:445–50.

Oranje A, De Waard-van der Spek F. Atopic dermatitis and diet. J Eur Acad Dermatol Venereol. 2000;14:437–8.

Orihara K, Nakae S, Pawankar R, Saito H. Role of regulatory and proinflammatory T-cell populations in allergic diseases. WAO J. 2008;1:9–14.

Ortonne JP, Perrot H, Thivolet J. Étude clinique et statistique d'une population de 100 vitiligos: facteurs étiologiques et étude clinique. Sem Hop Paris. 1976;52:679–86.

Owada Y, Takano H, Yamanaka H, Kobayashi H, Sugitani Y, Tomioka Y, Suzuki I, Suzuki R, Terui T, Mizugaki M, Tagami H, Noda T, Kondo H. Altered water barrier function in epidermal-type fatty acid binding protein-deficient mice. J Invest Dermatol. 2002;118(3):430–5.

Ozkaya E. Adult-onset atopic dermatitis. J Am Acad Dermatol. 2005;52:579–82.

Pajno GB, Vita D, Barberio E, Salzano G, Lombardo F, et al. Sublingual immunotherapy in mite-sensitized children with atopic dermatitis: a randomized, double-blind placebo-controlled study. J Allergy Clin Immunol. 2007;120:164–70.

Pallas S, Huss-Marp J, Ring J, Behrendt H, Eberlein B. Charakterisierung von Patienten mit umweltbezogenen Gesundheitsstörungen an einer dermatologisch-allergologischen Klinik. Umweltmed Forsch Prax. 2010;15:135–47.

Paller A, Eichenfield LF, Leung DY, et al. A 12-week study of tacrolimus ointment for the treatment of atopic dermatitis in pediatric patients. J Am Acad Dermatol. 2001;44:S47–57.

Paller AS, Lebwohl M, Fleischer AB, Antaya R, Langley RG, Kirsner RS, Blum RR, Rico MJ, Jaracz E, Crowe A, et al. Tacrolimus ointment is more effective than pimecrolimus cream with a similar safety profile in the treatment of atopic dermatitis: results from 3 randomized comparative studies. J Am Acad Dermatol. 2005;52:810–22.

Palmer CN, Irvine AD, Terron-Kwiatkowski A, et al. Common loss-of-function variants of the epidermal barrier protein filaggrin are a major predisposing factor for atopic dermatitis. Nat Genet. 2006;38:441–6.

Papoiu ADP, Wang H, Coghill RC, Chan Y-H, Yosipovitch G. Contagious itch in humans: a study of visual "transmission" of itch in atopic dermatitis and healthy subjects. Br J Dermatol. 2011;164:1299–303.

Papp K, Cather JC, Rosoph L, Sofen H, Langley RG, Matheson RT, Hu C, Day RM. Efficacy of apremilast in the treatment of moderate to severe psoriasis: a randomised controlled trial. Lancet. 2012; 380(9843):738–46.

Papp KA, Griffiths CE, Gordon K, Lebwohl M, Szapary PO, Wasfi Y, Chan D, Hsu MC, Ho V, Ghislain PD, Strober B, Reich K, PHOENIX 1 Investigators; PHOENIX 2 Investigators; ACCEPT Investigators. Long-term safety of ustekinumab in patients with moderate-to-severe psoriasis: final results from 5 years of follow-up. Br J Dermatol. 2013;168(4): 844–54.

Park J, Kim B-J, Kwon J-W, Song YH, Yu J, Kim H-B, Lee S-Y, Kim WK, Jee HM, Kim KW, Kim K-E, Hong S-J, Shin Y-J. Patterns of psychosocial adaptation and allergic disorders in Korean schoolchildren. Int Arch Allergy Immunol. 2011;154:249–57.

Paternoster L, Zhurov AI, Toma AM, Kemp JP, St Pourcain B, Timpson NJ, McMahon G, McArdle W, Ring SM, Smith GD, Richmond S, Evans DM. Genome-wide association study of three-dimensional facial morphology identifies a variant in PAX3 associated with nasion position. Am J Hum Genet. 2012;90:478–85.

Paul C, Lahfa M, Bachelez H, Chevret S, Dubertret L. A randomized controlled evaluator-blinded trial of intravenous immunoglobulin in adults with severe atopic dermatitis. Br J Dermatol. 2002;147: 518–22.

Penders J, Gerhold K, Stobberingh EE, Thijs C, Zimmermann K, Lau S, Hamelmann E. Establishment of the intestinal microbiota and its role for atopic dermatitis in early childhood. J Allergy Clin Immunol. 2013;132:601–7.

Pepys J. Atopy. In: Gell PG, Coombs RRA, Lachmann PF, editors. Clinical aspects of immunology. 3rd ed. Oxford: Blackwell; 1975. p. 877.

Peserico A, Stadtler G, Sebastian M, Fernandez RS, Vick K, Bieber T. Reduction of relapses of atopic dermatitis with methylprednisolone aceponate cream twice weekly in addition to maintenance treatment with emollient: a multicentre, randomized, double-blind, controlled study. Br J Dermatol. 2008;158:801–7.

Petermann F, Warschburger P, editors. Neurodermitis. Göttingen: Hogrefe; 1999.

Petermann F, Gulyas AF, Nieband K, Warschburger P. Effects of allergen avoidance at high altitude on children with asthma or atopic dermatitis. Pediatr Asthma Allergy Immunol. 2004;17:15–24.

Pfab F, Huss-Marp J, Gatti A, Fuqin J, Athanasiadis GI, Irnich D, Raap U, Schober W, Behrendt H, Ring J, Darsow U. Influence of acupuncture on type I hypersensitivity itch and the wheal and flare response in adults with atopic eczema – a blinded, randomized, placebo-controlled, crossover trial. Allergy. 2010a;66:903–10.

Pfab F, Valet M, Sprenger T, Huss-Marp J, Athanasiadis GI, Baurecht HJ, Konstantinow A, Zimmer C, Behrendt H, Ring J, Tölle TR, Darsow U. Temperature-modulated histamine-itch in nonlesional skin in atopic eczema – a combined psychophysical and neuroimaging study. Allergy. 2010b;65:84–94.

Pfab F, Valet M, Napadow V, Tölle TR, Behrendt H, Ring J, Darsow U. Itch and the brain. Chem Immunol Allergy. 2012;98:253–65.

Pflugshaupt C. Eigenwirkungen von Vehikeln. Systematik und Gedanken zur Vehikelwahl. Dt Dermatol. 1992;8:1144–55.

Pichler W, Bircher AA, Wüthrich B. Spezialistenkommission der Schweizer Gesellschaft für Allergolo-gie und Immunologie. Allergologie und Alternativmedizin. Stellungnahme zu paramedizinischen Verfahren, speziell Bioresonanz. Schweiz Ärztezeitung, nachgedruckt in. Allergologie. 1996;19:158–61.

Piérard GE. What do you mean by dry skin? Dermatologica. 1989;179:1–2.

Pilette C, Jacobson MR, Ratajczak C, Detry B, Banfield G, VanSnick J, et al. Aberrant dendritic cell function conditions Th2-cell polarization in allergic rhinitis. Allergy. 2013;68:312–21.

Pion IA, Koenig KL, Lim HW. Is dermatologic usage of coal tar carcinogenic? A review of the literature. Dermatol Surg. 1995;21:227–31.

Platts-Mills T, Mitchell E, Rowntree S, Chapman M, Wilkins S. The role of dust mite allergens in atopic dermatitis. Clin Exp Dermatol. 1983;8:233–47.

Plaut M, Tinkle SS. Risks of smallpox vaccination: 200 years after Jenner. J Allergy Clin Immunol. 2003;112:683–5.

Plötz SG, Simon HU, Darsow U, Simon D, Vassina E, Yousefi S, Hein R, Smith T, Behrendt H, Ring J. Use of anti-interleukin-5 antibody in hypereosinophilic syndrome with eosinophilic dermatitis. N Engl J Med. 2003;349:2332–7.

Plötz SG, Wiesender M, Todorova A, Ring J. What is new in atopic dermatitis/eczema? Expert Opin Emerg Drugs. 2014;19:9–18.

Pluut OA, Bianco C, Jakasa I, Visser MJ, Krystek P, Larese-Filon F, et al. Percutaneous penetration of silver from al silver containing garment in healthy volunteers and patients with atopic dermatitis. Toxicol Lett. 2015;235:116–22.

Prausnitz C, Kästner H. Studien über die Überempfindlichkeit. Zentralbl Bakteriol Parasitenkt Infekti-onskr Hygiene. 1921;86:160.

Premerlani M, Ludewig Y, Schnopp C, Ring J. Eczema school: practical approaches in an efficient module of tertiary prevention programs. In: Ring J, Przybilla B, Ruzicka T, editors. Handbook of atopic eczema. 2nd ed. Berlin/New York/Tokio: Springer; 2006. p. 576–81.

Prescott S. Early origins of allergic disease: a review of processes and influences during early immune development. Curr Opin Allergy Clin Immunol. 2003;3: 125–32.

Prescott SL, MacAubas C, Smallacombe T, Holt BJ, Sly PD, Holt PG. Development of allergen-specific T-cell memory in atopic and normal children. Lancet. 1999;353:196–200.

Prinz B, Nachbar F, Plewig G. Treatment of severe atopic dermatitis with extracorporal photophoresis. Arch Dermatol Res. 1994;287:48–52.

Prochazka B. Sensibilität und Abgrenzung bei Neurodermitikern. Wiesen: Porch; 1994.

Proksch E, Jensen JM, Elias PM. Skin lipids and epidermal differentiation in atopic dermatitis. Clin Dermatol. 2003;21:134–44.

Proksch E, Fölster-Holst R, Jensen M. Skin barrier function, epidermal proliferation and differentiation in eczema. J Dermatol Sci. 2006;43:159–69.

Prucha H, Chen W, Traidl-Hoffmann C, Todorova A, Akdis C, Lauener R, Ring J. Atopic eczema and allergies: practical relevance for diagnostic work-up. Community Based Med J. 2013;2:15–24.

Przybilla B, Ring J. Food allergy and atopic eczema. Semin Dermatol. 1990;9:220–5.

Przybilla B, Enders F, Ring J, Winkelmann H. Stigmata of atopic constitution in patients with atopic eczema or atopic respiratory disease. Acta Derm Venereol. 1991;71:407–10.

Przybilla B, Eberlein-König B, Rueff F. Practical management of atopic eczema. Lancet. 1994;343:1342–6.

Pugh SM, Rhodes J, Mayberry JF, Roberts DL, Heatley RV, Newcombe RG. Atopic disease in ulcerative colitis and Crohn's disease. Clin Allergy. 1979;9(3):221–3.

Purohit A, Duvernelle C, Melac M, Pauli G, Frossard N. Twenty-four hours of activity of cetirizine and fexofenadine in the skin. Ann Allergy Asthma Immunol. 2001;86:387–92.

Purvis DJ, Thompson JM, Clark PM, et al. Risk factors for atopic dermatitis in New Zealand children at age 3,5 years of age. Br J Dermatol. 2005;152:742–9.

Purwar R, Werfel T, Wittmann M. Regulation of IL-13 receptors in human keratinocytes. J Invest Dermatol. 2007;127:1271–4.

Quaranta M, Knapp B, Garzorz N, et al. Intraindividual genome expression analysis reveals a specific molecular signature of psoriasis and eczema. Sci Transl Med. 2014;6:244.

Queille-Roussel C, Raynaud F, Saurat JH. A prospective computerized study of 500 cases of atopic dermatitis in childhood. Acta Derm Venerol (Stockh). 1985;114(Suppl):87–92.

Raap U, Werfel T, Jaeger B, Schmid-Ott G. Atopische Dermatitis und psychischer Stress. Hautarzt. 2003;54:925–9.

Raap U, Ikoma A, Kapp A. Neurophysiology of pruritus. Hautarzt. 2006;57:379–84.

Rabinowitz LG, Esterly NB. Atopic dermatitis and ichthyosis vulgaris. Pediatr Rev. 1994;15:220–6; quiz 226.

Rajka G. Itch and IgE in atopic dermatitis. Acta Derm Venereol. 1980;92:38–43.

Rajka G. Essential aspects of atopic dermatitis. Berlin/New York/Heidelberg: Springer; 1989.

Rajka G, Winkelmann RK. Atopic dermatitis and Sézary Syndrome. Arch Dermatol. 1984;120:83–4.

Ramirez de Knott HM, McCormick TS, Kalka K, Skandamis G, Ghannoum MA, Schluchter M, Cooper KD, Nedorost ST. Cutaneous hypersensitivity to Malassezia sympodialis and dust mite in adult atopic dermatitis with a textile pattern. Contact Dermatitis. 2006;54:92–9.

Ramsay CA, Savoie JM, Gilbert M, Gidon M, Kidson P. The treatment of atopic dermatitis with topical fusidic acid and hydrocortisone acetate. J Eur Acad Dermatol Venerol. 1996;7(Suppl I):15–22.

Ravens-Sieberer U, Bullinger M. Assessing health-related quality of life in chronically ill children with the German KINDL: first psychometric and content analytical results. Qual Life Res. 1998;7:399–407.

Ravens-Sieberer U, Bullinger M. KINDL – Fragebogen zur Erfassung der gesundheitsbezogenen Le-bensqualität bei Kindernund Jugendlichen – Revidierte Form – Manual. 2000.

Rechardt E. An investigation in the psychosomatic aspects of Prurigo Besnier. Helsinki: Psych Clinic d. Univ Helsinki; 1970.

Reekers R, Beyer K, Niggemann B, et al. The role of circulating food antigen-specific lymphocytes in food allergic children with atopic dermatitis. Br J Dermatol. 1996;135:935–41.

Reese I, Werfel T (Hrsg). Nahrungsmittelallergie – Diätetische Gesichtspunkte und aktuelle Positionspapiere. 2 aktualisierte Auflage. Deisenhofen: Dustri Verlag; 2006.

Reinhard T, Ruzicka T, Sundmacher R. Pathogenese, Klinik und Therapie der Augenbeteiligung bei Atopie. Ophthalmologe. 1999;96:473–88.

Reitamo S. Tacrolimus: a new topical immunomodulatory therapy for atopic dermatitis. J Allergy Clin Immunol. 2001;107:445–8.

Reitamo S. European Tacrolimus Ointment Study Group: 0.1 % Tacrolimus ointment twice a day is an effective treatment for adults with moderate to severe atomic dermatitis. JEADV. 2003;17:180.

Reitamo S, Rissanen J, Remitz A, et al. Tacrolimus ointment does not affect collagen synthesis results of a single-center randomized trial. J Invest Dermatol. 1998;111:396–8.

Reitamo S, Van Leent EJ, Ho V, Harper J, Ruzicka T, Kalimo K, Cambazard F, Rustin M, Taïeb A, Gratton D, Sauder D, Sharpe G, Smith C, Junger M, de Prost Y. Efficacy and safety of tacrolimus ointment compared with that of hydrocortisone acetate ointment in children with atopic dermatitis. J Allergy Clin Immunol. 2002;109(3):539–46.

Reitamo S, Ortonne JP, Sand C, et al. A multicentre, randomized, double-blind, controlled study of long-term treatment with 0.1 % tacrolimus ointment in adults with moderate to severe atopic dermatitis. Br J Dermatol. 2005;152:1282–9.

Reitamo S, Ortonne JP, Sand C, Bos J, Cambazard F, Bieber T, Gronhoj-Larsen C, Rustin M, Fölster-Holst R, Schuttelaar M. Long-term treatment with 0.1 % tracrolimus ointment in adults with atopic der-matitis: results of a two-year, multicentre, non-comparative study. Acta Derm Venereol. 2007;87:406–12.

Reitamo S, Remitz A. An update on current pharmacotherapy options in atopic dermatitis. Expert Opin Pharmacother. 2014;15:1517–24.

Remy W, Rakoski J, Siebenwirth J, Ulm K, Wiesenauer M. Classical homeopathic treatment in atopic dermatitis. Allergologie. 1995;18:246–52.

Renz H, Hahn C, Schuhmann B, Kerzel S, Nassenstein C, Braun A, Päth G, Virchow C, Nockher WA. Neurotrophins in allergic bronchial asthma. In: Lowenstein H, Bienenstock J, Ring J, editors. From genes to phenotypes. Goettingen: Hogrefe Huber; 2006. p. 133–6.

Reuter J, Wölfle U, Weckesser S, Schempp C. Which plant for which skin disease? Part 1: atopic dermatitis, psoriasis, acne, condyloma and herpes simplex. J Dtsch Dermatol Ges. 2010;8:788–96.

Reynolds NJ, Franklin V, Gray JC, Diffey BL, Farr PM. Narrow-band ultraviolet B and broad-band ultraviolet. A phototherapy in adult atopic eczema: a randomised controlled trial. Lancet. 2001;357(9273):2012–6.

Ricci G, Patrizi A, Specchia F. Mite allergen (Der p 1) levels in houses of children with atopic dermatitis: the relationship with allergometric tests. Br J Dermatol. 1999;140:651–5.

Ricci G, Patrizi A, Specchia F, et al. Effect of house dust mite avoidance measures in children with atopic dermatitis. Br J Dermatol. 2000;143:379–84.

Ricci G, Patrizi A, Bendandi B, Menna G, Varotti E, Masi M. Clinical effectiveness of a silk fabric in the treatment of atopic dermatitis. Br J Dermatol. 2004;150(1):127–31.

Richter R, Ahrens S. Psychosomatische Aspekte der Allergie in Manuale allergologicum (Fuchs E, Schulz KH) Dustri-Verlag. München Deisenhofen. 1990;8:1–16.

Richter R, Dahme B. Psychosomatische Aspekte des Asthma bronchiale. Prax Klin Pneumol. 1987;60:1–16.

Riedler J, Braun-Fahrländer C, Eder W, Schreuer M, Waser M, Maisch S, Carr D, Schierl R, Nowak D, von Mutius E. Exposure to farming in early life and development of asthma and allergy: a cross-sectional survey. Lancet. 2001;358:1129–33.

Rigopolous D, Gregoriou S, Charissi C, Kontochristopoulos G, Kalogeromitros D, Georgala S. Tacro-limus ointment 0,1 % in pityriasis alba: an open-label, randomized, placebo-controlled study. Br J Dermatol. 2006;155(1):152–5.

Ring J. Anaphylaktoide Reaktionen. Berlin: Springer; 1978.

Ring J. Atopic dermatitis. A disease of general vasoactive mediator dysregulation. Int Arch Allergy Appl Immunol. 1979;59:233–9.

Ring J. Angewandte Allergologie. Munich: MMW; 1982a.

Ring J. Successful hyposensitization treatment in atopic eczema: results of a trial monozygotic twins. Br J Dermatol. 1982b;107:597–602.

Ring J. Was ist Atopie? In: Braun-Falco O, Burk G, editors. Fortschritte der praktischen Dermatologie und Venerologie. Berlin/Heidelberg/New York: Springer; 1983. p. 103–11.

Ring J, Lutz J. Decreased release of lysosomal enzymes from peripheral leukocytes of patients with atopic dermatitis. J Am Acad Dermatol. 1983;8(3):378–85.

Ring J. Erstbeschreibung einer "atopischen Familien-Anamnese" im Julisch-Claudischen Kaiserhaus: Augustus, Claudius, Britannicus. Hautarzt. 1985; 36:470–4.

Ring J. Endogenous versus exogenous eczema. Semin Dermatol. 1990;9:195–6.

Ring J, editor. Epidemiologie allergischer Erkrankungen. Munich: MMV; 1991a.

Ring J. Atopy: condition, disease, or syndrome? In: Ruzicka T, Ring J, Przybilla B, editors. Hand-book of atopic eczema. Berlin/Heidelberg/New York: Springer; 1991b. p. 3–8.

Ring J, editor. Neurodermitis. Expertise zur gesundheitlichen Versorgung und Vorsorge bei Kindern mit atopischem Ekzem. Landsberg: Ecomed; 1998.

Ring J. Allergy in practice. Berlin/Heidelberg/New York: Springer; 2005.

Ring J, Kunz B. Unsaturated fatty acids in the treatment of atopic eczema. In: Ring J, Ruzicka T, Przybilla B (eds), Handbook of Atopic Eczema 2nd ed, Springer, Berlin, New York; 1991.

Ring J, Behrendt H. Allergie-Entstehung und Immunglobulin E-Bildung: Rolle von Infektionen und Umweltschadstoffen? Allergo J. 1993;2:27–30.

Ring J, Fröhlich HH. Wirkstoffe in der dermatologischen Therapie. Berlin: Springer; 1985.

Ring J, Landthaler M. Hyper-IgE syndromes. Curr Probl Dermatol. 1989;18:79–88.

Ring J, Merkel C. Hämatogenes Kontaktekzem (systemische Kontaktdermatitis): Was ist das? In: Wolff H, Thomas P, Prinz J, editors. Fortschritte prakt Dermatol Venerol 22 (Ruzicka T. Berlin: Springer; 2012. p. 125–8.

Ring J, Thomas P. Histamine and atopic eczema. Acta Derm Venereol. 1989;144:70–7.

Ring J, Mathison DA, O'Connor R. In vitro cyclic nucleotide responsiveness of leukocytes and platelets in patients suffering from atopic dermatitis. Int Archs Allergy Appl Immunol. 1981;65:1–7.

Ring J, Palos E, Zimmermann F. Psychosomatische Aspekte der Eltern-Kind-Beziehung bei atopischem Ekzem im Kindesalter. Erziehungsstil, Familiensituation im Zeichentest und strukturierten Inter-view. Hautarzt. 1986;37:560–7.

Ring J, Przybilla B, Schwab U, Steger O. Klinisches Spektrum der Überempfindlichkeitsreaktionen gegen Sulfite. Allergologie. 1987;10:100–6.

Ring J, Kunz B, Bieber T, Vieluf D, Przybilla B. The "atopy patch test" with aeroallergens in atopic eczema (abstract). J Allergy Clin Immunol. 1989;82.

Ring J, Brockow K, Abeck D. The therapeutic concept of "patient management" in atopic eczema. Allergy. 1996;51:206–15.

Ring J, Darsow U, Gfesser M, Vieluf D. The ‚atopy patch test' in evaluating the role of aeroallergens in atopic eczema. Int Arch Allergy Immunol. 1997;113: 379–83.

Ring J, Darsow U, Behrendt H. Role of aeroallergens in atopic eczema: proof of concept with the atopy patch test. J Am Acad Dermatol. 2001a;45:49–52.

Ring J, Krämer U, Schäfer T, Behrendt H. Why are allergies increasing? Curr Opin Immunol. 2001b;13:701–8.

Ring J, Krämer U, Oppermann H, Ranft U, Behrendt H. Influence of pertussis/pertussis vaccination on asthma and allergy prevalence in East and West Germany. Allergy Clin Immunol Int J World Allergy Org. 2004;16(Suppl 1):17–24.

Ring J, Barker J, Behrendt H, et al. Review of the potential photococareinogenicity of topical calcineurin inhibitors. Position statement of the European Dermatology Forum. J Eur Acad Dermatol Venereol. 2005;19(6):663–71.

Ring J, Ruzicka T, Przybilla B, editors. Handbook of atopic eczema. 2nd ed. Berlin/New York: Springer; 2006.

Ring J, Möhrenschlager M, Henkel V. The US FDA "black box" warning for topical calcineurin inhibitors. Drug Saf. 2008;31:185–98.

Ring J, Abraham A, de Cuyper C, Kim K, Langeland T, Parra V, Pigatto P, Reunala T, Szcepanski R, Möhrenschlager M, Bräutigam M, Rossi AB, Meents-Kopecky E, Schneider D. Control of atopic eczema with pimecrolimus cream 1 % under daily practice conditions: results of a >2000 patient study. J Eur Acad Dermatol Venereol. 2009;22:195–203.

Ring J, Bachert C, Bauer P, Czech W (eds) Whitebook Allergy in germany 3rd ed. Urban Vogel, Munchen 2010.

Ring J, von Zumbusch M. Neurodermitis. Beck, Munchen 2002.

Ring J, Alomar A, Bieber T, Deleuran M, Fink-Wagner A, Gelmetti C, Gieler U, Lippozencic J, Luger T, Oranje AP, Schwerfer T, Schwenisson T, Seidenari

S, Simon D. Ständer S, Stingel G, Schaller Sza-lais, Szepietowski JC, Taïeb A, Werfel T, Wollenberg A, Darsow U. Guidelines for treatment of atopic eczema (atopic dermatitis). J Eur Acad Dermatol Venereol. 2012;26:1176–93 and 1045–60.

Roberts IF, West M, Ogilvie D, Dillon MJ. Malnutrition in infants receiving cult diets: a form of child abuse. Br Med J. 1979;I:296–8.

Rodriguez E, Baurecht H, Herberich E, Wagenpfeil S, Brown SJ, Cordell BA, Heather J. Meta-analysis of filaggrin polymorphisms in eczema and asthma: robust risk factors in atopic disease. J Allergy Clin Immunol. 2009;123:1361–70.

Roduit C, Frei R, Loss G, Büchele G, Weber J, Depner M, Loeliger S, Dalphin ML, Roponen M, Hyvärinen A, Riedler J, Dalphin JC, Pekkanen J, von Mutius E, Braun-Fahrländer C, Lauener R, Protection Against Allergy–Study in Rural Environments study group. Development of atopic dermatitis according to age of onset and association with early-life exposures. J Allergy Clin Immunol. 2012;130:130–6.

Roelofzen JHJ, Aben KKH, Oldenhof UTH, Coenraads P-J, Alkemade HA, van de Kerkhof PCM, van der Valk PGM, Kiemeney LALM. No increased risk of cancer after coal tar treatment in patients with psoriasis or eczema. J Invest Dermatol. 2010;130: 953–61.

Rokugo M, Tagami H, Usuba Y, Tomita Y. Contact sensitivity to Pityrosporum ovale in patients with atopic dermatitis. Arch Dermatol. 1990;126:627–32.

Romanos M, Gerlach M, Wamke A, Schmitt J. Association of attention-deficit/hyperactivity disorder and atopic eczema modified by sleep disturbance in a large population-based sample. J Epidemiol Community Health. 2010;64:269–73.

Rombold S, Lobisch K, Katzer K, Grazziotin TC, Ring J, Eberlein B. Efficacy of UVA1 phototherapy in 230 patients with various skin diseases. Photodermatol Photoimmunol Photomed. 2008;24:19–23.

Rosenfeldt V, Benfeldt E, Nielsen SD, Michaelsen KF, Jeppesen DL, Valerius NH, Paerregaard A. Effect of probiotic Lactobacillus strains in children with atopic dermatitis. J Allergy Clin Immunol. 2003;111(2):389–95.

Rosenwasser L, Klemm D, Dresback J, Inamura H, Mascali J, Klinnert M, Borish L. Promoter polymorphismus in the chromosome 5 gene cluster in asthma and atopy. Clin Exp Allergy. 1995;25 Suppl 2:74–8.

Rost GA. Allergische Disposition und Status exsudativus. Klin Wochenschr. 1929;8:2009–13.

Rost GA, Marchionini A. Asthma-Ekzem, Asthma-Prurigo und Neurodermitis als allergische Hautkrankheiten. Würzb Abh Gesamtgeb Prakt Med. 1932;27:10.

Rothenberg ME, Klion AD, Roufosse FE, Kahn JE, Weller PF, Simon HU, Schwartz LB, Rosenwasser L, Ring J, Griffin EF, Haig AE, Frewer PIH, Parkin JM, Gleich G. Treatment of patients with the hypereosinophilic syndrome with mepolizumab. N Engl J Med. 2008;358:1215–28.

Ruzicka T. Atopic eczema between rationality and irrationality. Arch Dermatol. 1998;134:1462–9.

Ruzicka T, Ring J. Enhanced releasability of prostaglandin E2 and leukotrienes B4 and C4 from leukocytes of patients with atopic eczema. Acta Derm Venereol. 1987;67:469–75.

Ruzicka T, Ring J, Przybilla B, editors. Handbook of atopic eczema. 1st ed. Berlin/Heidelberg/New York: Springer; 1991. p. 429–34.

Ruzicka T, Bieber T, Schopf E, Rubins A, Dobozy A, Bos JD, Jablonska S, Ahmed I, Thestrup-Pedersen K, Daniel F, Finzi A, Reitamo S. A short-term trial of tacrolimus ointment for the treatment of atopic dermatitis. European Tacrolimus Multicenter Atopic Dermatitis Study Group. N Engl J Med. 1997;337(12):816–21.

Rycroft RJG, Menné T, Frosch PJ, Benezra C. Textbook of contact dermatitis. 1st ed. Berlin: Springer; 1991.

Rysted I. Work-related hand eczema in atopics. Contact Dermatitis. 1985;12:164–71.

Rystedt I. Prognosis factors in atopic dermatitis. Acta Dermatol Venereol. 1985;65:206–13.

Rystedt I. Long-term follow-up in atopic dermatitis. Acta Dermatol Venereol [Suppl]. 1986;114:117–20.

Sakaguchi S, Wing K, Miyara M. Regulatory T cells – a brief history and perspective. Eur J Immunol. 2000;37 Suppl 1:S116–23.

Salob SP, Laverty A, Atherton DJ. Bronchial hyperresponsiveness in children with atopic dermatitis. Pediatrics. 1993;91:13–6.

Sampson HA. Utility of food-specific IgE concentrations in predicting symptomatic food allergy. J Allergy Clin Immunol. 2001;107:891–6.

Sampson HA. The evaluation and management of food allergy in atopic dermatitis. Clin Dermatol. 2003;21:183–92.

Samrao A, Berry TM, Goreshi R, Simpson EL. A pilot study of an oral phosphodiesterase inhibitor (apremilast) for atopic dermatitis in adults. Ach Dermatol. 2012;148:890–7.

Sandstrom MH, Faergemann J. Prognosis and prognostic factors in adult patients with atopic dermatitis: a long-term follow-up questionnaire study. Br J Dermatol. 2004;150:103–10.

Santamaria Babi LF, Picker LJ, Perez Soler MT, Drzimalla K, et al. Circulating allergen-reactive T cells from patients with atopic dermatitis and allergic contact dermatitis express the skin-selective homing receptor, the cutaneous lymphocyte-associated antigen. J Exp Med. 1995;181:1935–40.

Sanz ML, Maselli JP, Gamboa PM, Garcia-Aviles MC, Oehling A, Diéguez I, de Weck AL. Flow-cytometric basophil activation test. A review. J Investig Allergol Clin Immunol. 2002;12:143–54.

Sapolsky RM. Stress, the aging brain, and the mechanisms of neuron death. Cambridge, MA: MIT Press; 1992.

Sasagawa S. Studies on the dry form of eczema in childhood patchy pityriasiform lichenoid eczema (Kitamura-Takahashi-Sasagawa) Jpn. J Dermatol. 1967;77:62–87.

Saunders SP, Moran T, Floudas A, Wurlod F, Kaszlikowska A, Salimi M, Quinn EM, Oliphant CJ, Núñez G,

McManus R, Hams E, Irvine AD, McKenzie AN, Ogg GS, Fallon PG. Spontaneous atopic dermatitis is mediated by innate immunity, with the secondary lung inflammation of the atopic march requiring adaptive immunity. J Allergy Clin Immunol. 2015;pii: S0091-6749(15)01022-2. doi:10.1016/j.jaci.2015.06.045. [Epub ahead of print].

Saurat JH. Eczema in primary immune deficiencies. Clues to the pathogenesis of atopic dermatitis with special reference of the Wiskott-Aldrich syndrome. Acta Derm Venereol. 1985;114:125–8.

Saurat J-H, Woodley D, Helfer N. Cutaneous symptoms in primary immunodeficiencies. Curr Probl Dermatol. 1985;13:50–91.

Sawada E, Yoshida N, Sugiura A, Imokawa G. Th1 cytokines accentuate but Th2 cytokines attenuate ceramide production in the stratum corneum of human epidermal equivalents: an implication for the disrupted barrier mechanisms in atopic dermatitis. J Dermatol Sci. 2012;68:25–35.

Saxon A, Diaz-Sánchez D. Air pollution and allergy: you are what you breathe. Nat Immunol. 2005;6:223–6.

Schadewaldt H. Geschichte der Allergie. Bände 1–4, Munich: Dustri; 1980–1984.

Schaefer J, Rustenbach SJ, Zimmer L, Augustin M. Prevalence of skin diseases in a cohort of 48. 665 employees in Germany. Dermatology. 2008; 217:169–72.

Schaekel K, Kannagi R, Kniep B, Goto Y, Mitsuoka C, Zwirner J, Soruri A, von Kietzell M, Rieber E. 6-Sulfo LacNAc, a novel carbohydrate modification of PSGL-1, defines an inflammatory type of human dendritic cells. Immunity. 2002;17:289.

Schäfer T. Evidence-based Medicine (EBM) und Allergie-Prävention. Gibt es Evidenzbasierte Empfeh-lungen zur Prävention allergischer Krankheiten? Allergo J. 2002;11:312–9.

Schäfer T, Ring J. The possible role of environmental pollution in the development of atopic dermatitis. In: Williams HC, editor. Atopic dermatitis. Cambridge: Cambridge University Press; 2000. p. 155–68.

Schäfer T, Przybilla B, Ring J, Kunz B, Greif A, Überla K. Manifestation of atopy is not related to patients' month of birth. Allergy. 1993;48:291–4.

Schäfer T, Vieluf D, Behrendt H, Krämer U, Ring J. Atopic eczema and other manifestations of atopy: results of a study in East and West Germany. Allergy. 1996;51:532–9.

Schäfer T, Dirschedl P, Kunz B, Ring J, Überla K. Maternal smoking during pregnancy and lactation increases the risk for atopic eczema in the offspring. J Am Acad Dermatol. 1997a;36: 550–6.

Schäfer T, Nienhaus A, Haupt G, Vieluf D, Nagel S, Berger J, Ring J. Befunde der Hautuntersuchung und allergologischen Diagnostik. In: Epidemiologische Untersuchungsprogramm Bille-Siedlung, Behörde für Arbeit, Gesundheit und Soziales (BAGS) der Freien und Hansestadt Hamburg (Hrsg.), Bd. 1. Frankfurt/Berlin/Bern/New York/Paris/Wien: Peter Lang; 1997b.

Schäfer T, Vieluf D, Berger J, Ring J. Epidemiologie von Insektengiftallergien. Allergo J. 1997c;6:4–6.

Schäfer T, Heinrich J, Wjst M, Krause C, Adam H, Ring J, Wichmann HE. Indoor risk factors of atopic eczema in school children from East Germany. Environ Res. 1999;81:151–8.

Schäfer T, Staudt A, Ring J. Entwicklung des Deutschen Instruments zur Erfassung der Lebensqualität bei Hauterkrankungen (DIELH). Hautarzt. 2001;52: 492–8.

Schäfer T, Riehle A, Wichmann HE, Ring J. Alternative medicine in allergies – prevalence, patterns of use, and costs. Allergy. 2002;57:694–700.

Schäfer T, Krämer U, Behrendt H, Ring J. Epidemiologie des atopischen Ekzems. Allergo J. 2003a;12:430–8.

Schäfer T, Ruhdorfer S, Weigl L, Wesner D, Heinrich J, Döring A, Wichmann HE, Ring J. Intake of unsaturated fatty acid and HDL cholesterol levels are associated with manifestations of atopy in adults. Clin Exp Allergy. 2003b;33:1360–7.

Schäfer T, Borowski C, Diepgen T, et al. Evidenz-basierte und konsentierte Leitlinie "Allergieprävention". Allergo J. 2004a;13:252–60.

Schäfer T, Hölscher B, Ring J, Wichmann E, Heinrich J. Worm infestations reduce the risk for atopic eczema. Allergo J. 2004b;13:527–30 [in German].

Schäfer T, Merkl J, Klemm E, Wichmann HE, Ring J. We and our pets: allergic together? Acta Vet Hung (Separatum). 2008;56:153–61.

Schauber J, Dorschner RA, Coda AB, Büchau AS, Liu PT, Kiken D, et al. Injury enhances TLR2 function and antimicrobial peptide expression through a vitamin D-dependent mechanism. J Clin Invest. 2007;117:803–11.

Schauber J, Gallo RL. Antimicrobial peptides and the skin immune system. JACL. 2008;122:261–6.

Scheewe S, Warschburger P, Clausen K, Skusa-Freemann B, Petermann F. Neurodermitis-Verhaltenstrainings für Kinder, Jugendliche und Eltern. Munich: MMW-Quintessenz; 1997.

Schempp C, Emde M, Wölfle U. Dermatology in the Darwin anniversary. Part 1: evolution of the integument. J Dtsch Dermatol Ges. 2009;7:750–8.

Scheynius A, Johansson C, Buentke E, Zargari A, Linder MT. Atopic eczema/dermatitis syndrome and Malassezia. Int Arch Allergy Immunol. 2002;127:161–9.

Schlaud M, Atzpodien K, Thierfelder W. Allergic diseases. Results from the German Health Interview and Examination Survey for Children and Adolescents (KiGGS). Bundesgesundheitsblatt Gesundheitsforschung Gesundheitsschutz. 2007;50:701–10.

Schmid-Grendelmeier P, Simon D, Simon HU, Akdis CA, Wüthrich B. Epidemiology, clinical features, and immunology of the "intrinsic" (non-IgE-mediated) type of atopic dermatitis (constitutional dermatitis). Allergy. 2001;56:841–9.

Schmid-Grendelmeier P, Fischer B, Wüthrich B. IgE to Malassezia furfur/M. sympodialis. A serologic marker for the atopic eczema/dermatitis syndrome? Allergy Clin Immunol Int. 2002;14:140–2.

Schmid-Grendelmeier P, Doe P, Pakenham-Walsh N. Teledermatology in sub-Saharan Africa. Curr Probl Dermatol. 2003;32:233–46.

Schmidt T, Abeck D, Boeck K, Mempel M, Ring J. UVA1 irradiation is effective in treatment of chronic vesicular dyshidrotic hand eczema. Acta Derm Venereol. 1998;78:318–9.

Schmidt-Ott G, Kuensebeck HW, Jaeger B, Werfel T, Frahm K, Ruitman J, Kapp A, Lamprecht F. Validity study fort he stigmatisation experience in atopic dermatitis and psoriasis patients. Acta Derm Venereol. 1999;79:443–7.

Schmidt-Ott G, Burchard R, Neiderauer HH, Lambrecht F, Kunsebeck HW. Stigmatisation and quality of life of patients with psoriasis and atopic dermatitis. Hautarzt. 2003;54:852–7.

Schminke LF, Sawalle-Belohradsky J, Roesler J, Wollenberg A, Rack A, Borte M, et al. Diagnostic approach to the hyper-IgE syndrome: immunologic and clinical key findings to differentiate hyper-IgE syndrome from atopic dermatitis. J Allergy Clin Immunol. 2010;126:611–7.

Schmitt J, Meurer M, Klon M, Frick KD. Assessment of health state utilities of controlled and uncontrolled psoriasis and atopic eczema – a population-based study. Br J Dermatol. 2007a;158:351–9.

Schmitt J, Schmitt N, Meurer M. Cyclosporin in the treatment of patients with atopic eczema – a systematic review and meta-analysis. J Eur Acad Dermatol Venereol. 2007b;21:606–19.

Schmitt J, Csotonyi F, Bauer A, Meurer M. Determinants of treatment goals and satisfaction of patients with atopic eczema. J Dtsch Dermatol Ges. 2008;6: 458–65.

Schmitt J, Romanos M, Pfennig A, Leopold K, Meurer M. Psychiatric comorbidity in adult eczema. Br J Dermatol. 2009a;161:878–83.

Schmitt J, Romanos M, Schmitt NM, Meurer M, Kirch W. Atopic eczema and attention-deficit/hyperactivity disorder in a population-based sample of children and adolescents. JAMA. 2009b;301:724–6.

Schmitt J, Kirch W, Meurer M. Effects of the introduction of the German "Praxisgebühr" on outpatient care and treatment of patients with atopic eczema. J Dtsch Dermatol Ges. 2009c;7:879–87.

Schmitt J, Apfelbacher C, Chen CM, Romanos M, Sausenthaler S, Koletzko S, Bauer CP, Hoffmann U, Krämer U, Berdel D, von Berg A, Wichmann HE, Heinrich J. Infant eczema, infant sleeping problems, and mental health at 10 years of age: the prospective birth cohort study (German Infant Nutrition Intervention plus). J Allergy Clin Immunol. 2010;125:404–10.

Schmoeckel C, von Liebe V. [Acneiform exanthema caused by azathioprine] (Article in German). Hautarzt. 1983;34:413–5.

Schneider I, Harangi F, Sebök B. Clinical and pathological aspects of atopic dermatitis. Budapest: Akademiai Kiado; 2011.

Schnopp C, Ring J. Therapiestrategien bei atopischem Ekzem. J Med. 2003;3/4:16–20.

Schnopp C, Holtmann C, Stock S, et al. Topical steroids under wet-wrap dressings in atopic dermatitis – a vehicle-controlled trial. Dermatology. 2002;204: 56–9.

Schnopp C, Grosch J, Ring J, Ollert M, Mempel M. Microbial allergen-specific IgE is not suitable to identify the intrinsic form of atopic eczema in children. J Allergy Clin Immunol. 2008;121: 267–9.

Schnuch A, Uter W, Reich K. Allergic contact dermatitis and atopic eczema. In: Ring J, Przybilla B, Ruzicka T, editors. Handbook of atopic eczema. 2nd ed. Berlin/New York/Tokio: Springer; 2006. p. 178–201.

Schnyder UW. Neurodermitis – Asthma – Rhinitis. Eine genetisch-allergologische Studie. Suppl ad Acta Genetica et Statistica vol 10; Int Arch Allergy. 1960; 17: (keine Seitenangabe).

Schnyder UW, Borelli S. Neurodermitis constitutionalis sive atopica. In: Miescher G, Storck H, editors. Entzündliche Dermatosen I, Handbuch der Haut-und Geschlechtskrankheiten, vol. 2/1. Berlin/Heidelberg/New York: Springer; 1962. p. 228.

Schnyder UW, Klunker W. Über das phänotypische familienpathologische Verhalten der Atopien. Hautarzt. 1957;8:510–1.

Schoenecker I, Grübl A, Bartels P, Ulm K, Bauer CP. Klinische Effekte der Allergenreduktion durch Encasing – eine Metaanalyse. Allergo J. 2001;10: 95–9.

Schöni MH, Nikolaizik WH, Schöni-Afolter F. Efficacy trial of bioresonance in children with atopic dermatitis. Int Arch Allergy Immunol. 1997;112:238–46.

Schöpf E, Mueller JM, Ostermann T. Stellenwert der adjuvanten Basistherpaie bei chronisch-rezidivierenden Hauterkrankungen. Neurodermitis atopica/Psoriasis vulgaris. Hautarzt. 1995;46:451–4.

Schram ME, Roekevisch E, Leeflang MMG, Bos JD, Schmitt J, Spuls PI. A randomized trial of methotrexate versus azathioprine for severe atopic eczema. J Allergy Clin Immunol. 2011;128:353–9.

Schuh A, Nowak D. Evidence-based acute and long-lasting effects of climatotherapy in moderate altitudes and on the seaside. Dtsch Med Wochenschr. 2011;136:135–9.

Schuh A, Kneist W, Schnizer W, Senn E, Streicher U. Änderungen der Schweiß- und peripheren Durchblutungsregulation. Hautnah. 1989;1:57–8.

Schultz Larsen F. Atopic dermatitis: a genetic-epidemiologic study in a population-based twin sample. J Am Acad Dermatol. 1993;28:719–23.

Schultz Larsen F, Hanifin JM. Secular change in the occurrence of atopic dermatitis. Acta Derm Vernereol Suppl. 1992;176:7–12.

Schultz Larsen FV, Holm NV. Atopic dermatitis in a population based twin series. Concordance rates and heritability estimation. Acta Derm Venereol Suppl. 1985;114:159.

Schultz Larsen F, Holm NV, Henningsen K. Atopic dermatitis. A genetic-epidemiologic study in a population-based twin sample. J Am Acad Dermatol. 1986;15:487–94.

Schultz-Larsen F. Atopic eczma. Etiological studies based on a twin population. Dissertation, Legefo-reningens, Copenhagen; 1985.

Schultze-Werninghaus G. Should asthma management include sojourns at high mountain altitude? Chem Immunol Allergy. 2006;91:16–29.

Schut C, Weik U, Tews N, Gieler U, Deinzer R, Kupfer J. Psychophysiological effects of stress management in patients with atopic dermatitis: a randomized controlled trial. Acta Derm Venereol. 2013;93:57–61.

Schwanitz HJ. Diagnostik und Therapie von Handekzemen. Dtsch Med Wochenschr. 1992;117:343–8.

Seidenari S, Belletti B, Schinri ME. Skin reactivity to sodium lauryl sulfate in patients with respiratory atopy. J Am Acad Dermatol. 1996;35:47–52.

Selye H. A Syndrome Produced by Diverse Nocuous Agents. Nature. 1936;113:32.

Sheehan MP, Atherton DJ. A controlled trial of traditional Chinese medicinal plants in wide-spread non-exudative atopic eczema. Br J Dermatol. 1992;126:179–84.

Shenefelt PD. Hypnosis in dermatology. Arch Dermatol. 2000;136:393–9.

Sidbury R, Hanifin JM. Systemic therapy of atopic dermatitis. Clin Exp Dermatol. 2000;25:559–66.

Siebenwirth J, Lüdtke R, Remy W, Rakoski J, Borelli S, Ring J. Wirksamkeit von klassisch-homöopathischer Therapie bei atopischem Ekzem. Forsch Komplement Med. 2009;16:315–23.

Sigurgeirsson B, Boznanski A, Todd G, Vertruyen A, Schuttelaar ML, Zhu X, et al. Safety and efficacy of pimecrolimus in atopic dermatitis: a 5-year randomized trial. Pediatrics. 2015;135:597–606.

Silberberg I, Baer I, Rosenthal SA. The role of Langerhans cells in contact allergy. I. An ultrastructural study in actively induced contact dermatitis in guinea pigs. Acta Derm Venereol. 1974;54:321–31.

Silny W, Czarnecka-Operacz M. Spezifische Immuntherapie bei der Behandlung von Patienten mit atopischer Dermatitis. Ergebnisse einer placebokontrollierten Doppelblindstudie. Allergologie. 2006;29:171–83.

Simon FA. The allergen of human dander present in the skin of the general body surface. J Invest Dermatol. 1947;9:329–32.

Simon D, Braathen LR, Simon HU. Eosinophils and atopic dermatitis. Allergy. 2003;59:561–70.

Simon D, Hösli S, Kostylina G, Yawalkar N, Simon HU. Anti-CD20 (rituximab) treatment improves atopic eczema. J Allergy Clin Immunol. 2008;121:122–8.

Simon D, Bieber T. Systemic therapy of atopic dermatitis. Allergy. 2014;69:46–55.

Simons E. Drug therapy. Advances in H1-antihistamines. N Engl J Med. 2004;351:2203–17.

Simons FER, Johnston L, Simons KJ. Clinical pharmacology of the H1-receptor antagonists cetirizine and loratadine in children. Pediatr Allergy Immunol. 2000;11:116–9.

Simpson EL, Chalmers JR, Hanifin JM, Thomas KS, Cork MJ, McLean WH, et al. Emollient enhancement of the skin barrier from birth offers effective atopic dermatitis prevention. J Allergy Clin Immunol. 2014;134:818–23.

Skudlik C, Schöne D, Disch R. Klimatherapie. Allergologie. 1999;22:12–4.

Skudlik C, Weisshaar E, Wulfhorst B, et al. Multi-Center-Studie "Medizinisch-Berufliches Rehabilitationsverfahren Haut – Optimierung und Qualitätssicherung des Heilverfahrens (ROQ)" – Konzeption und Einbindung in das Stufenverfahren Haut. J Dtsch Dermatol Ges. 2009;7:122–6.

Smith FJ, Irvine AD, Terron-Kwiatkowski A, et al. Loss-of-function mutations in the gene encoding filaggrin cause ichthyosis vulgaris. Nat Genet. 2006;38:337–42.

Sokel B, Kent CA, Lansdown R, Atherton D, Glover M, Knibbs J. A comparison of hypnotherapy and biofeedback in the treatment of childhood atopic eczema. Contemp Hypnosis. 1993;10:70–5.

Sonkoly E, Muller A, Lauerma AI, Pivarcsi A, Soto H, Kemeny L, Alenius H, Dieu-Nosjean MC, Meller S, Rieker J, Steinhoff M, Hoffmann TK, Ruzicka T, Zlotnik A, Homey B. IL-31: a new link between T cells and pruritus in atopic skin inflammation. J Allergy Clin Immunol. 2006;117:411–7.

Soumelis V, Liu YJ. Human thymic stromal lymphopoietin: a novel epithelial cell-derived cytokine and a potential key player in the induction of allergic inflammation. Springer Semin Immunopathol. 2004;25:325–33.

Staab D, Diepgen TL, Fartasch M, Kupfer J, Lob-Corzilius T, Ring J, Scheewe S, Scheidt R, Schmid-Ott G, Schnopp C, Szczepanski R, Werfel T, Wittenmeier M, Wahn U, Gieler W. Age related, structured educational programmes for the management of atopic dermatitis in children and adolescents: multicentre, randomised controlled trial. BMJ. 2006;332:933–8.

Stachow R. Neurodermitis (atopische Dermatitis) Leitlinie der Fachgesellschaft Rehabilitation in der Kinder- und Jugendmedizin. AWMF-Leitlinie – Register Nr. 070/005, letzte Überarbeitung; 2002.

Stalder JF, Sourisse M. La dermatite atopique et l'infection staphylococcique. Ann Dermatol Venereol. 1989;16:341–5.

Stalder JF, Fleury M, Sourisse M, et al. Comparative effects of two topical antiseptics (chlorhexidine vs KMn04) on bacterial skin flora in atopic dermatitis. Acta Derm Venereol Suppl. 1992;176:132–4.

Stalder F, Taïeb A, ETFAD. Severity scoring of atopic dermatitis: the SCORACD index. Consensus Report of the European Task Force on Atopic Dermatitis. Dermatology. 1993;186:23–31.

Stalder JF, Bernier C, Ball A, De Raeve L, Gieler U, Deleuran M, Marcoux D, Eichenfield LF, Lio P, Lewis-Jones S, Gelmetti C, Takaoka R, Chiaverini C, Misery L, Barbarot S, Oriented Patient-Education Network in Dermatology (OPENED). Therapeutic patient education in atopic dermatitis: worldwide experiences. Pediatr Dermatol. 2013;30(3):329–34.

Ständer M. Ein neuer Weg der Psoriasisbehandlung: Die Thermalsole Phototherapie (TSPT). Dtsch Derm. 1976;36:149–53.

Ständer S, Zeidler C, Magnolo N, Raap U, Mettang T, Kremer AE, Weisshaar E, Augustin M. Clinical management of pruritus. J Dtsch Dermatol Ges. 2015;13:101–15.

Ständer S, Schäfer I, Phan NQ, Blome C, Herberger K, Heigel H, Augustin M. Prevalence of chronic pruritus in Germany: results of a cross-sectional study in a sample working population of 11,730. Dermatology. 2010;221:229–35.

Stangier U. Hautkrankheiten und körperdysmorphe Störung. Fortschritte der Psychotherapie. Göttingen: Hogrefe; 2001.

Stangier U, Gieler U, Ehlers A. Autogenes Training bei Neurodermitis. Z Allgemeinmed. 1992;68: 392–400.

Stangier U, Gieler U, Ehlers A. Neurodermitis bewältigen. Verhaltenstherapie, dermatologische Schulung, autogenes Training. Berlin: Springer; 1996.

Stauder A, Kovacs M. Anxiety symptoms in allergic patients: Identification and risk factors. Psychosom Med. 2003;65:816–23.

Staudt A, Ring J, Schäfer T. Deutsches Instrument zur Erfassung der Lebensmittelqualität bei Hauter-krankungen (DIELH) – Analyse nach Erkrankungsgruppen und Domänen. Allergo J. 2002;11:445–6.

Steinhoff M, Neisius U, Ikoma A, Fartasch M, Heyer G, Skov S, et al. Proteinase-activated receptor-2 mediates itch: a novel pathway for pruritus in human skin. J Neurosci. 2003;23:6176–80.

Steinke M, Fiocchi A, Kirchlechner V, et al. Perceived food allergy in children in 10 European nations. A randomized telephone survey. Int Arch Allergy Immunol. 2007;143:290–5.

Stickl H, Hochstein-Mintzel V, Mayr A, Huber HC, Schafer H, Holzner A. MVA vaccination against smallpox: clinical tests with an attenuated live vaccinia virus strain (MVA) (author's translation). Dtsch Med Wochenschr. 1974;99:2386–92.

Stiftung Warentest (Hrsg.). Handbuch Die andere Medizin. Nutzen und Risiken sanfter Heilmethoden. Berlin: Stiftung Warentest; 1994.

Stingl G, Wolff-Schreiner EC, Pickler WJ, Gschnait F, Knapp W, Wolff K. Epidermal Langerhans call bear Fc and C3 receptors. Nature. 1977;268:245.

Stingl G, Katz SI, Klement L, Green I, Shevach EM. Immunological functions of Ia bearing epidermal Langerhans cells. J Immunol. 1978;121:2005–13.

Storm van Leeuwen W, Bien Z, Varekamp H. Über die Hautreaktion mit Extrakten menschlicher Kopfhautschuppen bei allergischen Krankheiten. Klin Wochenschr. 1926;5:1023–5.

Strachan DP. Hay fever, hygiene, and household size. BMJ. 1989;299:1259–60.

Strachan DP. Allergy and family size: a riddle worth solving. Clin Exp Allergy. 1997;27:235–6.

Stuetz A, Grassberger M, Meingassner JG. Pimecrolimus (Elidel, SDZ ASM 981) preclinical pharmacologic profile and skin selectivity. Semin Cutan Med Surg. 2001;20:233–41.

Suárez AL, Feramisco JD, Koo J, Steinhoff M. Psychoneuroimmunology of psychological stress and atopic dermatitis: pathophysiologic and therapeutic updates. Acta Derm Venereol. 2012;92:7–15.

Suarez-Farinas M, Dhingra N, Gittler J, Shemer A, Cardinale I, de Guzman Strong C, Krueger Y, Guttman-Yassky E. Intrinsic atopic dermatitis shows similar Th2 and higher Th17 immune activation compared with extrinsic atopic dermatitis. J Allergy Clin Immunol. 2013;132:361–70.

Suetonius Gaius Tranquillus. De vita caesarum. Libri VIII. Ihm M, editor. Editio minor. Stuttgart: Teubner; 1958.

Sugiura H, Maeda T, Uehara M. Mast cell invasion of peripheral nerve in skin lesions of atopic dermatitis. Acta Derm Venereol. 1992;90:613–22.

Sulzberger MB, Witten VH. The effect of topically applied compound F in selected dermatoses. J Invest Dermatol. 1952;19:101–2.

Sun XD, You Y, Zhang L, Zheng S, Hong Y, Li J, Gao XH. The possible role of TRPC6 in atopic dermatitis. Med Hypotheses. 2012;78:42–4.

Susitaival P, Hannuksela M. The 12-year prognosis of hand dermatosis in 896 Finnish farmers. Contact Dermatitis. 1995;32:233–7.

Synnerstad I, Fredrikson M, Ternesten-Bratel A, Rosdahl I. Low risk of melanoma in patients with atopic dermatitis. J Eur Acad Dermatol Venereol. 2008;22(12): 1423–8. doi:10.1111/j.1468-3083.2008.02888.x. Epub 2008 Aug 14.

Szczepanowska J, Reich A, Szepietowski JC. Emollients improve treatment results with topical corticosteroids in childhood atopic dermatitis: a randomized comparative study. Pediatr Allergy Immunol. 2008;19: 614–8.

Szczepanski R, Gebert N, Hümmelink R, Könning J, Schmidt S, Runde B, Wahn U. Ergebnis einer strukturierten Asthmaschulung im Kindes- und Jugendalter. Pneumologie. 1996;50:544–8.

Szentivanyi A. The beta adrenergic theory of the atopic abnormality in bronchial asthma. J Allergy. 1968;42:203–32.

Szentivanyi A, Heim O, Schultze P, Szentivanyi J. Adrenoceptor binding studies with 3 H (dihydroalprenolol) and 3 h (dihydroergocryptine) on membranes of lymphocytes from patients with atopic disease. Acta Derm Venerol (Stockh). 1980;92:19–21.

Tada T. Regulation of reaginic antibodies information in animals. Prog Allergy. 1975;19:122.

Tada T, Kubo S, Nakayama T. Self-tolerance: multiple strategies for peripheral unresponsiveness of T cell. In: Ring J, Behrendt H, Vieluf D, editors. New trends in allergy IV. Berlin/New York: Springer; 1997. p. 359–64.

Taïeb A. Hypothesis: from epidermal barrier dysfunction to atopic disorders. Contact Dermatitis. 1999;41:177–80.

Taïeb A, et al. Dermatite atopique. In: Wallach D, Tilles G, editors. Histoire de la Dermatologie en France. Toulouse: Privat; 2002.

Talbot FB. Eczema in childhood. Med Clinics North Am. 1918;1:985–6.
Tan BB, Weald D, Strickland I, Friedmann PS. Double-blind controlled trial of effect of housedust-mite allergen avoidance on atopic dermatitis. Lancet. 1996;347:15–8.
Tan HT, Ellis JA, Koplin JJ, Matheson MC, Gurrin LC, Lowe AJ, Martin PE, Dang TD, Wake M, Tang ML, Ponsonby AL, Dharmage SC, Allen KJ. Filaggrin loss-of-function mutations do not predict food allergy over and above the risk of food sensitization among infants. Allergy Clin Immunol. 2012;130:1211–3.
Tanaka Y, Anan S, Yoshida H. Immunohistochemical studies in mite antigen-induced patch test sites in atopic dermatitis. J Dermatol Sci. 1990;1:361–8.
Tanaka A, Arita K, Lai-Cheong JE, Palisson F, Hide M, McGrath JA. New insight into mechanisms of pruritus from molecular studies on familial primary localized cutaneous amyloidosis. Br J Dermatol. 2009;161: 1217–24.
Temime P, Oddoze L. La chéilite exfoliatrice et la pulpite digitale keratosique craquelée récidivante peuvent être des manifestations atopiques. Bull Soc Fr Dermatol Syphiligr. 1970;77:150–6.
Tengvall Linder M, Johansson C, Scheynius A, Wahlgren C. Positive atopy patch test reactions to Pityrosporum orbiculare in atopic dermatitis patients. Clin Exp Allergy. 2000;30:122–31.
Terada N, Hamano N, Maesako KI, et al. Diesel exhaust particulates upregulate histamine receptor mRNA and increase histamine-induced IL-8 and GM-CSF production in nasal epithelial cells and en-dothelial cells. Clin Exp Allergy. 1999;29:52–9.
Terhoorst D, Kalali BN, Ollert M, Ring J, Mempel M. The role of toll-like receptors in host defenses and their relevance to dermatologic diseases. Am J Clin Dermatol. 2010;11:1–10.
Tey HL, Yosipovitch G. Itch in ethnic populations. Acta Derm Venereol. 2010;90:227–34.
Thijs J, Krastev T, Weidinger S, Buckens CF, de Bruin-Weller M, Bruijnzeel-Koomen C, Flohr C, Hijnen D. Biomarkers for atopic dermatitis: a systematic review and meta-analysis. Curr Opin Allergy Clin Immunol. 2015;15(5): 453–60. doi:10.1097/ACI.0000000000000198.
Thoma K. Topical vehicles: composition, principles of application and action. In: Ruzicka T, Ring J, Przybilla B, editors. Handbook of atopic eczema. Berlin/Heidelberg/New York: Springer; 1991. p. 364–74.
Thomas KS, Dean T, Gilbert C, Sach TH, Koller K, Frost A, Williams HC; the SWET Trial Team. A randomized controlled trial of ion-exchange water softeners for the treatment of eczema in children (ISRCTN: 71423189). PLoS Med 2011;8:e1000395.
Thum D, Seidl HP, Hein R, Ring J, Andres C, Mempel M. Current resistance patterns of Staphylococcus aureus towards topical antibiotics and relevant antiseptics in patients with atopic dermatitis and impetigo. J Dtsch Dermatol Ges. 2013;11:875–8.
Thyssen JP, Carlsen BC, Johansen JD, Meldgaard M, Szecsi PB, Stender S, Menné T. Filaggrin null-mutations may be associated with a distinct subtype of atopic hand eczema. Acta Derm Venereol. 2010;90:528.
Thyssen JP. The association between filaggrin mutations, hand eczema and contact dermatitis: a clear picture is emerging. Br J Dermatol. 2012;167:1197–8.
Tokura Y. Extrinsic and intrinsic types of atopic dermatitis. J Dermatol Sci. 2010;58:1–7.
Traidl-Hoffmann C, Mariani V, Hochrein H, et al. Pollen-associated phytoprostanes inhibit dendritic cell IL12 production and augment helper type II cell polarization. J Exp Med. 2005;201:627–36.
Traidl-Hoffmann C, Münster I, Ring J, Behrendt H. Impact of desloratadine on the crosstalk between human keratinocytes and leukocytes: implications for anti-inflammatory activity of antihistamines. Int Arch Allergy Immunol. 2006;140:315–20.
Traidl-Hoffmann C, Jakob T, Behrendt H. Determinants of allergenicity. J Allergy Clin Immunol. 2009;123: 558–66.
Trautmann A, Akdis M, Kleemann D, Altznauer F, Simon HU, Graeve T, Noll M, Bröcker EB, Blaser K, Akdis CA. T cell-mediated Fas-induced keratinocyte apoptosis plays a key pathogenetic role in eczematous dermatitis. J Clin Invest. 2000;106:25–35.
Troncone R, Merrett TG, Ferguson A. Prevalence of atopy is unrelated to presence of inflammatory bowel disease. Clin Allergy. 1988;18(2):111–7.
Tudhope SJ, Catley MC, Fenwick PS, et al. The role of I[kappa]B Kinase 2, but not activation of NF[kappa]B, in the release of CXCR3 ligands from IFN-[gamma]-stimulated human bronchial epithelial cells. J Immunol. 2007;179:6237–45.
Tuft LA. Importance of inhalant allergen in atopic dermatitis. J Invest Dermatol. 1949;12:211–9.
Tupker RA, De Monchy JG, Coenraads PJ, Homan A, van der Meer JB. Induction of atopic dermatitis by inhalation of house dust mite. J Allergy Clin Immunol. 1996;97:1064–70.
Turpenen M. Absorption of hydrocortisone from the skin reservoir in atopic dermatitis. Br J Dermatol. 1991;124:358–60.
Überla K, Dirschedl P, Gries A, Kunz B, Letzel H, Oed I, Ring J, Schotten K, Stickl H, Vogl-Voswinckel AE. Die Innenraumbelastung mit SO2 und NOx, allergische Symptome und die Keimbesiedelung der Gaumenmandeln bei 5-6jährigen. Projektbericht der Arbeitsgruppe "Gesundheitsmonitoring in der Oberpfalz". Inst. f. Med. Informationsverarbeitung, Biometrie und Epidemiologie, Munich; 1988
UCB, Institute of Allergy. Allergic diseases as a public health problem. Brussels: European Allergy White Paper; 1997.
Uehara M. Infraorbital fold in atopic dermatitis. Arch Dermatol. 1981;117:627–9.
Uehara M. Clinical and histological features of dry skin in atopic dermatitis. Acta Derm Venereol. 1985;114:82–6.
Uehara M, Kimura C. Descendant family history of atopic dermatitis. Acta Derm Venereol. 1993;73:62–3.

Uehara M, Ofuji S. Patch test reaction to human dander in atopic dermatitis. Arch Dermatol. 1976;112: 151–4.

Uehara M, Sawai T. A longitudinal study of contact sensitivity in patients with atopic dermatitis. Arch Dermatol. 1989;125:366–8.

Uehara M, Amemiya T, Arai M. Atopic cataracts in a Japanese population. Dermatologica. 1995;170:180.

Uehara M, Sugiura H, Omoto M. Paternal and maternal atopic dermatitis have the same influence on development of the disease in children. Acta Derm Venereol. 1999;79:235.

Undre NA, Moloney FJ, Ahmadi S, Stevenson P, Murphy GM. Skin and systematic pharmacokinetics of tacrolimus following topical application of tacrolimus ointment in adults with moderate to severe atopic dermatitis. Br J Dermatol. 2009;160:665–9.

Urbach E. Klinik und Therapie der allergischen Krankheiten. Wien: Maudrich; 1939.

Valenta R, Seiberler S, Natter S, Mahler V, Mossabeb R, Ring J, Stingl G. Autoallergy: a pathogenetic factor in atopic dermatitis? J Allergy Clin Immunol. 2000;105:432–7.

Van Bever HP, Docx M, Stevens WJ. Food and food additives in severe atopic dermatitis. Allergy. 1989;44: 588–94.

van den Bogaard EH, Bergboer JG, Vonk-Bergers M, van Vlijmen-Willems IM, Hato SV, van der Valk PG, Schröder JM, Joosten I, Zeeuwen PL, Schalkwijk J. Coal tar induces AHR-dependent skin barrier repair in atopic dermatitis. J Clin Invest. 2013;123(2): 917–27.

van Leeuwen S. Allergische Krankheiten, Asthma Bronchioli, Heufieber, Urticaria und Andere. Berlin: Springer; 1926.

Van Reijsen FC, Bruijnzeel-Koomen CA, Kalthoff FS, et al. Skin-derived aeroallergen-specific T-cell clones of Th2 phenotype in patients with atopic dermatitis. J Allergy Clin Immunol. 1992;90(2):184–93.

Vandenplas Y, Hauser B, van den Borre C, et al. The long-term effect of a partial whey hydrolysate formula on the prophylaxis of atopic disease. Eur J Pediatr. 1995;154:488.494.

Vanslow NA, Yamate M, Adams MS, Callies Q, Arbor A. The increased prevalence of atopic diseases in anhidrotic congenital ectodermal dysplasia. J Allergy. 1970;45:302–9.

Verbow J. Juvenile plantar dermatosis (JPD). Acta Derm Venereol Suppl. 1989;144:153–4.

Verbow J, Hart A. Severe varicella in a child with atopic eczema and ichthyosis. Practitioner. 1986;230:15–6.

Vercelli D. Discovering susceptibility genes for asthma and allergy. Nat Rev Immunol. 2008;8:169–82.

Verhagen J, Akdis M, Traidl-Hoffmann C, Schmid-Grendelmeier P, Hijnen DJ, Knol EF, Behrendt H, Blaser K, Akdis C. Absence of T-regulatory cell expression and function in atopic dermatitis skin. Allergy Clin Immunol. 2006;117:1176–83.

Verhoef CM, van Roon JA, Vianen ME, Bruijnzeel-Koomen CA, Lafeber FP, Bijlsma JW. Mutual antagonism of rheumatoid arthritis and hay fever; a role for type 1/type 2 T cell balance. Ann Rheum Dis. 1998;57:275–80.

Verhoeven EW, de Klerk S, Kraaimaat FW, van de Kerkhof PC, de Jong EM, Evers AM. Biopsychosocial mechanisms of chronic itch in patients with skin diseases: a review. Acta Derm Venereol. 2008;88:211–8.

Vickers CF. The natural history of atopic eczema. Its incidence and course. Acta Derm Venereol (Stockh). 1980;92:113–5.

Vickers CFH. The natural history of atopic eczema. Acta Derm Venereol Suppl (Stockh). 1989;92:113–5.

Vieluf D, Korting HC, Braun-Falco O, Belohradsky BH. Eczematous skin lesions in X-linked immunodeficiency with hyper-IgM. In: Fritsch P, Schuler G, Hintner H, editors. Immunodeficiency and skin, Current problems in dermatology, vol. 18. Basel: Karger; 1989. p. 60–5.

Vieluf D, Kunz B, Bieber T, Przybilla B, Ring J. "Atopy patch test" with aeroallergens in patients with atopic eczema. Allergo J. 1993;2:9–12.

Vieluf D, Wieben A, Ring J. Oral provocation tests with food additives in atopic eczema. Int Arch Allergy Immunol. 1999;118:232–3.

Vieths S, Holzhauser T, Erdmann S, et al. Neue Deklarationspflicht für Nahrungsmittelallergene in Lebensmitteln – Stellungnahme der Arbeitsgruppe Nahrungsmittelallergie der Deutschen Gesellschaft für Allergologie und Klinische Immunologie und des Ärzteverbandes Deutscher Allergologen. Allergo J. 2006;15:114–23.

Vigo PG, Girgis KR, Pfuetze BL, Critchlow ME, Fisher J, Hussain I. Efficacy of anti-IgE therapy in patients with atopic dermatitis. J Am Acad Dermatol. 2006;55(1): 168–70.

Vocks E, Borelli S, Rakoski J. Climatotherapy in atopic dermatitis. Allergologie. 1994;17:208–13.

Vocks E, Borelli S, Busch R, Düngemann H, Ring J. Biometrische Studie zur Wetterabhängigkeit und Wetterempfindlichkeit beim atopischen Ekzem. Act Dermatol. 2002;28:363–9.

von Berg A, Koletzko S, Gruebl A, et al. The effect of hydrolysed cow's milk formula for allergy prevention in the first year of life: The German Infant Nutritional Intervention Study, a randomized double-blind trial. J Allergy Clin Immunol. 2003;111:533–40.

von Berg A, Filipiak-Pittroff B, Krämer U, et al. Preventive effect of hydrolyzed infant formula persists until age 6 years: Long-term results from the German Infant Nutritional Intervention Study (GINI). Allergy Clin Immuno. 2008;121:1442–7.

Von Buboff D, Bausinger H, Matz H, Koch S, Hacker G, Takikawa O, Bieber T, Hanau D, de la Salle H. Human epidermal langerhans cells express the immunoregulatory enzyme indoleamine 2,3-dioxygenase. J Invest Dermatol. 2004;123:298.

von Ehrenstein OS, von Mutius E, Ili S, Baumann L, Bohm O, von Kries R. Reduced risk of hay fever and asthma among children of farmers. Clin Exp Allergy. 2000;30:187–90.

von Eiff AW. Psychologie und Klinikstress. Therapiewoche. 1984;34:S7192–6.

Von Hertzen L, Haahtela T. Prevention of allergic diseases. In: Pawankar R et al., editors. Allergy frontiers: therapy and prevention. Berlin/New York/Tokio: Springer; 2010. p. 447–64.

Von Kobyletzki G, Freitag M, Herde M, Hoxtermann S, Stucker M, Hoffmann K, Altmeyer P. Photo-therapy of atopic dermatitis: comparison between conventional UVA1 phototherapy, UVA1 cold light phototherapy and combined UVA-UVB phototherapy. Hautarzt. 1999;50(1):27–33.

von Mutius E, Vercelli D. Farm living: effects on childhood asthma and allergy. Nat Rev Immunol. 2010;10:861–86.

von Mutius E, Martinez FD, Fritzsch C, et al. Prevalence of asthma and atopy in two areas of West and East Germany. Am J Respir Crit Care Med. 1994a;49:358–64.

von Mutius E, Martinez FD, Fritzsch C, Nicolai T, Reitmeir P, Thiemann HH. Skin test reactivity and number of siblings. Br Med J. 1994b;308:692–5.

von Mutius E, Weiland SK, Fritzsch C, Duhmen H, Keil U. Increasing prevalence of hay fever and atopy among children in Leipzig, East Germany. Lancet. 1998;351:862–6.

von Mutius E, Braun-Fahrländer C, Schierl R, Riedler J, Ehlermann S, Maisch S, Waser M, Nowak D. Exposure to endotoxin or other bacterial components might protect against the development of atopy. Clin Exp Allergy. 2000;30:1230–4.

Von Pirquet C. Allergy. MünchMed Wschr. 1906; 30:1457–8.

von Sonnenburg F, Perona P, Schunk M, Sbornik M, Darsow U, Ring J, von Krempelhuber A, Vollmar J, Rösch S, Baedeker N, Sobek V, Chaplin P. Safety and immunogenicity of the third generation smallpox vaccine IMVAMUNE® (MVA-BN®) in atopic dermatitis patients. (in prep).

Voorhoorst R, Spieksma-Boezeman MIA, Spieksma FTM. Is a mite (Dermatophagoides sp.) the producer of the housedust allergen? Allergie Asthma. 1964;10:329–34.

Vourch-Jourdain M, Barbarot S, Taïeb A, Diepgen T, Ambonati M, Durosier V, Sibaud V, Stalder JF. Patient-oriented SCORAD: a self-assessment score in atopic dermatitis. Dermatology. 2009;218:246–51.

Waersted A, Hjorth N. Pityrosporum orbiculare – a pathogenic factor in atopic dermatitis of the face, scalp and neck? Acta Derm Venereol Suppl. 1985;114:146–8.

Wahlgren CF, Hagermark O, Bergstrom R. The antipruritic effect of a sedative and a non-sedative antihistamine in atopic dermatitis. Br J Dermatol. 1990;122(4):545–51.

Wahn U, von Mutius E. Childhood risk factors for atopy and the importance of early intervention. J Allergy Clin Immunol. 2001;107:567–74.

Wahn U, Wichmann HE. Spezialbericht Allergien: Gesundheitsberichterstattung des Bundes. Stuttgart: Statistisches Bundesamt; 2000. p. 1–147.

Wahn U, Bos JD, Goodfield M, Caputo R, Papp K, Manjra A, Dobozy A, Paul C, Molloy S, Hultsch T, Graeber M, Cherill R, de Prost Y, for the Flare Reduction in Ekzema with Elidel (Children) Multicenter Investigator Study Group. Efficacy and safety of pimecrolimus cream in the long-term management of atopic dermatitis in children. Pediatrics. 2002;110:1–8.

Waite DA, Eyles EF, Tonkin SI, O'Donnell TV. Asthma prevalence in Tokelauan children in two environments. Clin Allergy. 1980;10:71–5.

Wakita H, Ohkuro M, Ishii N, Hishinuma I. A putative antipruritic mechanism of the phosphodiesterase-4 inhibitor E6005 by attenuating capsaicin-induced depolarization of C-fibre nerves. Exp Dermatol. 2015;24:215–6.

Wallach D, Taïeb A, Tilles G, editors. Histoire de la dermatite atopique. Paris: Masson; 2004.

Walzer M. Studies in absorption of undigested proteins in human beings: I. A simple direct method of studying the absorption of undigested protein. J Immunol. 1927;14:143–74.

Wandtke F, Stanek KW, Götz M, Jarisch R. Bioresonanz – Allergietest versus Pricktest und RAST. Allergologie. 1993;16:144–5.

Wang B, Rieger A, Kilgus O, Ochiai K, Maurer D, Födinger D, Kinet J, Stingl G. Epidermal Langerhans cells from normal human skin bind monomeric IgE via FceRI. J Exp Med. 1992;175:1353–65.

Wang IJ, Hsieh WS, Wu KY, Guo YL, Hwang YH, Jee SH, Chen PC. Effect of gestational smoke exposure on atopic dermatitis in the offspring. Pediatr Allergy Immunol. 2008;19:580–6.

Warndorff JA. The response of sweat gland to acetylcholine in atopic subjects. Br J Dermatol. 1970;83:306 ff.

Warnecke J, Wendt A. Anti-inflammatory action of pale sulfonated shale oil (ICHTHYOL pale) in UVB erythema test. Inflamm Res. 1998;47:75–8.

Warner JO. Obesity and allergic disease: closely related epidemics of the 21st century. Pediatr Allergy Immunol. 2009;20:305–6.

Warschburger P, Buchholz HAT, Petermann F. Psychological adjustment in parents of young children with atopic dermatitis: which factors predict parental quality of life? Br J Dermatol. 2004;150:304–11.

Watkins CDB. Pityriasis alba: a form of atopic dermatitis. Arch Dermatol. 1961;83:915–9.

Weber A, Lau S, Wahn U. Möglichkeiten und Nutzen der Innenraumallergenanalyse. Allergo J. 1997;6:139–44.

Wedi B, Raap U, Lewrick H, Kapp A. Delayed eosinophil programmed cell death in vitro: a common feature of inhalant allergy and extrinsic and intrinsic atopic dermatitis. J Allergy Clin Immunol. 1997;100(4):536–43.

Weidinger S, Klopp N, Wagenpfeil S, et al. Association of a STAT 6 haplotype with elevated serum IgE levels in a population based cohort of white adults. J Med Genet. 2004a;41:658–63.

Weidinger S, Schäfer T, Malek B, von Schmiedeberg S, Schill WB, Ring J, Köhn FM. Association between atopy and cryptorchidism. J Allergy Clin Immunol. 2004b;114:192–3.

Weidinger S, Klopp N, Rummler L, Wagenpfeil S, Novak N, Baurecht HJ, et al. Association of NOD1

polymorphisms with atopic eczema and related phenotypes. J Allergy Clin Immunol. 2005;116:177–84.
Weidinger S, Mayerhofer A, Raemsch R, Ring J, Köhn FM. Prostate-specific antigen as allergen in human seminal plasma allergy. J Allergy Clin Immunol. 2006;117(1):213–5.
Weidinger S, Rodriguez E, Stahl C, et al. Filaggrin mutations strongly predispose to early-onset and extrinsic atopic dermatitis. J Invest Dermatol. 2007; 127:724–6.
Weidinger S, Gieger C, Rodriguez E, et al. Genome-wide scan on total serum IgE levels identifies FCER1A as novel susceptibility locus. PLoS Genet. 2008a;4:e10001166. Epub 2008 Aug 22.
Weidinger S, O'Sullivan M, Illig T, et al. Filaggrin mutations, atopic eczema, hay fever, and asthma in children. J Allergy Clin Immunol. 2008b;121:1203–9.
Weiland SK, von Mutius E, Hirsch T, et al. Prevalence of respiratory and atopic disorders among children in East and West of Germany five years after unification. Eur Respir J. 1999;14:862–70.
Weinberg E, Fourie B, Allmann B, Toerien A. The use of cefadroxil in superinfected atopic dermatitis. Curr Ther Res Clin Exp. 1992;52(5):671–6.
Werfel T. Allergenspezifische T-Zell-Antwort bei Ekzemkrankheiten. Munich: Dustri-Verlag; 2000.
Werfel T, Breuer K. Role of food allergy in atopic dermatitis. Curr Opin Allergy Clin Immunol. 2004;4(5):379–85.
Werfel T, Kapp A. T-cells in atopic dermatitis. In: Leung D, Bieber T, editors. Atopic dermatitis. St. Louis: Marcel Decker; 2002. p. 241–66.
Werfel T, Reese I. Diätetik in der Allergologie. 2nd ed. Munich: Dustri; 2009.
Werfel T, Morita A, Grewe M, et al. Allergen specificity of skin-infiltrating T cells is not restricted to a type-2 cytokine pattern in chronic lesions of atopic dermatitis. J Invest Dermatol. 1996;107:871–6.
Werfel T, Breuer K, Rueff F, et al. Usefulness of specific immunotherapy in patients with atopic dermatitis and allergic sensitization to house dust mites: a multicentre, randomized, dose-response study. Allergy. 2006;61:202–5.
Werfel T, Ballmer-Weber B, Eigenmann PA, Niggemann B, Rancé F, Turjanmaa K, Worm M. Eczematous reactions to food in atopic eczema: position paper of the EAACI and GA2LEN. Allergy. 2007; 62(7):723–8.
Werfel T, Aberer W, Augustin M, et al. Leitlinie Neurodermitis. AWMF reg. 013/027 AWMF online 2008,
Werfel T, Erdmann S, Fuchs T, et al. Vorgehen bei vermuteter Nahrungsmittelallergie bei atopischer Dermatitis. Allergo J. 2008b;17:476–83, (AWMF Leitlinienregister Nr. 061/010, www.awmf-online.de).
Werfel T, Lotte C, Scheewe S, Staab D, editors. Manual Neurodermitisschulung. Munich/Orlando: Dustri; 2008c.
Werfel T, Aberer W, Augustin M, et al. Neurodermitis S2-Leitlinie. J Dtsch Dermatol Ges. 2009;7:s1–46.
Werfel T, Heratizadeh A, Niebuhr M, Kapp A, Roesner LM, Karch A, Erpenbeck VJ, Lösche C, Jung T, Krug N, Badorrek P, Hohlfeld JM. Exacerbation of atopic dermatitis on grass pollen exposure in an environmental challenge chamber. J Allergy Clin Immunol. 2015;136(1):96–103.e9. doi:10.1016/j.jaci.2015.04.015. Epub 2015 Jun 1.
Weymayr C, Heissmann, N. Die Homöopathie-Lüge – so gefährlich ist die Lehre von den weißen Kügelchen. Munich: Piper; 2012.
Whitfield A. On the white reaction (white line) in dermatology. Br J Dermatol. 1938;50:71–82.
Whitlock A. Psychophysiologic aspects of skin disease. Toronto: Saunders; 1976.
Wichmann HE, Schlipköter HW, Füllgraf G, editors. Handbuch der Umweltmedizin, 3 Bände, 18. Er-gänzungslieferung. Landsberg: Ecomed; 1995–2000.
Wiesenauer M, Gaus W, Häussler S. Behandlung der Pollinosis mit Galphimia glauca. Allergologie. 1990;13:359–63.
Wilhelm KP, Scholermann A. Efficacy and tolerability of a topical preparation containing 10 % urea in patients with atopic dermatitis. Akt Dermatol. 1998;24(1–2):26–30.
Wilkinson JD. Fusidic acid in dermatology. Br J Dermatol. 1998;139 Suppl 53:37–40.
Willan R. On cutaneous diseases. London: Johnson; 1808.
Williams HC, editor. Atopic Dermatitis. The epidemiology, causes and prevention of atopic eczema. Cambridge, UK: Cambridge University Press; 2000.
Williams HC. Clinical practice. Atopic dermatitis. N Engl J Med. 2005;352:2314–24.
Williams HC, Wüthrich B. The natural history of atopic dermatitis. In: Williams HC, editor. Atopic dermatitis. The epidemiology, causes and prevention of atopic eczema. Cambridge, UK: Cambridge University Press; 2000. p. 41–59.
Williams HC, Burney PG, Hay RJ, Archer CB, Shipley MJ, Hunter JJA, Bingham EA, Finlay AY, et al. The U.K. Working Party's Diagnostic Criteria for Atopic Dermatitis. I. Derivation of a minimum set of discriminators for atopic dermatitis. Br J Dermatol. 1994a;131:383–96.
Williams HC, Burney PGJ, Hay RJ, Strachan D, Hay RJ. The U.K. working party's diagnostic criteria for atopic dermatitis. II. Observer variation of clinical diagnosis and signs of atopic dermatitis. Br J Dermatol. 1994b;131:397–405.
Williams HC, Pembroke AC, Forsdyke H, Boodoo G, Hay RJ, Burney GJ. London-born black Caribbean children are at increased risk of atopic eczema. J Am Acad Dermatol. 1995;32:212–7.
Williams HC, Burney PG, Pembroke AC, Hay RJ. Validation of the U.K. diagnostic criteria for atopic dermatitis in a population setting. U.K. Diagnostic Criteria for Atopic Dermatitis Working Party. Br J Dermatol. 1996;135:12–7.
Winge MCG, Bilcha KD, Liedén A, Shibeshi D, Sandilands A, Wahlgren C-F, McLean WHI, Nordenskjöld M,

Bradley M. Novel filaggrin mutation but no other loss-of-function variants found in Ethiopian patients with atopic dermatitis. Br J Dermatol. 2011;165: 1074–80.

Wise F, Sulzberger MB. Editor's remarks. In: Yearbook of dermatology and syphilology. Chicago: Year Book Medical; 1933.

Wistokat-Wülfing A, Schmidt P, Darsow U, Ring J, Kapp A, Werfel T. Atopy patch test reactions are associated with T-lymphocyte mediated allergen-specific immune responses in atopic dermatitis. J Allergy Clin Immunol. 1998;101:196–7.

Wohlrab W. Bedeutung von Harnstoff in der externen Therapie. Hautarzt. 1989;40(Suppl IX):35–41.

Wohlrab W. Neurodermitis und Harnstoff. Hautarzt. 1992;43(Suppl XI):1–4.

Wollenberg A, Kraft S, Hanau D, Bieber T. Immunomorphological and ultrastructural characterization of Langerhans cells and a novel, inflammatory dendritic epidermal cell (IDEC) population in lesional skin of atopic ecyema. J Invest Dermatol. 1996;106:446.

Wollenberg A, Sharma S, von Bubnoff D, Geiger E, Haberstok J, Bieber T. Topical tacrolimus (FK506) leads to profound phenotypic and functional alterations of epidermal antigen-presenting dentritic cells in atopic dermatitis. J Allergy Clin Immunol. 2001;107:219–525.

Wollenberg A, Wetzel S, Burgdorf WH, Haas J. Viral infections in atopic dermatitis: pathogenic aspects and clinical management. J Allergy Clin Immunol. 2003a;112:667–74.

Wollenberg A, Zoch C, Wetzel S, Plewig G, Przybilla B. Predisposing factors and clinical features of eczema herpeticum: a retrospective analysis of 100 cases. J Am Acad Dermatol. 2003b;49(2):198–205.

Wollenberg A, Reitamo S, Atzori F, Lahfa M, Ruzicka T, Healy E, Giannetti A, Bieber T, Vyas J, Deleuran M. Proactive treatment of atopic dermatitis in adults with 0.1 % tacrolimus ointment. Allergy. 2008;63:742–50.

Wollenberg A, Oranje A, Deleuran M, Simon D, Szalai S, et al. ETFAD/EADV eczema task force 2015 position paper on diagnosis and treatment of atopic dermatitis. J Eur Acad Dermatol Venereol, in press.

Wong RC, Fairley JA, Ellis CN. Dermographism: a review. J Am Acad Dermatol. 1984;11:643–52.

Woodfolk JA, Wheatley LM, Piyasena RV, Benjamin DC, Platts-Mills TAE. Trichophyton antigens associated with IgE antibodies and delayed type hypersensitivity: Sequence homology to two families of serine proteinases. J Biol Chem. 1998;273:29489–96.

Worm M, Ehlers I, Sterry W, Zuberbier T. Clinical relevance of food additives in adult patients with atopic dermatitis. Clin Exp Allergy. 2000;30:407–14.

Worm M, Forschner K, Lee HH, Roehr CC, Edenharter G, Niggemann B, Zuberbier T. Frequency of atopic dermatitis and relevance of food allergy in adults in Germany. Acta Derm Venereol. 2006;86(2): 119–22.

Wright RJ. Stress and atopic disorders. J Allergy Clin Immunol. 2005;116:1301–6.

Wüthrich B. Zur Immunpathologie der Neurodermitis constitutionalis. Bern: Huber; 1975.

Wüthrich B. Neurodermitis atopica sive consitutionalis. Ein pathogenetisches Modell aus der Sicht des Allergologen. Aktuel Dermatol. 1983;9:1–7.

Wüthrich B. Neurodermitis atopica. Wien Med Wochenschr. 1989;139:156–65.

Wüthrich B, editor. The atopy syndrome in the third millennium. Basel: Karger; 1999a.

Wüthrich B. Clinical aspects, epidemiology, and prognosis of atopic dermatitis. Ann Allergy Asthma Immunol. 1999b;83:464–70.

Wüthrich B. Epidemiologie der Allergien in der Schweiz. Ther Umsch. 2001;58:253–8.

Wüthrich B, Schmid-Grendelmeier P. The atopic eczema/dermatitis syndrome. Epidemiology, natural course, and immunology oft he IgE-associated ("extrinsic") and the nonallergic 8 "intrinsic") AEDS. J Invest Allergol Clin Immunol. 2003;13:1–5.

Wüthrich B, Schnyder UW. Eine wenig bekannte Ausdrucksform der Neurodermitis atopica: Das patchy pityriasiform lichenoid eczema ("Kitamura-Takahashi-Sasagawa"). Akt Dermatol. 1981;7:85–7.

Wüthrich B, Frei PC, Bircher A, et al. Bioresonanz – diagnostischer und therapeutischer Unsinn. Allergologie. 2006;29:244–9.

Wüthrich B, Schmid-Grendelmeier P, Schindler C, Imboden M, Bircher A, Zemp E. Probst-Hensch N and the SAPALDIA team: prevalence of atopy and respiratory allergic diseases in the elderly SAPALDIA population. Int Arch Allergy Immunol. 2013;162:143–8.

Yaghmaie B, Koudelka CW, Simpson EL. Mental health comorbidity in patients with atopic dermatitis. J Allergy Clin Immunol. 2013;131:428–33.

Yamaguchi J, Aihara M, Kobayashi Y, Kambara T, Ikezawa Z. Quantitative analysis of nerve growth factor (NGF) in the atopic dermatitis and psoriasis horny layer and effect of treatment on NGF in atopic dermatitis. J Dermatol Sci. 1991;53:48–54.

Yamamoto M, Haruna T, Ueda C, Asano Y, Takahashi H, Iduhara M, Takaki S, Yasui K, Matsuo Y, Arimura A. contribution of itch-associated scratch behavior to the development of skin lesions in Dermatophagoides farina-induced dermatitis model in NC/Nga mice. Arch Dermatol Res. 2009;301:739–46.

Yanase DJ, David-Bajar K. The leukotriene antagonist montelukast as a therapeutic agent for atopic dermatitis. J Am Acad Dermatol. 2001;44(1):89–93.

Yang Q. Acupuncture treatment of 139 cases of neurodermatitis. J Tradit Chin Med. 1997;17:57–8.

Yin H, He R, Oyoshi M, Geha RS. Animal models of atopic dermatitis. J Invest Dermatol. 2009;129: 31–40.

Yosipovitch G, Bernard JD. Chronic pruritus. N Engl J Med. 2013;368:126–63.

Young SH, Rubin JM, Daman HR, editors. Psychobiological aspects of allergic disorders. New York: Praeger; 1986.

Yun JW, Seo JA, Young WH, Koh HJ, Bae IH, Part YH, Lim KM. Antipruritic effects of TRPV1 antagonist in murine atopic dermatitis and itching models. J Invest Dermatol. 2011;131:1576–9.

Zachariae H, Cramers M, Herlin T, Jensen J, et al. Non-specific immunotherapy and specific hyposensitization in severe atopic dermatitis. Acta Derm Venereol Suppl. 1985;114:48–54.

Zink A, Gensbaur A, Zirbs M, Seifert F, Suarez IL, Mourantchanian V, Weidinger S, Mempel M, Ring J, Ollert M. Targeting IgE in severe atopic dermatitis with a combination of immunoadsorption and omalizumab. Acta Derm Venereol. 2015. doi:10.2340/00015555-2165.

Zollner TM, Wichelhaus TA, Hartung A, et al. Colonization with superantigen-producing Staphylococcus aureus is associated with increased severity of atopic dermatitis. Clin Exp Allergy. 2000;30:994–1000.

Zuberbier T, Edenharter G, Worm M, et al. Prevalence of adverse reactions to food in Germany – a population study. Allergy. 2004;59:338–45.

Zuberbier T, Aberer W, Asero R, Bindslev-Jensen C, Brzoza Z, Canonica GW, Church MK, Ensina LF, Giménez-Arnau A, Godse K, Gonçalo M, Grattan C, Hebert J, Hide M, Kaplan A, Kapp A, Abdul Latiff AH, Mathelier-Fusade P, Metz M, Nast A, Saini SS, Sánchez-Borges M, Schmid-Grendelmeier P, Simons FE, Staubach P, Sussman G, Toubi E, Vena GA, Wedi B, Zhu XJ, Maurer M, European Academy of Allergy and Clinical Immunology, Global Allergy and Asthma European Network, European Dermatology Forum, World Allergy Organization. The EAACI/GA(2)LEN/EDF/WAO Guideline for the definition, classification, diagnosis, and management of urticaria: the 2013 revision and update. Allergy. 2014;69:868–87.

Zurbriggen B, Wüthrich B, Cachelin AB, Wili PB, Kägi MK. Comparison of two formulations of cyclosporin A in the treatment of severe atopic dermatitis. A double-blind, single-centre, cross-over pilot study. Dermatology. 1999;198:56–60.

Index

J. Ring, *Atopic Dermatitis: Eczema*, DOI 10.1007/978-3-319-22243-1